Outdoor Emergency Care

Comprehensive First Aid for Nonurban Settings

8307

Outdoor Emergency Care

Comprehensive First Aid for Nonurban Settings

Warren D. Bowman, Jr., M.D.

CREDITS

Education Director: Judy Over
Editor: Alicia Leppert
Medical Editor: Diana Copsey
Art Director/Illustrator: Reata Bitter, Bitter-Sweet Studio
Cover Design: Roxie Speer, Twelfth Street Design
Paste-up: Sandi Daley
Typography: Bradford/Will Graphics
Printer: American Web
Cover Photo: © 1988 Mark Heifner
Contributing Editor: Patricia Beagle
Contributing Illustrator: Ed Zilberts

Printed in the United States of America

TABLE OF CONTENTS

PART I

TABLE OF CONTENTS

PART II

PART III

ACKNOWLEDGEMENTS

Producing a textbook of this magnitude would have been impossible without many useful suggestions and contributions from members of the National Ski Patrol and others interested in outdoor emergency care. The entire manuscript has been reviewed in depth by members of the National Ski Patrol's Winter Emergency Care Program Administration Committee, the National First Aid and Medical Advisory committees, and Winter Emergency Care supervisors, in addition to a special Expert Medical Review Committee composed of physicians who are experts in outdoor emergency care.

The author wishes to cite the following persons in particular for their contributions to the review of the textbook and in coordinating pilot instructional programs before this first edition printing:

National Ski Patrol Winter Emergency Care Program Administration Committee

Marlén Guell
John Clair
Carol Smith
William Simonsen
John Chandler, M.D.
Jack Mason
Jeff Olsen
*Diana Penwell

National Medical Advisory Committee

John Mues, M.D., Alaska Division
James J. Hamilton, M.D., Central Division
*William Diefenbach, M.D., Eastern Division
Fred Spannaus, M.D., Eastern Division
David L. Chittenden, M.D., Far West Division
*Robert J. Gilbert, M.D., Far West Division
T.W. McCowin, M.D., Intermountain Division
Jon Anderson, M.D., Northern Division
David W. Allen, M.D., Ph.D., Pacific Northwest Division
H. Rolan Zick, M.D., Rocky Mountain Division
John Chandler, M.D., Southern Division

National First Aid Committee

Sandy Henry, Alaska Division
Kathy Ferrigan, Central Division
*Sandra Scull, Eastern Division
*William McCollum, Far West Division
Jack Wright, Intermountain Division
Herb Seaton, International Division
*William Lay, Northern Division
John Poundstone, Northern Division
Carol Fountain, Pacific Northwest Division
*Denise Gruebel, Rocky Mountain Division
Dr. French Moore, Southern Division

Expert Medical Review Committee

Paul Auerbach, M.D.
Robert Meisterling, M.D.
Harvey A. Ries, M.D.
Joseph B. Serra, M.D.
Noel E. Sloan, M.D.
Richard Withington, M.D.

Winter Emergency Care Supervisors

Sandy Henry, Alaska Division
*Marc Bond, Alaska Division
Sue Gormley, Central Division
*Jeff Olsen, Central Division
*Douglas Jamieson, Central Division
Kathy Ferrigan, Central Division
Richard Hampel, Eastern Division
Mary Davis, Eastern Division
David Tauber, Eastern Division
Clinton (Bud) Dow, Far West Division
*Jack Ross, Far West Division
Jack Wright, Intermountain Division
Herb Seaton, International Division
*Harley Schwarz, Northern Division
John Poundstone, Northern Division
David L. Allen, M.D., Ph.D., Pacific Northwest Division
Greg Horstman, Professional Division
*Frankie Stuart, Rocky Mountain Division
Luann Dodge, Rocky Mountain Division
*John Chandler, M.D., Southern Division
Jim Hunter, Southern Division

*former committee members

The efforts and evaluations of NSP instructor trainers, instructors, and patrollers who participated in pilot programs were extremely valuable in writing the first edition.

Special thanks are owed to former National First Aid Advisor Diana Penwell, National Winter Emergency Care Supervisor Jeff Olsen, Assistant National Chairman John Clair, and Assistant National Chairman Jack Mason.

The following persons contributed to or reviewed specific sections of the text: Alton L. Thygerson, Ed.D., Dave Decker, William Schneiderman, Arthur J. Varley, Jr., M.D., Alexander Butman, RoseAnn Jankowski, Garrett Nanninga, Walter Gregg, Goeffrey Keller, Norman Lauson, Sheriff Greg Noose (Stillwater County., MT), William Giles, Dr. Richard Weingart, Hilbert (Huck) Finn, and Patricia Beagle.

Exceptional thanks are owed to Judy Over, National Ski Patrol Education Director; Alicia Leppert, National Ski Patrol Communications Director; Diana Copsey, medical editor; Reata Bitter, textbook art director, and illustrator; Roxie Speer, textbook cover designer; and Sandi Daley, pasteup artist.

Another special thanks to the Billings Clinic for their support of the project and for granting me the time to work on the text.

ABOUT THE AUTHOR

Warren D. Bowman, Jr., M.D. specializes in internal medicine and hematology and has special interests in wilderness and mountain medicine. Dr. Bowman has been a member of the Department of Internal Medicine, Billings Clinic, Billings, Montana, since 1960. He is a clinical associate professor of medicine at the University of Washington Medical School.

Dr. Bowman has served the National Ski Patrol as its national medical advisor since 1970 and has been an active member of the Beartooth Ski Patrol at Red Lodge Mountain, Montana, since 1964.

He is a fellow of the American College of Physicians and a former governor of the Montana Chapter of ACP. Dr. Bowman also belongs to the International Society for Ski Safety, the Beartooth Mountain Rescue Group, and is a founding member of the Wilderness Medical Society. He is a member of the medical committee of the American Alpine Club and of the medical commission of the Union International des Associations d'Alpinisme (UIAA). Dr. Bowman also is medical director and chairman of the medical committee for the National Association for Search and Rescue (NASAR), and a former board chairman of the Midland Empire Chapter of the American Red Cross.

As a ski patroller, Dr. Bowman also has served as Northern Division ski mountaineering advisor, and has twice received the national award as outstanding administrative patroller. He is a nationally registered avalanche and ski mountaineering instructor and holds National #3537.

Dr. Bowman is a member of the editorial advisory board of *Response* magazine and the editorial board of *Journal of Wilderness Medicine*. He has written many journal articles on medical subjects, textbook chapters on cold injury and wilderness survival, and first aid manuals, including the National Ski Patrol's *Winter First Aid Manual.*

*This textbook is dedicated to the thousands of ski patrollers
past and present who have spent untold hours in the wind and cold
ministering to the injured and ill in the snowy mountains.*

Introduction

Things can never be as they once were; be sad and rejoice.

—*Author unknown*

The discovery of sulfa drugs and antibiotics during the 1930s was the beginning of a revolution in medical care. As ancient scourges such as syphilis, tuberculosis, leprosy, smallpox and malaria were controlled or eliminated, infection – once the greatest killer of mankind – was superceded by trauma and degenerative diseases. Hospital care also improved dramatically as new techniques of diagnosis and treatment were introduced and breakthroughs in technology led to the marvels of open-heart surgery, organ transplantation, and the artificial kidney. The care of the critically ill improved markedly with the development of the intensive care unit. (However, it remains to be seen whether the latest epidemic, AIDS, will yield as easily to our efforts.)

Despite these advances, by the 1960s it was obvious that *care of the patient prior to reaching the hospital* had not kept pace with improvements in in-hospital care. Injuries were the leading cause of death and disability in children and young people, and the poor quality of prehospital care was a national disgrace.

In 1966, the National Research Council produced a landmark report, *Accidental Death and Disability: The Neglected Disease of Modern Society*, that stimulated a national effort to create the Emergency Medical Services (EMS) system, a closely-linked, interdependent network of emergency departments and emergency vehicles manned by trained emergency medical technicians (EMTs), prepared to reach patients rapidly, provide modern emergency care and transport them to the hospital.

During this time, the American Academy of Orthopaedic Surgeons produced the EMT "bible," *Emergency Care and Transportation of the Sick and Injured*, based on the National EMS Standard Curriculum developed by the National Highway Traffic Safety Administration, United States Department of Transportation (DOT).

The EMS system has dramatically improved prehospital care but, as noted by the National Research Council in 1985, every year one in every three Americans is injured and more than 140,000 die from trauma. There still is much to be done.

Before 1985, the National Ski Patrol (NSP) required its members to be trained in basic first aid by taking the American Red Cross Advanced First Aid and Emergency Care Course. Patrollers also had to complete a special course in winter first aid that emphasized training in high-altitude and cold-weather illnesses and injuries, ski injuries, and the special equipment and techniques used by patrollers.

The National Ski Patrol has always been in a unique position compared to other providers of prehospital care. In addition to caring for seldom-seen illnesses and injuries such as deep frostbite and acute mountain sickness, its members often serve in locations far from hospitals and frequently must provide care for an hour or more before patients can be turned over to the EMS system. Nordic ski patrollers and ski mountaineers can be many hours or even days from a doctor or hospital.

In the fall of 1985, the National Ski Patrol reexamined available first aid training courses. The American Red Cross Advanced First Aid and Emergency Care Course was designed primarily for urban laypersons with quick access to the EMS system. EMT training, primarily oriented toward heart attacks and auto accidents in an urban setting, was designed for ambulance attendants, and, in some cases, was dependent upon radio support from emergency room physicians. Without extensive modification, neither of these two major training systems was suited to the needs of ski patrollers. These findings motivated the National Ski Patrol to develop its Winter Emergency Care (WEC) program, a new program in emergency care that reflects the NSP's primary concern with the winter environment.

Outdoor Emergency Care is designed as a textbook for the NSP Winter Emergency Care program. The knowledge and skills presented here are fundamental; they differ only as appropriate to the outdoor environment and closely follow the DOT's National EMT Standard Curriculum, 1984 revision. The WEC program's main purpose is to prepare ski patrol candidates without previous first aid or EMT training to handle the prehospital emergency care problems seen at an alpine or nordic ski area. However, because patient care in nonurban settings generally has lagged behind aid available in urban settings, this textbook is designed to be useful to *any* person who may need to provide first aid outdoors. The contents are not limited to cold-weather emergency situations. This textbook covers all types of outdoor problems, including patient care when definitive medical help may be hours or days away because of distance, adverse travel conditions, or communication difficulties.

Outdoor Emergency Care uses a carefully selected, minimal number of medical terms. The terms are defined when first used and are listed in the glossary. They are a form of shorthand: each one replaces several words or a sentence of nontechnical English, and all are commonly used in the EMS system. Serious rescuers who coordinate with the EMS system will find them useful and time-saving.

Other terms used in this textbook also need to be explained. First, the word "rescuer" is used to designate a ski patroller, backcountry search and rescue group member, leader of a backcountry recreational party, or any other person who provides care in an emergency. The word "patient" applies to the ill or injured person who requires such care. The author believes that this word, which in the past has referred only to persons cared for by physicians and nurses, is better than the alternatives. "Patient" has replaced "victim" in the EMS literature and is defined by Webster's New Collegiate Dictionary as "the recipient of any of various personal services." The term "victim" has unattractive implications of causation, the term "subject" is nonspecific, and the term "casualty"–commonly used in British Commonwealth countries–connotes trauma alone.

"Definitive medical care" refers to care given in a hospital or physician's office. An "emergency medical technician," or "EMT," is a person who has passed a basic or advanced EMT course sanctioned by his or her state and the U.S. Department of Transportation. "EMS system" refers to the interconnected network of hospitals, emergency departments, ambulances, helicopters, physicians, nurses, and EMTs that provides most prehospital emergency care. The terms "first aid" and "emergency care" will be used somewhat interchangeably, but the author prefers to use "first aid" for simpler techniques that do not require much equipment and that rely on speedy coordination with the EMS system, and to use "emergency care" for more sophisticated, EMT-level techniques where EMS interaction may be delayed.

In-depth material on anatomy and physiology is included to stimulate interest in understanding human body function and the location of important body parts, although some of this information may not be immediately applicable in emergency care.

Although specific descriptions of emergency care techniques are provided in this textbook, the student should understand that there is never only one "correct" way of managing a specific problem. Any technique that is consistent with well-recognized principles of anatomy, physiology and emergency care, does the job well, and does not injure the patient is acceptable.

The student will not become an expert care provider simply by studying this textbook nor by successfully completing the National Ski Patrol Winter Emergency Care course or other similar course. However, this course will furnish the groundwork for the continuing study, practice, and review necessary to be "worthy to serve the suffering." One aim of this textbook is to prepare the student to analyze and devise rational emergency care for unusual situations not specifically covered in training. To this end, special emphasis will be given to a solid foundation in anatomy, physiology, in-depth patient assessment for both injuries and medical illnesses, and improvisation of first aid equipment and techniques.

The textbook is divided into three parts. Part I contains the material covered in the National Ski Patrol's Winter Emergency Care program. Part II includes other important topics of outdoor emergency care not covered in the WEC program. Part III includes important legal considerations, a discussion of wilderness emergency care, and lists of suggested items to include in emergency care kits.

Warren D. Bowman, Jr., MD, FACP
National Medical Advisor
National Ski Patrol

Billings Clinic
Billings, Montana
January 1988

1

Adapting to the Outdoor Environment

If the external air is of a high temperature, it does not take up the superfluous heat of the body fast enough, and we complain of too much heat: if it is very cold, it absorbs the heat too fast and produces the sensation of cold. To remedy this, we interpose a covering, which acting as a strainer, lets less air come into contact with the body, and checks the escape of the vital heat. As the atmospheric air becomes colder, more heat is conducted from the body. As it would be inconvenient in the day to be burthened with a mass of clothing entirely equivalent to great degrees of cold, we have to resort to fire and warm rooms to correct the state of the atmosphere, as a supplement to our clothing.

> —*Thomas Jefferson*
> *Notes on the State of Virginia*

Modern, civilized people spend most of their lives in artificial cocoons, where indoor temperatures can be regulated; food, water, and clothing are easy to obtain; and shelter is always available. The underpinnings of technology that support this existence are fragile, as can be seen when a natural or manmade disaster occurs: the amenities of civilization collapse, and basics such as food, water and shelter are difficult or impossible to obtain. Even a temporary power outage illustrates the thinness of civilization's veneer. Modern man is at a loss when electric stoves, refrigerators, air conditioners, and automatic garage doors cease to function.

Increased leisure time and a growing interest in outdoor activities are leading more and more persons outside, at times into actual wilderness. When modern conveniences are left behind, life is reduced to the basics and individuals become completely dependent on their own resources. Our ancestors' hard-won knowledge of how to survive must then be relearned, sometimes at considerable cost. The outdoor environment, particularly the wilderness, is often called "hostile" when, in fact, it is merely indifferent and impartial. Training, experience, knowledge, proper equipment, and the development of at least rudimentary backcountry common sense permit relatively safe enjoyment of nonurban areas.

For basic survival, the body requires food, water, a constant supply of oxygen, and a core temperature regulated within the relatively narrow limits of 75 degrees to 107 degrees Fahrenheit (°F) or 24 degrees to 42 degrees Centigrade or Celsius (°C). For comfort and optimum performance, the body must be in top physical condition and free from disease or injury. Each of these requirements will be examined in turn.

Table 1.1

SURVIVAL REQUIREMENTS

Oxygen
Maintenance of body temperature
Water
Food
Physical integrity

OXYGEN

Air at sea level has a barometric pressure of 760 millimeters of mercury (mm Hg) and is composed of 21 percent oxygen and 78 percent nitrogen. The remaining 1 percent is made up of a small amount of carbon dioxide and trace amounts of rare gases such as argon. From the standpoint of human survival and well-being, the most important physical property of oxygen is its **partial pressure**, i.e., the percentage of total air pressure accounted for by oxygen. At sea level, this is 160 mm Hg (21 percent of 760 mm Hg). Inhaled air travels to the most distant parts of the respiratory tract, the **alveoli** (smallest air sacs of the lungs), where it is diluted by the carbon dioxide and water vapor found there. This dilution lowers the partial pressure of oxygen (PO2) in the alveolar air to 100 mm Hg (Fig. 1.1).

Fig. 1.1 *The partial pressure of oxygen varies as air is taken into the body.*

The exchange of carbon dioxide and oxygen between the air and the blood occurs in the alveoli. The blood in the alveolar capillaries is separated from the alveolar air by two thin membranes: the walls of the capillaries and the walls of the alveoli, which together have a thickness of only a few microns (one micron = .000039 inches or .001 millimeter). (The anatomy of the lung is described in more detail in Chapter 2.)

An important law of the behavior of gases states that any gas tends to diffuse from an area of higher pressure into an area of lower pressure. Thus, the higher PO_2 in the alveoli drives oxygen across the thin intervening membranes into the unoxygenated capillary blood, increasing its PO_2 from 40 mm Hg to 95 mm Hg, or just slightly below the 100 mm Hg PO_2 of alveolar air. As this oxygenated arterial blood circulates through the body, cells extract 58 percent of its oxygen (55 mm Hg), so that deoxygenated (venous) blood has a PO_2 of 40 mm Hg.

If the circulatory and respiratory systems are normal, a sea level PO_2 of 160 mm Hg is more than adequate for normal body function. However, under certain circumstances, oxygen in the air is insufficient or normal transport pathways are interrupted. Common examples are listed in Table 1.2.

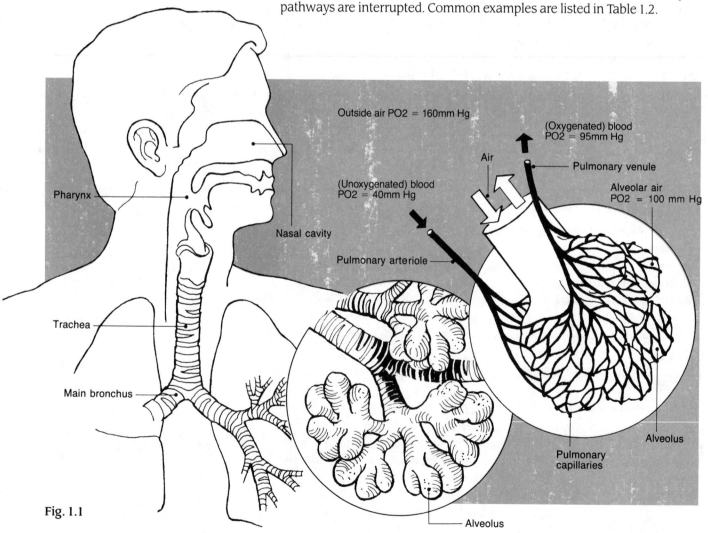

Fig. 1.1

Outside air PO2 = 160mm Hg

(Oxygenated) blood PO2 = 95mm Hg

Air

(Unoxygenated) blood PO2 = 40mm Hg

Pulmonary venule

Alveolar air PO2 = 100 mm Hg

Pharynx

Nasal cavity

Pulmonary arteriole

Trachea

Main bronchus

Alveolus

Pulmonary capillaries

Alveolus

Table 1.2

WAYS IN WHICH OXYGEN SUPPLY MAY BE INTERRUPTED

1. Insufficient Oxygen in the Air Entering the Body
   a. High altitude.
   b. Burial in a snow or dirt avalanche.
   c. Poorly ventilated snow cave.
   d. Malfunction of underwater breathing apparatus.
   e. Near drowning.
2. Upper-airway Obstruction
   a. Relaxation of the tongue or tissues of the pharynx in an unconscious person.
   b. Aspirated food, vomitus, false teeth, or other foreign material.
   c. Injury to the face or neck.
3. Lower-airway Obstruction
   a. Foreign body.
   b. Pus, blood, or mucus.
4. Interference with Lung Function
   a. Acute
      (1) Filling of the alveoli with pus, blood or fluid, as in pneumonia, lung hemorrhage, or pulmonary edema.
      (2) Partial or total collapse of the lung because of pressure from blood, fluid, or air in the pleural space.
   b. Chronic
      (1) Thickening of the walls of the alveoli, as in pulmonary fibrosis.
      (2) Loss of some alveoli, enlargement of others, and narrowing of the bronchi, as in emphysema.
      (3) Replacement of lung tissue by cancer.
5. Interference with Thoracic Cage Function or Pleural Space Integrity
   a. Paralysis of the nerve supply to the diaphragm and intercostal muscles in spinal cord injury.
   b. Crushing injury to the chest resulting in flail chest caused by broken ribs.
   c. Open chest wound.
6. Interference with the Brain's Control of Breathing
   a. Head injury.
   b. Meningitis.
   c. Stroke.
7. Abnormal Function of the Circulatory System
   a. Illness
      (1) Heart attack.
      (2) Chronic heart failure.
      (3) Fluid in the sac around the heart.
      (4) Blood clot in the lung (pulmonary embolus).
   b. Injury
      (1) Shock, hemorrhagic or other.
      (2) Direct injury to the heart.
8. Interference with the Blood's Oxygen-carrying Capacity
   a. Anemia.
   b. Carbon monoxide poisoning.

Emergency care in each of these situations includes administering oxygen. Care for the individual conditions is described in detail in later sections of this textbook.

As one ascends from sea level, the barometric pressure drops by 20 mm Hg for each 1,000 feet (305 meters) of elevation. At 10,000 feet (3,048 meters), the barometric pressure is two-thirds that at sea level; at 18,000 feet (5,486 meters), it is only half. The percent of oxygen in the air remains constant at 21 percent, but the partial pressure drops along with the barometric pressure.

The lowest alveolar PO2 at which an unacclimatized individual can survive without losing consciousness is 37 to 40 mm Hg, equivalent to an altitude of about 18,000 feet. Despite this limitation, humans have reached the summit of Mt. Everest (29,028 feet or 8,848 meters, 253 mm Hg barometric pressure) without supplemental oxygen, and there are permanent human habitations at altitudes close to 18,000 feet in the Chilean Andes and in Tibet.

The body adjusts to high altitudes by **acclimatization**, a process that takes several weeks or longer to complete. The first stage of acclimatization is rapid, deep breathing, or **hyperventilation**, which removes carbon dioxide and adds oxygen rapidly enough to raise the alveolar PO2. Later, the rate and depth of breathing are reset at a permanently higher level, the body produces more red blood cells to deliver oxygen to the tissues, and the action of the heart and skeletal muscles becomes more efficient. People who live at high altitude eventually develop larger chests and lungs and have higher pulmonary artery pressures. They also have thicker blood because of increased numbers of red blood cells.

Table 1.3

SUMMARY OF ACCLIMATIZATION

Hyperventilation occurs.
Changes occur in the blood's oxygen-uptake capacity.
Changes occur in the blood's oxygen-carrying capacity.
The heart and skeletal muscle action becomes more efficient.

Mountaineers and high-altitude skiers can use this information to better enjoy their stays at high altitude and to avoid the diseases of altitude (Chapter 19).

Hypoxia (lack of oxygen) is an important stress factor at high altitude, but its effects are often hard to separate from the effects of cold, high winds, dehydration, exhaustion, and hypothermia. Travelers to high altitude should be in good physical condition, well nourished, well rested, and free of illness or injury. To encourage acclimatization, allow enough time for a *slow ascent to altitude*. Provide a rest day after ascending from sea level to 10,000 feet (3,048 meters) and limit altitude gains above 10,000 feet to 1,000 to 1,500 feet (305 to 457 meters) per day. Mountaineers should "carry high and sleep low," i.e., ferry loads of supplies to a high cache and return to a lower camp for the night. Dehydration and hypothermia should be anticipated and avoided; meals and snacks should be frequent and nourishing.

During acute exposure to high altitude, the decrease in oxygen can cause fatigue, weakness, headache, loss of appetite, nausea, insomnia, shortness of breath on exertion, and Cheyne-Stokes respirations (waxing and waning of the depth of breathing with regular periods during which breathing ceases). These symptoms probably occur to some extent in everyone who goes rapidly from sea level to 8,000 feet (2,438 meters) or above.

REGULATION OF BODY TEMPERATURE

Humans are called **homeotherms** because they are warm-blooded creatures who maintain a relatively constant body temperature despite changes in environmental temperature. Homeothermy is required for optimum functioning of the body's enzyme systems, which work best at 98.6 to 100°F (37 to 37.8°C). The human body can be thought of as a *heat-generating machine* whose internal temperature is the net result of opposing mechanisms which tend to increase or decrease **body heat production**, increase or decrease **body heat loss**, and increase or decrease the accumulation of heat from the outside.

Basal heat production, which averages 50 kilocalories per square meter of body surface per hour, is the result of internal metabolic processes. Heat production can be increased by muscular activity such as shivering and exercise, by eating, by fever, and by exposure to cold, which increases hunger and the release of hormones that stimulate heat production. Shivering increases basal heat production four to five times; violent exercise increases basal heat production up to 10 times. The body also can draw heat from external sources such as the sun, fire, and hot food and drink.

Table 1.4

METHODS OF AVOIDING DANGEROUS DEGREES OF COOLING

Increase heat production.
Add heat from the outside.
Decrease heat loss.*

*Most energy-efficient method

Table 1.5

METHODS OF INCREASING HEAT PRODUCTION

Involuntary	*Voluntary*
Shivering	Muscular activity
Foot stamping and other semiconscious activity	Eating Heat from hot food and drink
Non-shivering thermogenesis Thyroxin Epinephrine Norepinephrine	Food energy Stove, fire, sun

Heat is lost from the body in five ways: by **conduction**, **convection**, **evaporation**, **radiation**, and **respiration**. To illustrate the relative importance of these mechanisms, a resting body in still air of average humidity and a temperature of 70°F (21°C) loses 70 percent of its heat by radiation, conduction, and convection; 27 percent by evaporation; and only 3 percent

Fig. 1.2 *Core and Shell Concept in Body Temperature Regulation*

Table 1.6

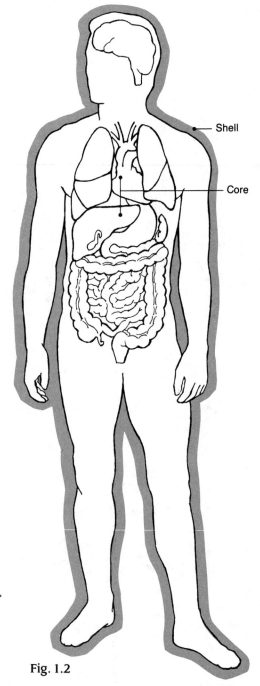

Fig. 1.2

through urine, feces, and the lungs. However, during hard exercise, evaporation can account for up to 85 percent of heat loss, while conduction, convection, radiation, and respiration together account for only about 15 percent.

MECHANISMS OF HEAT LOSS

Conduction
Convection
Evaporation
Radiation
Respiration

Conduction is the direct transfer of heat by contact of a warm body to a cooler object. The amount of heat transferred depends on the temperature difference and the speed with which the heat is conducted. Contact with metal or other materials that conduct heat rapidly may cause frostbite at low temperatures or burns at high temperatures.

Convection refers to the transfer of heat when air that is cooler than body temperature moves across the body's surface. The amount of heat transferred depends on the speed and temperature of the air. When the air temperature is low and there is no shelter, exposure to high winds can cause dangerous heat loss.

Evaporation is the loss of heat when water or another volatile liquid on the body's surface is converted into vapor. Because of the high **heat of vaporization** of water (540 calories of heat are consumed during the evaporation of 1 gram of water), considerable heat can be lost through evaporation of water from skin or wet clothing. Evaporation is increased in the presence of wind and low humidity and is decreased in high humidity. This is a major source of beneficial heat loss in hot, dry climates. Frostbite caused by conduction and evaporation can occur when gasoline or other volatile organic liquids with freezing points below 32°F (0°C) are spilled on the skin.

Radiation refers to heat lost from the body through infrared waves. Major amounts of heat are lost by radiation from uncovered skin. This may be beneficial in hot climates, but individuals exposed to cold temperatures require adequate clothing, including warm head gear, to prevent dangerous loss of body heat by radiation.

Body heat is lost through **respiration** as inhaled air is warmed to body temperature before being exhaled. The amount of heat lost depends on the outside air temperature and the rate and depth of breathing.

The **human brain** is the most important organ for regulating body temperature. Conscious activities such as adding or removing clothing, seeking shelter from the sun or from cold and wind, eating and drinking, and regulating the amount of heat produced by muscular activity are more important than the body's automatic adjustments to excessive heat or cold.

When studying body temperature regulation, it is convenient to think of the body as being composed of a **core**, which includes the central nervous system, heart, lungs, liver and other important internal organs, and a **shell**, composed of the skin, muscles and extremities (Fig. 1.2).

The extremities can gain or lose large amounts of heat because their surface areas are large in relation to their volumes. At moderate, comfortable temperatures, the core temperature is kept stable by constant, small adjustments in metabolic rate, muscular activity, and skin circulation. When the body is chilled, **heat production** is augmented by a slight increase in the metabolic rate, by shivering, and by semiconscious activities such as foot stamping. At the same time, the body decreases **heat loss** by reducing sweat production and restricting circulation of blood to the skin and extremities. Also, as body temperature falls, an individual tends to curl up into a ball so that a smaller surface area is exposed to the environment. These adjustments preserve the core temperature, at the expense of the shell temperature, if necessary.

When the body overheats, there is a tendency to reverse these mechanisms. In response to heat, a person will feel sluggish and languid and will find a cool place to rest. This decreases the amount of heat produced by muscular activity. Heat loss may be increased by fanning oneself or by removing clothing. Circulation to the skin and extremities increases, allowing heat to be lost by radiation and convection. Sweating increases heat loss by evaporation. If these mechanisms fail to maintain body heat within the optimum range, injury can occur because of frostbite and hypothermia at one extreme or heat stroke at the other.

Regulating Body Heat Gain and Loss

Stay in the best possible physical condition by exercising regularly. The body also must be properly rested, fed, and hydrated for the mechanisms of heat production and heat loss to function well.

Table 1.7

METHODS OF CONSERVING HEAT

Involuntary	Voluntary
Decrease sweating	Add clothing
Shunt blood away from the shell	Seek shelter
Decrease body surface area (curl into a ball)	

Table 1.8

METHODS OF DECREASING BODY HEAT LOSS

Use optimal insulation made of proper fabrics and proper lofting materials: wool, polypropylene, down, Dacron, polyester pile, foam.

Use the layering principle so that clothing can be added and warm air can be trapped.

Protect yourself from the wind to prevent the windchill effect.

Use adequate coverings for body parts with a large surface-area-to-volume ratio. Avoid getting wet.

Avoid contact with cold substances.

Avoid excessive respiratory heat loss.

Avoid alcohol and nicotine.

Use a personal flotation device in water-related sports.

COLD WEATHER

Insulating garments can prevent heat loss caused by conduction, convection, and radiation. Because air has extremely low thermal conductivity, the best garments for cold climates are those made of materials that trap a layer of still, warm air around the body and maintain this microclimate despite extremes of wind and cold temperatures. Some insulating ability is lost when garments are wet or when air spaces are reduced because the garment has become compressed or matted.

Suitable materials fall into two general groups: woven fabrics and nonwoven fibers. Some nonwoven fibers, such as polyester pile, are incorporated into a fabric; others, such as down, are used in garments as a filler to provide loft. In some cases, a fiber, such as polyester, can be made into fabric or used as a filler.

Traditionally, the best and most practical insulating fabrics for cold-weather clothing have been wool, polyester, and acrylic; the best fibers have been down, Dacron, and foam. Wool has a special property; it remains warm even when wet because of its low wicking action and ability to suspend water droplets between its fibers without seriously affecting insulating ability. Cotton garments, particularly denim and corduroy, should not be worn in cold weather because of cotton's high wicking ability and poor insulating value, which is reduced even further when wet.

Down is unsurpassed for dry, very cold climates but is inferior to Dacron in damp, moderately cold climates because wet down balls up and is less warm and harder to dry than wet Dacron. Orlon and related acrylic fabrics were developed to mimic the properties of wool at a lower cost. These fabrics are almost as warm as wool and are lighter, easier to dry, and less itchy. Foam, a lightweight plastic material containing multiple small air bubbles, is used to insulate boots, mittens, and gloves.

Newer insulating materials include Hollofil II and Quallofil, which are hollow, synthetic fibers designed on the principle of reindeer hair; Thermolactyl, a fabric containing acrylic and polyester; Thermoloft, a combination of solid-core polyester and Quallofil fibers; and polyester pile. Polyester pile jackets are superior to wool sweaters because they are lighter, dry more easily, and stay warm when wet.

Thinsulate and Thermolite, which are thin fiberfill insulations, have higher insulating values because their fibers are small, more finely divided, and trap more air than other materials when made into garments of similar thickness.

Olefin and polypropylene are two popular newer materials with low thermal conductance, high insulating ability, and quick wicking action. Another recent arrival is Capilene, a type of polyester treated to increase wicking ability. These new fabrics are popular choices for thermal underwear and may be the best choice for persons who perspire heavily during cold-weather activities.

Clothing should be **layered** to prevent both chilling and overheating. Layering allows flexibility because one or more layers may be added or subtracted as necessary. Overheating is undesirable because excessive perspiration can saturate clothing and cause heat loss through conduction and evaporation. Because water conducts heat away from the body 32 times faster than does air at the same temperature, wet clothing causes rapid heat loss in cold weather.

Clothing should be selected with both climate and activity in mind. For example, an alpine skier who spends considerable time riding chairlifts and whose downhill speed generates significant windchill will need more layers of clothing than a nordic skier who generates more heat from muscular activity. Clothing should be easily adjustable. Sweaters, shells and jackets should have full-length zippers, and shells should have ventilation zippers near the armpits. Outer layers should be sized generously so that inner layers can expand to their full thicknesses.

Windproof and water-resistant outer garments of nylon, 60/40 cloth (60 percent nylon, 40 percent cotton), or Gore-Tex will prevent heat loss from convection, conduction, and evaporation. These garments should include a ski or mountain parka and wind pants or warm-up pants. The parka should be no shorter than fingertip length unless bib-style pants are worn.

As the wind velocity rises, the "effective" temperature drops (**windchill effect**). This concept refers to the *rate* of heat loss rather than the actual temperature reached as long as evaporation is not a factor. Figure 1.3 illustrates the relationship between actual temperature, wind velocity, and effective temperature at the skin surface and underscores the necessity for windproof outer clothing and for *seeking shelter during periods of cold and high wind*.

Because a body in motion tends to create its own wind, a skier or snowmobiler is more susceptible to frostbite when moving than when stationary (Fig. 1.4). There is a marked danger of frostbite when the windchill factor is 1400 or above (see Fig. 1.3), a range easily attained by a moving skier or snowmobiler when the temperature is -10°F (-23°C). However, many skiers have suffered frostbite just by riding a chairlift while wearing clothing inadequate to protect from the wind and cold.

When the weather is cold, windy and wet, such as during a blizzard at 32°F (0°C), evaporation, convection, radiation, and conduction combine to produce rapid heat loss. This can be a very dangerous situation for those caught unprepared (Fig. 1.5).

To reduce heat loss from **infrared radiation**, wear a hat. At 5°F (-15°C), up to 70 percent of the heat produced by the body can be lost from an uncovered head. This occurs partly because there is no reduction in blood flow to the head in response to cold. The adage "if your feet are cold, put on a hat" is true (Fig. 1.6).

Prevent loss of heat from respiration by avoiding overexertion and excessive heavy breathing. When temperatures are extremely cold, inhaled air can be warmed by pulling a hood or scarf in front of the face to form a frost tunnel (Fig. 1.7).

Avoid heat loss from conduction by sitting on a toboggan, pack or log, rather than in the snow or on a cold rock or metal object (Fig. 1.8). Because bare fingers can freeze to ski bindings, crampons and other metal objects, thin gloves (glove liners) should be worn. Avoid skin contact with gasoline or other volatile liquids with freezing points lower than water which will cause instant frostbite because of conduction and evaporation (Fig. 1.9).

People can lessen heat loss from conduction and evaporation by staying dry or drying off quickly when they get wet in cold weather. Ideally, outer

Fig. 1.3 *Windchill Chart*

clothing should be windproof, should not collect snow, and should shed water. However, outer clothing should not be waterproof because this would cause inner garments to become wet with perspiration. Designers who strive to create the ideal outer garment have a difficult task: to develop a fabric that will allow water to pass from the inside out but not from the outside in. At this time, Gore-Tex appears to do this best although other good fabrics are available. Gore-Tex also is highly windproof and is a good choice for outer garments.

Be sure to adequately cover the head, ears, hands, and feet. This counteracts the tendency of body parts with a high surface-area-to-volume ratio to lose heat rapidly by conduction, convection, and radiation. Coverings should not be so tight that they restrict blood circulation. If socks and mittens get wet, dry them or replace them with dry spares.

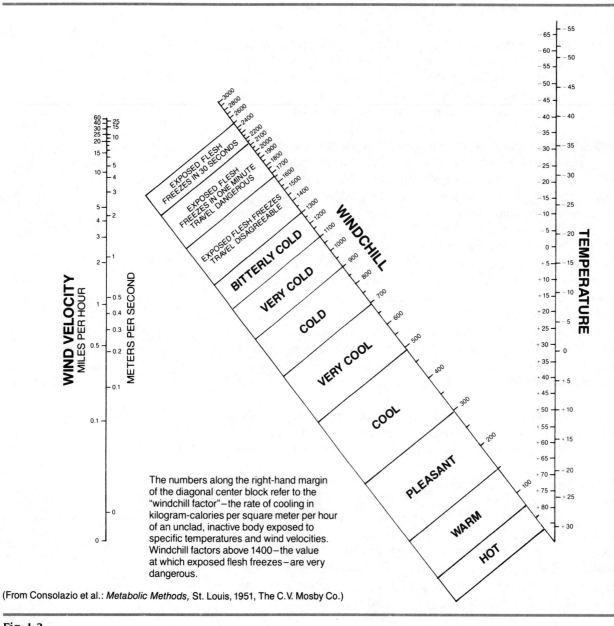

The numbers along the right-hand margin of the diagonal center block refer to the "windchill factor"—the rate of cooling in kilogram-calories per square meter per hour of an unclad, inactive body exposed to specific temperatures and wind velocities. Windchill factors above 1400—the value at which exposed flesh freezes—are very dangerous.

(From Consolazio et al.: *Metabolic Methods*, St. Louis, 1951, The C.V. Mosby Co.)

Fig. 1.3

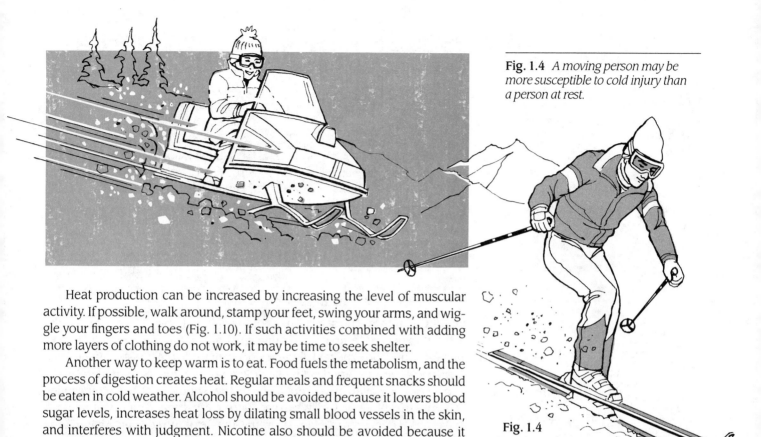

Fig. 1.4 *A moving person may be more susceptible to cold injury than a person at rest.*

Fig. 1.4

Heat production can be increased by increasing the level of muscular activity. If possible, walk around, stamp your feet, swing your arms, and wiggle your fingers and toes (Fig. 1.10). If such activities combined with adding more layers of clothing do not work, it may be time to seek shelter.

Another way to keep warm is to eat. Food fuels the metabolism, and the process of digestion creates heat. Regular meals and frequent snacks should be eaten in cold weather. Alcohol should be avoided because it lowers blood sugar levels, increases heat loss by dilating small blood vessels in the skin, and interferes with judgment. Nicotine also should be avoided because it constricts small blood vessels in the hands and feet, predisposing them to frostbite.

Know when to quit and seek shelter. The rescuer should know how to build a fire under adverse conditions and know the basics of emergency shelter construction (Fig. 1.11). Emergency survival equipment should always be carried in the wilderness.

Fig. 1.5 *The cold outdoor environment can be dangerous to those caught unprepared.*

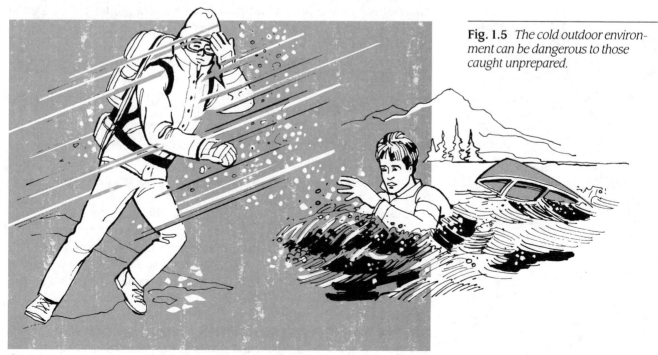

Fig. 1.5

Fig. 1.6 *Wear a hat in cold weather.*

Fig. 1.7 *A frost tunnel will warm inhaled air.*

Fig. 1.8 *Avoid unnecessary contact with cold objects.*

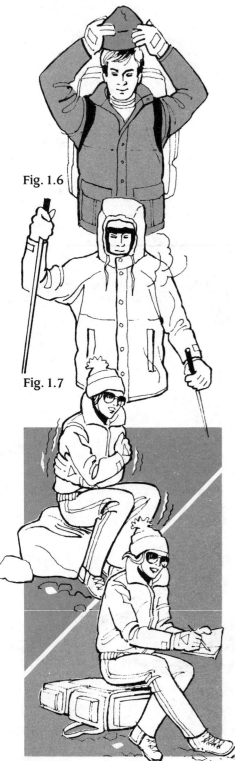

Fig. 1.6

Fig. 1.7

Fig. 1.8

Table 1.9

SAMPLE COLD-WEATHER SURVIVAL KIT

Waterproof matches	Emergency food
Candle	Toilet paper
Sunglasses	Fire starter
Plastic whistle	Sunscreen or sunblock
Signal mirror	Plastic or nylon tarp
Metal pot with bale	100 feet of 1/8-inch nylon cord
First aid kit	Lightweight snow shovel
Flashlight	Ski poles that convert
Extra clothing (at least	into an avalanche probe
two extra layers)	

Sample Cold-Weather Clothing (Fig. 1.12)

Outer Garments: The selection of cold-weather clothing depends upon the activity, expected temperature ranges, predicted amount and type of precipitation, and the expected altitude. For example, in the Coastal Alpine Zone (Cascades, Sierras, Appalachians), where temperatures are moderate and rain is common even in the winter, the rescuer should choose clothing made of fabrics that function well when wet, are easy to dry, and repel water (wool, polyester pile, polypropylene, Dacron, Gore-Tex). In the High Alpine Zone (Rocky Mountains and other inland ranges), where temperatures are lower and the rescuer is less apt to get wet, insulating value and windproofing are more of a concern, and down might be chosen over Dacron, nylon or 60/40 cloth over Gore-Tex).

Underwear: One-hundred-percent wool or 85-percent wool/15-percent nylon underwear is a good choice, but polypropylene, Thermax, and Capilene are probably the new standard. Net underwear is satisfactory if it is made of wool. Synthetic combinations are adequate for alpine skiers; however, waffle-weaves and other types of cotton underwear are inadequate and should be avoided.

Shirt: Wool and polypropylene shirts generally are the best choice; they should open completely in front, or at least have a half-zipper. Turtlenecks protect the neck, as do neck warmers; either can be pulled up to protect the face. Orlon, nylon, or polyester blends are suitable fabrics for shirts worn by alpine skiers.

Pants: Wool pants or knickers are preferable. The hard-finish wool pants found in military surplus stores are durable and reasonably priced. Downhill skiers should select wool or part-wool stretch or quilted pants or bibs. Cotton, particularly denim and corduroy, should be avoided.

Sweater/Jacket: A wool sweater is a good choice, but polyester pile jackets are better. The front should close with a full zipper, buttons, or snaps.

Parka: This garment can be a standard ski or mountain parka filled with down, Dacron, or another insulating material. A jacket or vest worn with a windproof and water-resistant shell is a more versatile combination. The parka or shell should have a hood with drawstring closure and, unless bibs are worn, should be fingertip length or longer to keep the hips and waist warm and to avoid exposing bare skin when bending over. Metal zipper pulls and metal snaps should be situated so they do not touch bare skin.

Wind Pants or Warm-up Pants: These types of pants are a must for cold windy weather, for digging a snow cave, and for working on a patient in wet or deep snow. They can be made of nylon or, preferably, Gore-Tex.

Socks: Wool and polypropylene socks are best. It is preferable to wear a pair of thin, polypropylene socks next to the skin topped with one or more pairs of heavy, wool socks.

Hat: The best hat choice is a wool, polypropylene, or acrylic stocking type that can be pulled down to cover the ears. Unless a neck warmer also is worn, choose a hat with a face mask or balaclava feature to protect the face from cold wind. A light eyeshade or tennis visor is useful for high-glare conditions. Caps with visors and ear protectors that can be pulled down also are popular.

Mittens or Gloves: Mittens tend to be warmer than gloves but are less useful when delicate finger movements are required. A good combination is to wear a pair of thin, polypropylene liners inside heavy, wool or wool/polypropylene mittens, topped by a windproof shell of nylon or Gore-Tex. Depending on temperature and type of activity, any combination of these three layers can be worn at one time. The light liners will protect the hands when ski bindings need adjustments or a splint must be applied. Alpine skiers may prefer leather mittens or gloves lined with foam, down, or Thinsulate. If shells are worn, they should be long enough to cover the wrists.

Boots: Boot choice will depend on both the form of activity and the expected temperature. Boots should be roomy enough to accommodate a pair of polypropylene socks plus one or two pairs of heavy wool socks. The boots must be large enough that the toes are neither cramped nor likely to strike the end of the boot during downhill travel. To avoid both cold feet and blisters, boots should be laced firmly enough so that the heel does not move but not so tightly that the toes cannot be easily wiggled. Use gaiters or overboots in snow country to keep snow out of the tops of the boots.

Fig. 1.9 *Avoid contact with cold liquids.*

Fig. 1.10 *Muscular activity increases heat production.*

Fig. 1.11 *Know when to quit and seek shelter.*

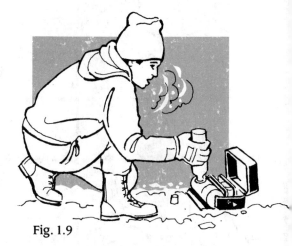

Fig. 1.9

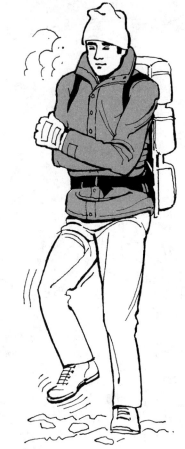

Fig. 1.10

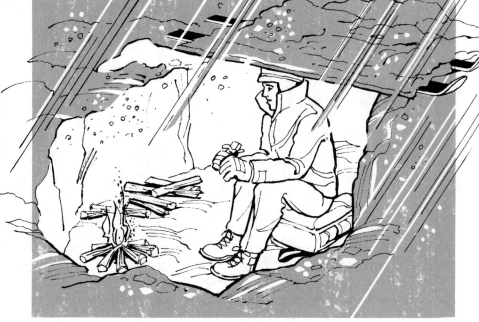

Fig. 1.11

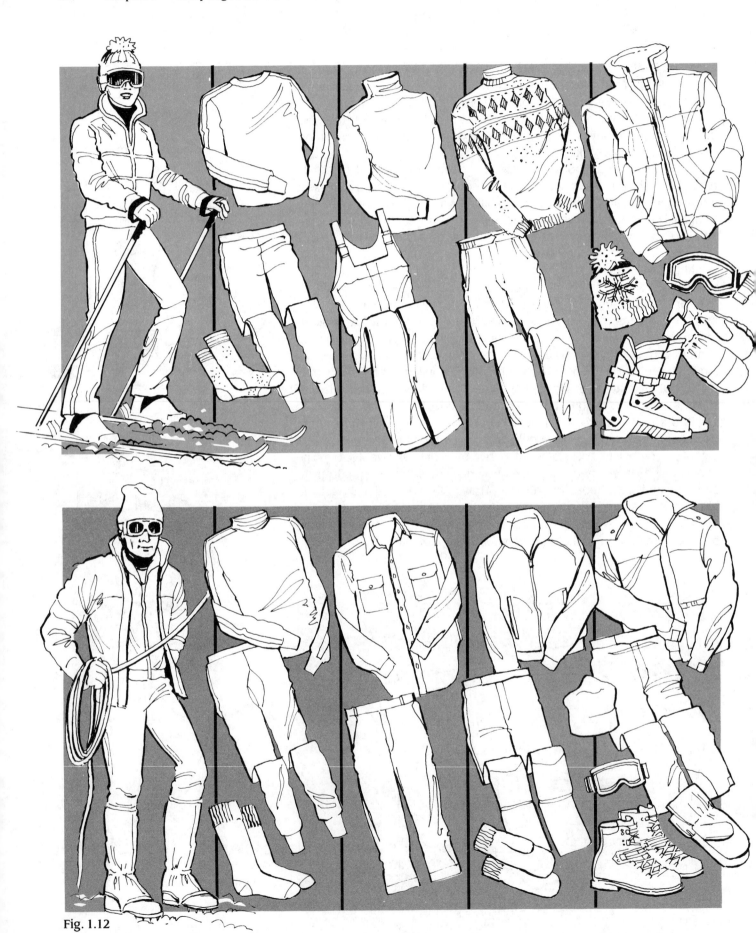

Fig. 1.12

For moderate temperatures, use sturdy full-thickness leather climbing boots 6 to 8 inches in height with rubber lug soles. Double mountaineering boots work well for winter mountaineering in colder temperatures. These boots consist of outer boots made of leather, plastic or nylon, and inner boots insulated with felt or foam. Boots used for ice climbing need to be quite stiff. Boots with a removable felt inner liner such as the Sorel work well for snow-shoeing and other types of non-technical activities. For ski touring and ski mountaineering, special single and double ski boots are available to fit either three-pin or mountaineering ski bindings. Special overboots or felt-lined gaiters are desirable for high-altitude mountaineering in cold weather.

Rain Gear: In moderate climates or very wet conditions where rain or wet snow may be encountered, waterproof outer garments may be preferable to garments made of Gore-Tex or other water-repellent fabrics.

Vapor Barrier Garments: Vapor barrier socks, underwear, and sleeping bag liners are becoming popular. The vapor barrier system consists of a waterproof garment worn either next to the skin or over a thin garment of polypropylene or similar material. This traps a warm film of moisture next to the skin, decreases water requirements by reducing sweating, and increases the insulating properties of outer garments by keeping them dry. This system seems to work better in very cold weather than at moderate temperatures and probably should be avoided by those who perspire excessively. Also, some people dislike the clammy feeling of these garments. Sufficient spare underclothing must be carried to ensure that a dry set will be available each day.

Fig. 1.12 *Alpine skiers and mountaineers should apply the layering principle when selecting cold weather clothing.*

HOT WEATHER

Conditions that predispose humans to serious heat stress occur throughout most of the temperate zone during the summer months and in the tropics year-round. Because heat stress depends on both temperature and humidity, a moderately warm tropical environment with high humidity can be just as dangerous as a hotter, drier desert environment. Death can occur when the body's core temperature rises above 104° to 105°F (40° to 40.6°C). In North America, serious heat stress can occur during marathon races run in hot weather, during long climbs on sun-exposed mountain faces, and during desert hikes. Vehicle breakdowns in isolated desert locations can be very hazardous to unprepared passengers.

Here are some ways to prevent problems from excessive heat:

A. Maximize heat loss
   1. Increase heat loss through conduction, convection, and radiation by exposing the maximum amount of bare skin to the outside air. When in the shade, remove as much clothing as possible. When in the sun, the skin must be protected from sunburn. Because heat loss and sweating may be impaired by sunscreens, a good compromise is to cover the face and hands with a sunscreen with a high SPF (sun protection factor) number (see Chapter 19) and wear a long-sleeved shirt and long pants of thin, loose-fitting, light-colored (preferably white) cotton. Hal Brody, an expert desert hiker, recommends providing additional ventilation by cutting 3-inch triangular holes in clothing at the groin and armpits (Tierney, Gloria, "Body Heat." *Backpacker*, July 1987, p. 26.). Wear a hat

Fig. 1.13 *Proper protective clothing is important in hot weather.*

Fig. 1.14 *Drink plenty of fluids in a hot environment.*

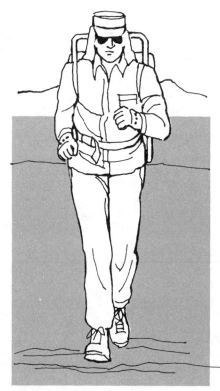

Fig. 1.13

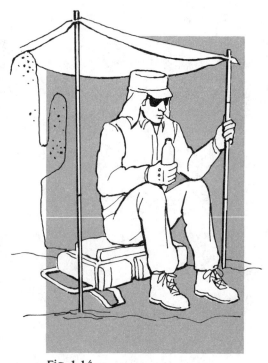

Fig. 1.14

with a wide brim or a Foreign-Legion-style cap with a neck protector and ventilation holes in the crown. Protect the hands with gloves. Sturdy hiking or climbing boots are necessary to protect the feet from hot ground, sharp rocks, and the spines of cacti. Use high-quality sunglasses to protect the eyes from glare (Fig. 1.13) and to block out damaging ultraviolet and infrared rays.

2. Maintain hydration by drinking adequate fluids (Fig. 1.14), some of which can contain electrolyte supplements. Enough water *must* be carried or be readily available in the field. Water bottles should be wrapped in clothing or other insulation and buried in a backpack to keep the water cool.

3. Use the layering principle of dressing so that layers can be taken off during the heat of the day and added at night when the dry desert soil cools rapidly.

4. Because of its high thermal conductivity, poor insulating ability and good wicking ability, cotton is the fabric of choice for hot-weather clothing. Clothing should be loose to improve air circulation.

B. Minimize heat gain

1. Use coverings to protect the head and body from the direct rays of the sun.

2. Seek shade during the hottest part of the day. Make a sun shelter by suspending a tarp from cacti or by laying the tarp on a framework of poles. Because desert air is much cooler a foot *above* or a few inches *below* the ground surface, the desert traveler should lie on a platform or in a scooped-out depression rather than directly on the ground.

3. Avoid muscular exertion during periods of high heat and high humidity.

4. Protect the skin by wearing shoes and avoiding contact with hot metal objects.

5. When traveling in hot weather, rest in the shade rather than in the sun.

Table 1.10

AVOIDING EXCESS BODY HEAT

Increasing Heat Loss:
  Wear cotton clothing.
  Expose bare skin to air.
  Aid evaporation by hydration and acclimatization to heat.
Reducing Heat Gain From Outside:
  Seek shade during the heat of the day.
  Wear protective clothing.
  Wear the proper type of hat, gloves, and boots.
  Avoid touching metal.
  Do not lie directly on the ground, but on a low platform or in a depression scooped out of the ground.
Decreasing Heat Production:
  Decrease muscular activity.

Table 1.11

SAMPLE DESERT SURVIVAL KIT FOR VEHICLES

Waterproof matches	Flashlight
Sturdy knife	Metal pot with bale
Candle	Map
Fire starter	Plastic or nylon tarp
Plastic whistle	Signal mirror
Nylon tarp	Toilet paper
Card with ground-to-air signals	First aid kit
Change for pay phone	50 feet of ⅛-inch nylon cord
Sunscreen or sunblock	CB radio
Compass	Lip salve
Spare sunglasses	Folding saw
Five-gallon water jug, full	Heavy gloves
Short-handled folding shovel	

Material for constructing four solar stills: four sheets of clear plastic, 6 feet x 6 feet, reinforced in the center by an X of duct tape; four pieces of surgical tubing, 6 to 8 feet long; four 1-quart plastic bowls (Fig. 1.15).

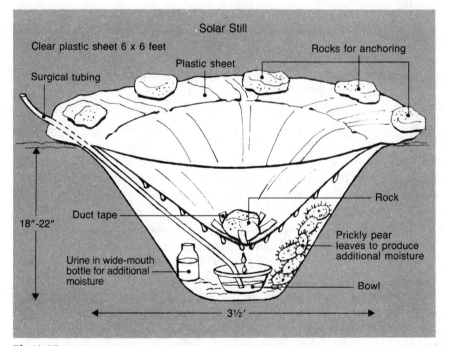

Fig. 1.15 *Solar Still*

Fig. 1.15

The body adapts better to heat and altitude than to cold. Acclimatization to heat includes an increase in blood volume and heart efficiency to carry heat from the body core to the surface. Perspiration increases, and the sweat contains less salt. After a week to 10 days, exposure to heat is noticeably less debilitating. On return to a cooler climate, these processes reverse. The most obvious change is a temporary increase in urine volume as the blood volume contracts and the excess liquid is excreted by the kidneys.

Table 1.12

ACCLIMATIZATION TO HEAT

The process takes seven to 10 days to complete.
Blood volume increases.
Sweating rate increases.
Less sodium and potassium is lost in sweat.
Efficiency of heart increases.

FOOD AND WATER

Nutrition must be a concern to outdoor travelers, especially members of res-cue groups who may engage in unplanned, heavy physical activity for long periods in severe weather without adequate food or rest. Performance can be increased if the principles of good nutrition are applied both before and dur-ing an outdoor experience. Proper nutrition is the bedrock of physical per-formance. In striving for physical fitness, the rescuer needs to emphasize nutrition as well as physical conditioning.

The six groups of nutrients are **carbohydrates**, **proteins**, **fats**, **minerals**, **vitamins**, and **water**.

Table 1.13

Fig. 1.16 *Sources of Carbohydrate*

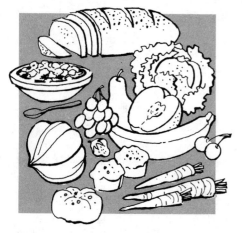

Table 1.14

FOOD SOURCES OF CARBOHYDRATE

Vegetables
Cereals
Fruits
Sugar

THE SIX GROUPS OF NUTRIENTS

Carbohydrates	Minerals
Proteins	Vitamins
Fats	Water

Carbohydrates: These organic compounds are composed of carbon, hydrogen, and oxygen. When oxidized in the body, they produce energy, heat, carbon dioxide, and water. They are present in food mainly as sugars and starches and are broken down during digestion into simple sugars that are converted into **glucose**. Carbohydrate is stored as **glycogen** in the liver and muscles and can be broken down quickly into glucose to provide a rapid source of energy. However, these glycogen stores are not large and are mark-edly depleted by a fast as short as 24 hours. Eating a high-carbohydrate diet for several days will double the glycogen stores and can increase endurance up to three times that of an ordinary balanced diet. Conversely, a low-car-bohydrate diet can decrease glycogen stores and reduce endurance by as much as 50 percent. The main dietary sources of carbohydrate are fruits, vegetables, cereals, and sugar (Fig. 1.16).

Fats: Fats are also made up of carbon, oxygen, and hydrogen and, when burned, they also produce heat, energy, water, and carbon dioxide. In cases of starvation, body fat tends to be broken down into acidic compounds. If these compounds accumulate in the blood faster than they can be burned, they cause the body tissues and blood to become excessively acidic (**acido-sis**). One type, cholesterol, has been implicated as a cause of **arterio-sclerosis**, a disease characterized by thickening and loss of elasticity of arterial walls. In general, vegetable (polyunsaturated) fats are less likely to cause arteriosclerosis than animal (saturated) fats. However, some vegetable fats, such as coconut oil, are highly saturated.

Common food sources of fat are butter, lard, cooking oil, mayonnaise, and ice cream. Fat also is found in lesser amounts in dairy products, meat, eggs, nuts, vegetables, and cereals (Fig. 1.17).

In the body, fat serves as the main storage form of energy. One gram of fat has the equivalent of nine calories of energy; a gram of protein or carbohydrate has only four. Fat in the subcutaneous tissues insulates against cold but interferes with heat loss in hot weather. During brief exercise, energy is derived equally from fat and carbohydrate. As the duration of the exercise lengthens, the percent of energy supplied by fat increases up to 80 percent.

Proteins: Proteins contain nitrogen, sulfur, and phosphorus in addition to carbon, hydrogen, and oxygen. They are complicated molecules composed of chains of **amino acids**. Common sources of protein are eggs, dairy products, meat, poultry, fish, legumes (peas and beans), nuts, and cereals (Fig. 1.18).

Animal products, especially eggs, are better sources of complete protein than vegetable products. Vegetarians should include eggs and dairy products in their diets or consume a wide variety of grains and legumes to obtain all essential amino acids as well as adequate calcium, phosphorus, and vitamin B12. There is no benefit from eating excessive amounts of protein, since the excess will be converted into energy that, if not used, is stored as fat.

Vitamins: Trace amounts of these substances are essential to the metabolic functioning of the body. Because vitamins cannot be made by the body, they must be supplied in food. Fortunately, a balanced diet will supply sufficient quantities of essential vitamins. Fourteen vitamins have been identified to date: the water-soluble vitamins, B_1, B_2, B_6, niacin, pantothenic acid, biotin, choline, folic acid, B_{12}, and C; and the fat-soluble vitamins, A, D, E, and K.

Water-soluble vitamins are not stored in the body and need to be consumed daily. Fat-soluble vitamins can be stored in the body. When too much vitamin A or D is ingested, a toxic condition called hypervitaminosis can develop. For example, eating seal or polar bear liver, which are extremely rich in vitamin A, can cause acute vitamin A toxicity.

A well-balanced diet contains adequate vitamins, making vitamin supplements unnecessary. A daily multivitamin tablet does no harm, but megadoses of vitamins (more than 10 times the recommended daily allowance) may be harmful. For example, too much vitamin C can cause gout, gastritis, and diarrhea; too much vitamin B_6, nerve damage, too much niacin, heart abnormalities; and too much vitamin E, headaches and weakness. In our society, vitamin supplements are overproduced, overpromoted, and overconsumed, making American sewers the world's most vitamin enriched.

Minerals: Four percent of body weight is made up of inorganic elements and simple inorganic compounds called minerals. The most common minerals in the body are compounds of calcium, phosphorus, magnesium, iron, sodium, potassium, sulfur, fluorine, and zinc.

There is little need to supplement a well-balanced diet with minerals, since they are abundant in common foods. However, iron is poorly absorbed from the digestive tract, and growing children and women of childbearing age may require iron supplements. People who do not get adequate calcium from sources such as dairy products should take calcium supplements to help prevent osteoporosis in later life.

Fig. 1.17 *Sources of Fat*

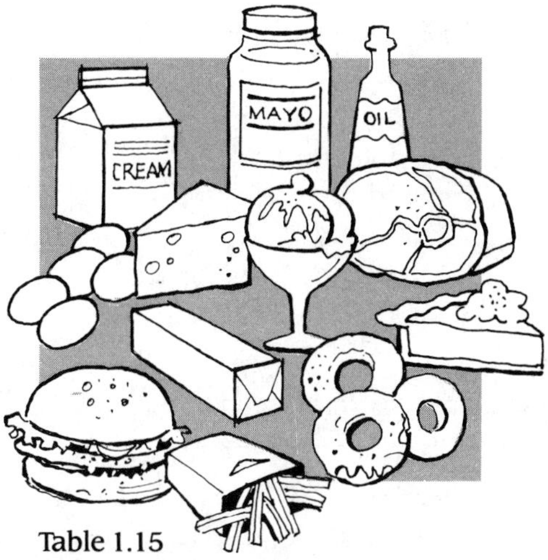

Table 1.15

FOOD SOURCES OF FAT

Butter	Dairy products
Lard	Meat
Cooking oil	Eggs
Mayonnaise	Nuts
Ice cream	Vegetables
Cereals	

Fig. 1.18 *Sources of Protein*

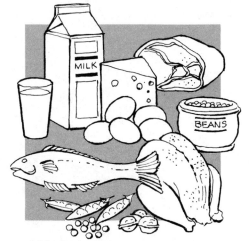

Table 1.16

FOOD SOURCES OF PROTEIN

Eggs	Fish
Dairy products	Peas
Meat	Beans
Poultry	Nuts
Cereals	

Table 1.17

THE FOURTEEN VITAMINS

Water Soluble   *Fat Soluble*
B_1, B_2, B_6, Niacin,   A, D, E, K
Pantothenic acid,
Biotin, Choline,
Folic acid, B_{12}, C

Table 1.18

ESSENTIAL MINERALS

Major	*Trace*
Calcium	Copper
Phosphorus	Iodine
Magnesium	Chromium
Iron	Selenium
Sodium	Zinc
Potassium	Fluorine
Sulfur	Molybdenum
	Cobalt
	Manganese

Table 1.19

During prolonged exertion in hot weather, sweating may deplete the body of sodium and potassium, leading to fatigue, muscle cramps or even heat exhaustion. Under these conditions, electrolytes and water should be replaced by drinking lightly salted, cold water (1/3 teaspoon salt per liter). Even though commercial electrolyte beverages contain electrolytes in slightly different amounts than needed, healthy individuals usually can excrete the excess in their urine. A normal diet contains so much potassium that potassium depletion is almost never a problem except when a potassium-depleting diuretic medication is taken for high blood pressure or heart disease.

In summary, the best diet is one that supplies adequate nutrients for heat and energy production and for tissue maintenance, repair, and growth. A person of average size should eat about 65 grams of protein daily, with two-thirds of that amount supplied by meat and dairy products and one-third by vegetables, fruits and whole grains, including bread. About 45 grams of fat should be eaten daily, mainly as meat and dairy products, plus the small amount found in vegetables, fruit, nuts, and whole grains. About 150 grams of carbohydrate should be consumed, mostly as fruits, vegetables, and whole-grain cereals.

These components will provide for the basic needs of the body but will total less than 1,300 calories. The additional 2,000 to 3,000 calories needed by an active individual may be obtained from a variety of foods, depending on individual choice. Foods that contain large amounts of refined sugar and/or saturated fat should be kept to a minimum (candy and other sweets, animal fat, lard, butter, cream, ice cream, coconut oil, egg yolks, shellfish, and organ meats).

COMPONENTS OF A PROPER DIET

Protein:	65 grams (two-thirds from meat and dairy products, one third from cereals, vegetables)
Fat:	45 grams (from meat, dairy products, vegetables, nuts, cereals)
Carbohydrate:	150 grams (from fruits, vegetables, cereals)
Calories:	2,000 to 5,000
Avoid:	Candy and other sweets, animal fat, lard, butter, cream, ice cream, coconut oil, egg yolk, shellfish, organ meats.

Those who expect to engage in strenuous physical activity should increase the percentage of carbohydrate in their diet to 70 to 80 percent for several days *beforehand* by eating large amounts of potatoes, rice, pasta, and other high-carbohydrate foods. This diet should be continued for several days *after* the activity to replenish muscle glycogen stores.

The number and size of servings can be increased to provide the calories necessary to support a given level of activity. This may be as high as 4,000 to 5,000 calories a day during a prolonged rescue effort or mountaineering expedition. Most additional calories should come from complex carbohydrates such as fruits, vegetables, and whole grains.

Table 1.20

MINIMUM REQUIREMENTS FOR ADEQUATE NUTRITION

Food Group	Servings (average size)
Milk and milk products	2
Meat and/or other high-protein food sources	2
Vegetables and fruits	4
Cereals and whole grains	4

Emergency food should be light in weight, high in energy, and should not require cooking or complicated preparation. Examples include cheese, sausage, candy bars, gorp, bread, nuts, cocoa, instant breakfast drink, fruitcake, and dried fruit. Living off the land is a romantic notion and may be possible for experienced persons in survival situations, but, in general, an untrained person cannot find enough wild food to replace the energy expended searching for it.

Water: Water makes up about 60 percent of the body weight of an average young adult male. In females, the percentage of water is somewhat lower and the percentage of fat somewhat higher. The average sedentary person excretes about 2,500 milliliters (2.7 quarts) of water each day. Of this total, 1,200 milliliters (1.3 quarts) is lost in the urine, 1,000 milliliters (1.1 quarts) through the skin and lungs, and 300 milliliters (10 ounces) in the stool. Therefore, to prevent dehydration, 2,500 milliliters (2.7 quarts) of water must be added daily. While 700 milliliters (24 ounces) of water is created during the metabolism of protein, fat, and carbohydrate, the remaining 1,800 milliliters (2 quarts) must come from liquids and the fluids contained in such foods as meat, vegetables, and fruits.

Table 1.21

WATER BALANCE

Gain	Loss
Metabolism = 700 ml	Urine = 1,200 ml
Liquids and water-containing foods = 1,800 ml	Skin and lungs = 1,000 ml
	Stool = 300 ml
Total = 2,500 ml	Total = 2,500 ml

At high altitude, in hot weather, and during strenuous exercise, the amount of water lost through skin and lungs increases greatly. These losses can total 1,000 milliliters (1.1 quarts) per hour during nordic ski racing.

Active efforts must be made to prevent dehydration in the outdoors, especially in very cold and very hot weather, and at high altitude. Cold weather decreases the sense of thirst, which may lead to a state of chronic, mild dehydration. At temperatures below freezing and at elevations above the snow line, the lack of liquid water and the time and effort required to melt snow compound the problem. In desert areas, water may be almost impossible to find.

Avoid or purify surface water contaminated by human or animal wastes. *Giardia lamblia*, an organism found in animal feces that is responsible for painful diarrhea, may contaminate surface water. Small streams and springs coming down from high, uninhabited areas at right angles to the main valley drainage are more apt to be safe than larger streams running in the valley floor. However, purification still is wise.

Purify water by boiling, filtration, or disinfection. Remove obvious dirt by straining the water through cloth. If water is boiled, boil it for five minutes plus one minute for each 1,000 feet (305 meters) of altitude above sea level. Several excellent brands of filters are available. Look for filters with pores small enough to remove bacteria and *Giardia* cysts; most will not remove viruses.

The most practical chemical disinfection is iodine-based. Tetraglycine hydroperiodide tablets (Potable Aqua) are widely available. However, there is some question whether this compound kills *Giardia* cysts. Newer agents are being developed and may be available soon.

Whenever open water is encountered on the trail in winter, drink plenty and fill all empty canteens. Take time in the morning to melt and purify enough snow to provide each party member with enough to drink plus a canteenful for the day. At night, drink enough water to satisfy thirst, and sleep with a full canteen to prevent it from freezing. It is more efficient to melt ice or hard snow than to melt light, powdery snow. On warm, sunny days, snow can be spread on a dark poncho to melt.

During hot weather, especially in desert areas, carry large amounts of water since natural water sources cannot be relied on. A desert survival kit should contain the materials to make several solar stills (see Fig. 1.15), and desert travelers should be familiar with the fundamentals of desert and hot-weather survival.

At high altitude and when working hard, drink at least 3 to 4 liters (3.2 to 4.2 quarts) of water; in deserts, as much as a liter per hour may be needed. Urine output is a good indicator of the state of hydration. Daily urine production should equal 1 to 1.5 liters (1.1 to 1.6 quarts), and the color should be light. Strenuous exercise may cause urine to be orange-brown, while vitamin supplements containing riboflavin (vitamin B1) will turn it bright yellow. Make water more palatable by adding fruit flavors or making hot drinks to encourage consumption. However, when working hard and perspiring heavily, it is better to drink small amounts of plain, cold water frequently. Adding sugar to water and overfilling the stomach by drinking large amounts of liquid at one time are counterproductive because they delay gastric emptying.

If water supplies are limited, sweat should be rationed by avoiding overexertion. In desert areas, the traveler should rest in the shade during the heat of the day and travel in the early morning or at night.

PHYSICAL CONDITIONING

Physical fitness and conditioning are important to members of any outdoor recreational or rescue group because outdoor travel imposes great physical demands and presents the possibility of severe, prolonged physical stress. Therefore, rescuers should maintain a superior level of physical fitness. Most rescuers participate in sports related to their rescue interests such as climbing, recreational skiing, caving, and kayaking. These activities require strong, supple, durable bodies for full enjoyment. Although the best training for any sport is to practice that sport, people with demanding urban jobs may have to substitute a carefully selected set of exercises that can be performed regularly in their spare time and close to home.

Proper physical conditioning improves the strength of muscles and tendons, enhances coordination, flexibility and endurance, and reduces the chance of injury. Conditioning allows individuals to exert harder and longer without tiring and to recover more rapidly after rest. Conditioning also increases the margin of safety in a survival situation.

Proper conditioning slows aging and helps maintain normal weight. The drop in U.S. mortality from cardiovascular disease in the past 20 years is probably due in part to increased participation in active sports by people of all ages. The fit rescuer performs better because the fit body functions better, is better able to avoid injury, and recovers faster if injured. Fitness can be divided into two parts: **cardiovascular** or **aerobic** (oxygen-requiring) **fitness**, which develops the heart and circulatory system to meet the body's changing demands for blood; and **motor fitness**, which develops and enhances strength, power, endurance, balance, agility, and flexibility. Suitable conditioning programs should develop both types of fitness.

Studies of skeletal muscle structure (histology) and function (physiology) indicate that there are two types of voluntary muscle fibers: Type I or "slow-twitch" fibers, which are designed for sustained, slow contractions and rely mainly on aerobic metabolic processes; and Type II or "fast-twitch" fibers, which are capable of rapid contractions, tend to rely on anaerobic (non-oxygen-requiring) metabolism, and form lactic acid readily.

Successful endurance athletes such as nordic ski racers, bicycle racers, marathon runners, and long-distance swimmers tend to have more slow-twitch than fast-twitch fibers. Athletes who engage in short, intense bursts of effort, such as sprinters, jumpers and weight lifters, do better if they have a predominance of fast-twitch fibers.

Fig. 1.19 *Three Types of Endurance Athletes*

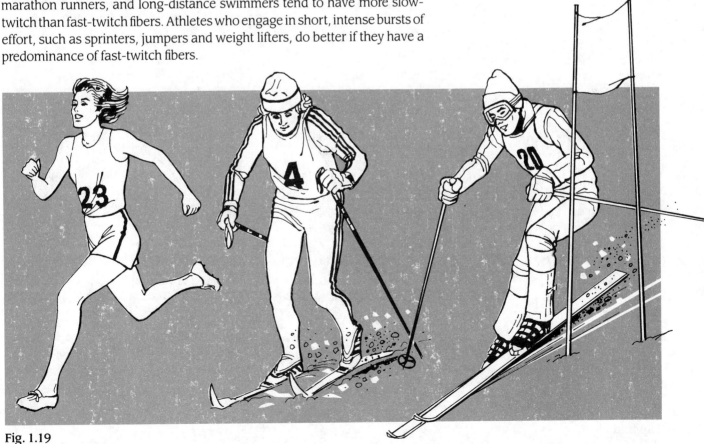

Fig. 1.19

Fig. 1.20 *A good physical conditioning program includes a warm-up and cool-down period, stretching exercises, calisthenics, and aerobic exercise.*

Although the proportion of fast-and slow-twitch fibers is determined at birth, selective development of one type over the other is possible to some extent. It is interesting that top alpine ski racers show wide individual variations in the relative numbers of fast- and slow-twitch fibers. This suggests that alpine skiers and ski racers employ both fiber types and that their training should emphasize aerobic techniques as well as strength, agility, and the other components of motor fitness. Training for backpacking and nordic skiing should emphasize both upper- and lower-body endurance.

The training goal for any endurance sport is to *maximize the body's ability to extract and use oxygen*. This ability can be measured by pulmonary function tests. The greatest ability to extract and use oxygen (VO2max) is produced by training that uses the upper and lower extremities *at the same time*, such as roller skiing and speed hiking with poles on dry land, nordic skiing on snow, and using a nordic skiing simulator.

A good training program should start off moderately but aim for an eventual minimum workout length of 45 minutes four times a week. The program should include a proper warm-up period with stretching exercises and selected calisthenics designed to develop the upper and lower extremities, back, and trunk (sit-ups, pull-ups, leg raises, push-ups, dips between parallel bars, barbell exercises, toe raises, hops over a box, etc.). Handball, racquetball, climbing boulders, gymnastics, wrestling and other vigorous games can be substituted for calisthenics.

The workout should build cardiovascular fitness and endurance with a period of rhythmical, nonstop training (swimming, jogging, bicycling, roller skiing, or using a rowing machine, exercise bicycle or nordic skiing simulator). For minimum effectiveness, these exercises must be vigorous enough to develop and maintain a heart rate of 75 percent of the subject's maximum age-related heart rate for at least 15 minutes. This rate is calcu-

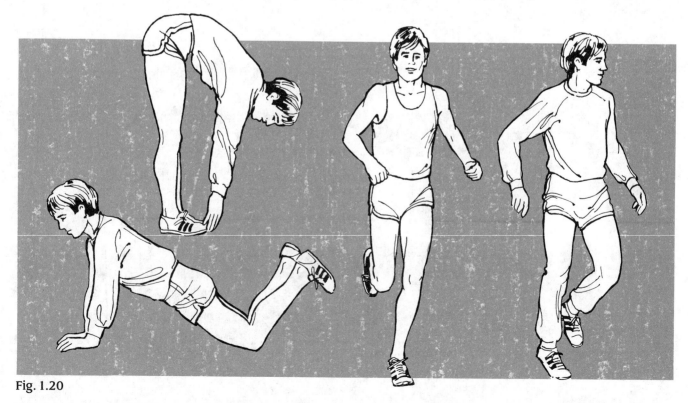

Fig. 1.20

lated by subtracting one's age from 220 and multiplying by .75. The last part of the workout is a cooling down period.

People who have not been exercising regularly should get a thorough checkup by a physician before embarking on a fitness program. Exercise should be progressive so that optimum fitness can be achieved by steadily increasing the demands made on the body. Excessive fatigue, inability to sleep the following night, a prolonged fast pulse, and persistent muscle and joint tenderness are signs that the workout has been too hard. Soon, however, the benefits of fitness become evident. The fit person feels less tired at the end of the day despite having expended more energy. Sleep is more restful, the body is less tense, and weight is maintained more easily. Individuals who follow a fitness program may not be transformed into Olympic athletes, but they will be better athletes than unfit individuals of equal natural ability and will be better able to enjoy the outdoors safely.

2

Overview of Human Anatomy and Physiology

The proper study of mankind is man.

–Alexander Pope
An Essay on Man

Fig. 2.1 *Typical Cell and its Parts*

INTRODUCTION

The basic unit of all living matter is the cell (Fig. 2.1). Individual cells group together to form tissues, tissues group together to form organs, and organs group together to form organ systems. The eight organ systems can be categorized as **primary**, **secondary**, and **supportive**, based on the importance of their contribution to basic body survival. The primary organ systems are the circulatory and respiratory, the secondary systems are the digestive and urinary, and the supportive systems are the cutaneous, nervous, musculoskeletal, and reproductive.

The primary organ systems function and interact with two major purposes: to carry oxygen, food and other essential materials *to* and remove waste products *from* each cell.

The **circulatory system** consists of a "pump," the heart; a set of "pipes," the blood vessels; and fluid to fill the pipes, the blood. It is a closed system, in which blood is pumped by the heart through increasingly smaller vessels to the smallest vessels, the capillaries, which transfer oxygen and nutrients directly to each cell and pick up carbon dioxide and other waste products. The blood then flows back to the heart through increasingly larger vessels and is cleansed of carbon dioxide and other wastes on the way.

The **respiratory system** brings air into the lungs, transfers oxygen to the red blood cells, and removes carbon dioxide from the blood.

The **digestive system** ingests food, breaks it down into simpler compounds that can be absorbed into the blood, and expels the residue.

The **urinary system** is the major cleanser of the blood. This system removes the waste products of cellular metabolism and excretes them in the urine.

The **skeletal system** provides protection, form and support to the body and permits an upright stance.

The **muscular system** acts together with the skeletal system to permit body movement.

The **skin and subcutaneous tissues** protect the internal body parts and keep them from drying out. This system also helps control body temperature

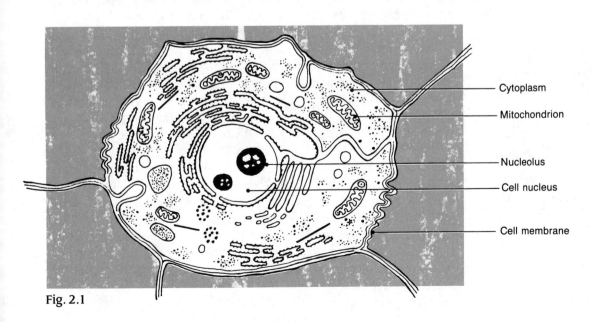

Fig. 2.1

Fig. 2.2 *Specialized Cells*

and contains the special organs responsible for sensations of pain, touch, and temperature.

The **nervous system** collects and processes stimuli from the environment and coordinates the activities of the other major organ systems.

The **reproductive system** provides the means for producing successive generations of offspring.

THE WORK OF THE CELL

Living cells have both **basic** and **specialized functions**. All cells convert food to **heat** and **energy** through a complex process that requires oxygen and breaks down carbohydrates, fats and proteins into water, carbon dioxide, and simple waste compounds. The same amount of water, carbon dioxide, heat, energy, and wastes would be produced if the food were set on fire outside the body. Cells use a series of complicated chemical reactions regulated by substances called enzymes to produce energy in small, usable amounts. Because these enzymes work best at or slightly above normal human body temperature (98.6°F or 37°C), body temperature must be carefully regulated to ensure optimum body functioning.

Energy is used by cells to fuel basic tasks such as the vital processes of growth, repair, reproduction, and storing energy as fat and carbohydrate.

Most cells also have specialized, energy-requiring functions (Fig. 2.2). For example, muscle cells contain contractile proteins that allow them to shorten, causing the muscle to contract and permitting body movement. Cells that line the stomach and small intestine produce enzymes and other substances that break down food so it can be absorbed into the bloodstream. The pancreas produces a hormone, **insulin**, essential for the use of glucose as fuel by the cells. Cells that line the respiratory tract produce mucus and have hair-like projections called cilia that move with a coordinated wave-like motion to clear the lungs of mucus.

All of these processes are part of the body's **metabolism**, i.e., the chemical reactions that produce or use energy. The major requirement for metabolism is **oxygen**, which is so vitally important that an oxygen-deprived cell can die within minutes. Different body cells may vary in sensitivity to lack of oxygen: heart cells are injured if deprived of oxygen for more than a few seconds, brain cells are injured within 4 to 6 minutes. Muscle cells can withstand oxygen deprivation much longer and can even incur an **oxygen debt.**

During short periods of very strenuous activity, the muscles use fuel so rapidly that the circulatory and respiratory systems cannot supply the muscles with enough oxygen to completely metabolize their principal fuel, carbohydrates. Without oxygen, carbohydrates are broken down into an intermediate product, lactic acid, which accumulates in the blood and the muscle tissues during exercise. This creates an oxygen debt that is paid after exercise when sufficient oxygen can be delivered to break down the lactic acid to carbon dioxide and water (Fig. 2.3). Although a certain amount of lactic acid accumulation is safe, it is one of the causes of muscle pain during and after strenuous exercise.

Because oxygen is so vital, techniques to assist and reestablish the function of the respiratory and circulatory systems assume central importance in emergency care.

Skin Cells

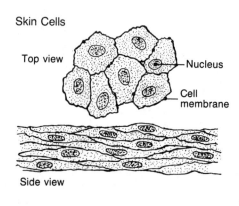

Trachea Cells

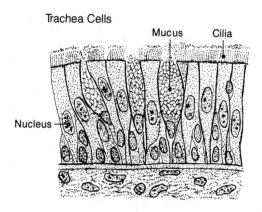

Striated Muscle Cells

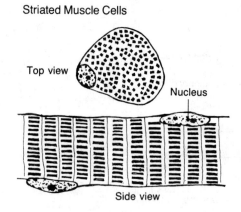

Fig. 2.2

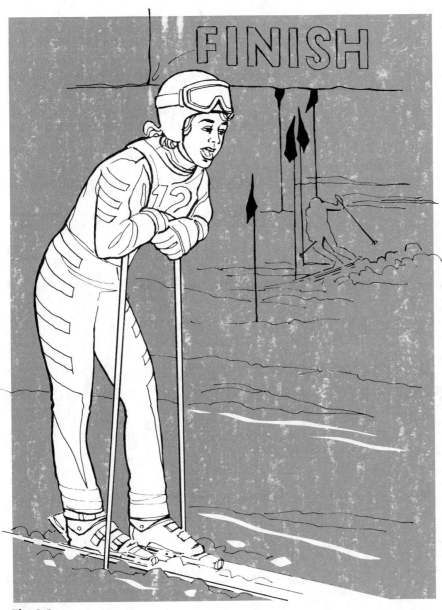

Fig. 2.3

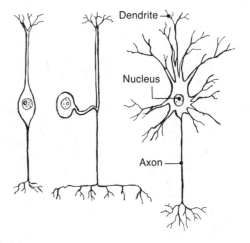

Fig. 2.3 *An oxygen debt must be paid after strenuous exercise.*

Nerve Cells

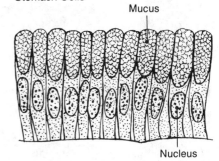

Stomach Cells

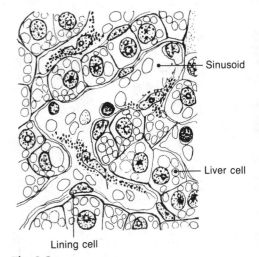

Liver Cells

Fig. 2.2

VOCABULARY

Before examining the eight organ systems in more detail, it is necessary to present a few important anatomical terms used in this text (Fig. 2.4). The terms refer to the human body standing *erect* and *facing* the examiner with the arms held so that the palms of the hands face forward. The terms permit the rescuer to talk intelligently with members of the EMS system, describe observations accurately, and avoid confusion.

The terms *right* and *left* refer to the *patient's* right and left. The body is considered to be divided into right and left halves by an imaginary plane, the **median plane**. The intersection of this plane with the surface of the body in front and in back is known as the **midline** of the body. Keeping this in mind, there are three pairs of relative terms that can be used to express the relationship of any given structure to another.

Fig. 2.4 *Anatomical Terms for the Human Body*

The term **anterior** means *nearer* to the *front* surface of the body, while **posterior** means *nearer* to the *back* surface of the body. **Medial** means *nearer* the **midline** of the body; **lateral** means *farther* from the midline of the body. **Superior** means *nearer* to the **top of the head**, while **inferior** means *nearer* to the **soles of the feet.**

One final pair of terms also is important: **proximal** means closer to the **trunk of the body**; **distal** means closer to the **tips of the extremities.**

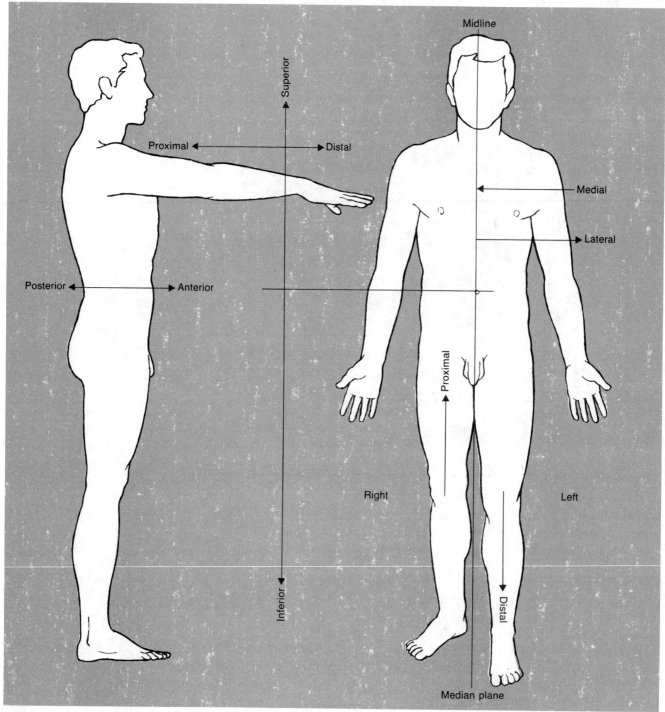

Fig. 2.4

THE CIRCULATORY SYSTEM

The circulatory system includes the **heart**, **arteries**, **capillaries**, **veins**, and **blood**. These are linked together to form a closed system (Fig. 2.5) of two loops, the **pulmonary** and **systemic circulations**. The heart (Figs. 2.5, 2.6) lies between the lungs in the thoracic cage. It is divided into a right and left side; each side contains two chambers, an **atrium** and a **ventricle**. The right side of the heart is smaller than the left because it pumps blood into the smaller, low-pressure pulmonary circulation.

Blood returning to the heart from the body enters the **right atrium**, passes into the **right ventricle**, and then flows to the **main pulmonary artery**, which divides into right and left branches that supply the respective lungs. These branches divide into progressively smaller arteries, terminating in the **pulmonary capillaries**, which line the walls of the smallest air sacs, the **alveoli.**

Reoxygenated blood collects in tiny veins, which join to form progressively larger veins to bring blood to the **left atrium** of the heart. The blood is pumped from the left atrium into the **left ventricle** and then into the major artery of the body, the **aorta.**

The aorta curves up over the heart and then runs down through the body branching off into a number of large **arteries** (Fig. 2.8a): the **coronaries**, which supply the heart; the **carotids**, which supply the head and neck; the **subclavians**, which supply the upper extremities; the **superior and inferior mesenterics**, which supply the digestive tract; the **renals**, which supply the kidneys; and the **iliacs**, which supply the lower extremities. These arteries divide into smaller and smaller branches, eventually forming capillaries that interlace so each cell is close enough to a capillary to be easily supplied with oxygen and nutrients.

Fig. 2.5 *Schema of the Heart and Circulatory System*

Fig. 2.6 *Anatomical Position of the Heart in the Thoracic Cage*

Fig. 2.7 *Heart and the Roots of the Great Vessels*

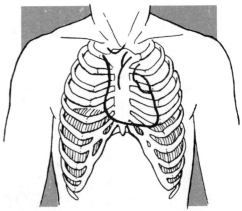

Fig. 2.6

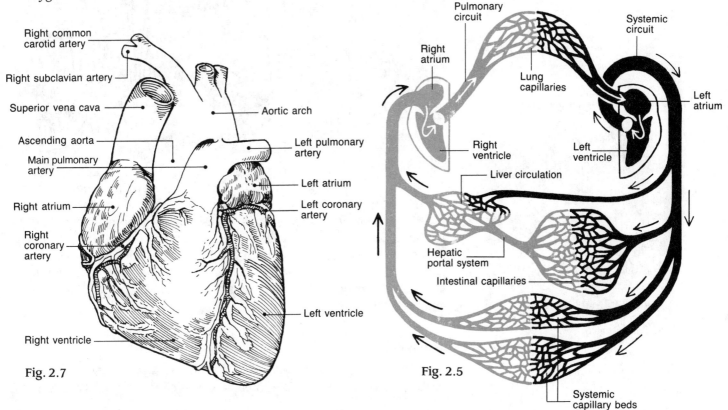

Fig. 2.7

- Right common carotid artery
- Right subclavian artery
- Superior vena cava
- Ascending aorta
- Main pulmonary artery
- Right atrium
- Right coronary artery
- Right ventricle
- Aortic arch
- Left pulmonary artery
- Left atrium
- Left coronary artery
- Left ventricle

Fig. 2.5

- Pulmonary circuit
- Right atrium
- Right ventricle
- Systemic circuit
- Lung capillaries
- Left atrium
- Left ventricle
- Liver circulation
- Hepatic portal system
- Intestinal capillaries
- Systemic capillary beds

Fig. 2.8 *Major Blood Vessels*

Fig. 2.9 *Microorganic Appearance of the Blood*

Deoxygenated blood containing waste products is conducted back to the heart through larger and larger veins, many named to correspond with the arteries (Fig. 2.8b). Eventually the returning blood empties into the two major veins of the body, the **inferior** and **superior venae cavae**. The superior vena cava drains the head, neck, and upper extremities; the inferior vena cava drains the abdomen, pelvis, and lower extremities. Both of these large veins drain into the **right atrium.**

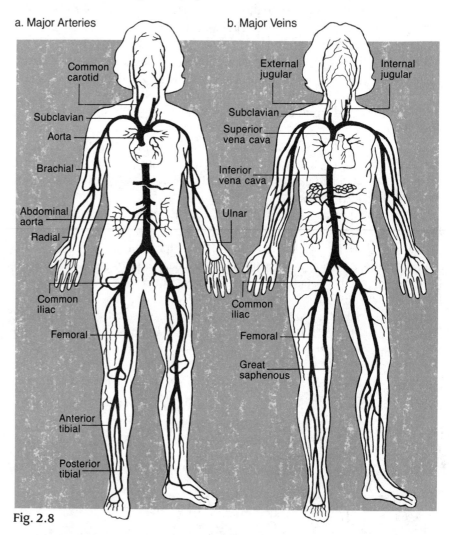

Fig. 2.8

In general, the deeper veins of the body run close to the corresponding arteries, while the veins of the skin do not.

Blood circulation is a continuous process. The heart normally beats 60 to 100 times a minute, pumping about 80 milliliters (2.5 ounces) of blood into the aorta with each beat. The heart of an average-sized adult male at rest pumps blood at the rate of about 5.5 liters per minute (1.5 gallons per minute). Major damage to the heart or a major artery can lead to rapid blood loss and death within minutes.

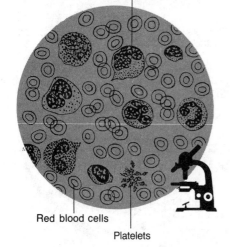

Fig. 2.9

The Blood

Blood is a thick, red fluid made up of cells and **plasma** (Fig. 2.9). There are three types of cells in blood: **red cells**, which carry oxygen; **white cells**, which fight infection; and **platelets**, which aid blood clotting. Plasma is a liquid that consists of water and a remarkable number of different minerals, inorganic compounds, and organic compounds such as proteins, simple sugars, and fats. It contains transient materials such as nutrients and waste materials that are transported to and from cells, and component materials such as proteins and other complex substances involved in immunity and blood clotting.

THE RESPIRATORY SYSTEM

The respiratory system includes the organs involved in bringing outside air into the body and placing it in close contact with the blood. From above downward, the components of the respiratory system (Fig. 2.10) are organized into the **upper airway**, which includes the nose, mouth and pharynx; and the **lower airway**, which includes the larynx, trachea, bronchi, and alveoli.

In emergency care, the use of the term "airway" usually refers to the upper airway (as in "clearing the airway"). The upper airway is located in the head and neck; the lower airway in the neck and chest. The chest contains the right and left **thoracic cavities**, separated by the **mediastinum**, which

Fig. 2.10 *Components of the Respiratory System*

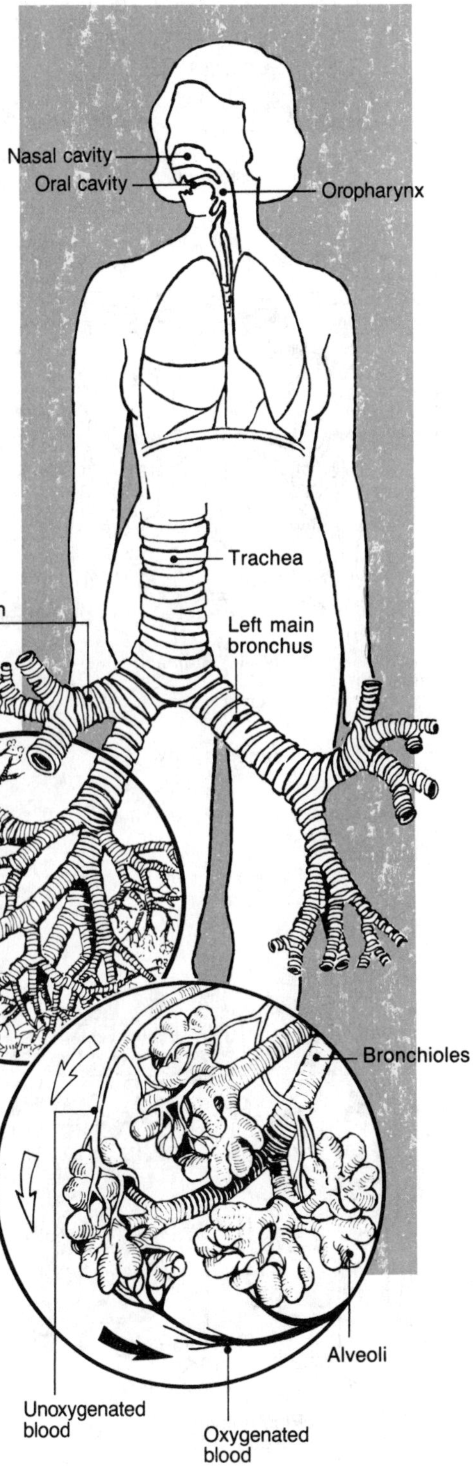

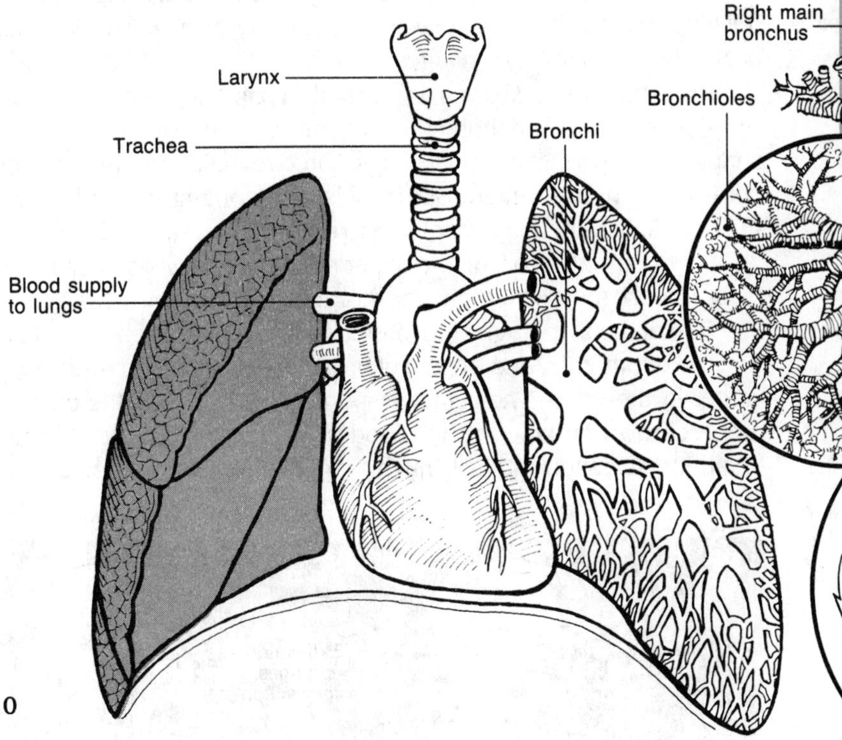

Fig. 2.10

contains the **trachea, esophagus, heart,** and **great vessels**. The thoracic cavities contain the right and left lungs. The trachea branches into the **right** and **left main bronchi**, which enter the roots of their respective lungs and branch into smaller bronchi and finally into the **bronchioles**. The **alveoli** are attached like bunches of grapes to the bronchioles. Lung capillaries in the walls of the alveoli bring the blood into close contact with the alveolar air so that oxygen and carbon dioxide can be easily exchanged between air and blood.

Fig. 2.11 *Chest Wall and Thoracic Cage*

Fig. 2.12 *Contents of the Thoracic Cage*

Fig. 2.13 *Mechanics of Breathing*

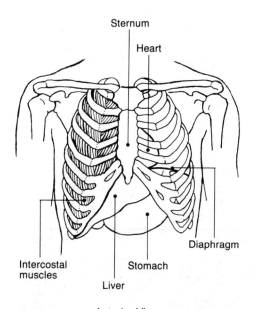

Sternum

Heart

Intercostal muscles

Stomach

Liver

Diaphragm

Anterior View

Fig. 2.11

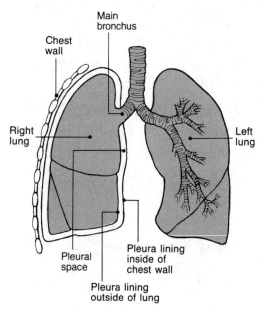

Main bronchus

Chest wall

Right lung

Left lung

Pleural space

Pleura lining inside of chest wall

Pleura lining outside of lung

Fig. 2.12

The Breathing Process

The chest wall (Fig. 2.11) is a semi-rigid unit containing 12 pairs of ribs that are attached to the spine in back and, except for the last two pairs, to the breastbone (sternum) in front. Between each pair of ribs are several layers of **intercostal muscle**. The outer intercostal muscles lift and rotate the ribs, thus increasing the chest size from front to back, while the inner intercostal muscles pull the ribs closer together. The ribs, vertebral column, and sternum enclose the **thoracic cage**, which blends with the neck above and is separated from the abdominal cavity by the **diaphragm**. Contracting the outer intercostal muscles and the diaphragm enlarges the space within the thoracic cage as the ribs move up and out and the diaphragm moves down.

The thoracic cage contains the right and left lungs (Fig. 2.12). A continuous thin membrane, the **pleura**, lines the inner wall of the thoracic cavity and covers the outer surface of the lung, forming a closed sac. The inside of the sac is called the **pleural space**. Normally, the pleura lining the rib cage and the pleura covering the outside of the lung are separated only by a thin film of fluid so that the pleural space is a *potential* rather than an *actual* space.

To **breathe in** (inhale), the thoracic cage enlarges, which tends to drop the pressure in the pleural space below that of the outside air so that air flows into the upper and lower airways and expands the lungs (Fig. 2.13). Note that the lungs expand because they are *pushed out from within* rather than *pulled out* as the thoracic cage enlarges.

Breathing out (exhaling) is normally a passive process since the elastic recoil of the lungs and thoracic cage returns them to their previous size and shape, driving the air out of the lungs. Forced exhalation can be performed by contracting the inner intercostal muscles or by forcing the diaphragm up (as in the Heimlich maneuver, Chapter 5) to decrease the size of the thoracic cage.

For breathing to occur, the upper and lower airways must be open, the pleural space must be airtight, the thoracic cage must move as a unit, and the function of the diaphragm and intercostal muscles must be coordinated.

The depth, rate, and rhythm of breathing is controlled by the respiratory center in the brain. The center responds to either too little oxygen or too much carbon dioxide in the blood by *increasing* the depth and rate of breathing. It responds to too much oxygen or too little carbon dioxide in the

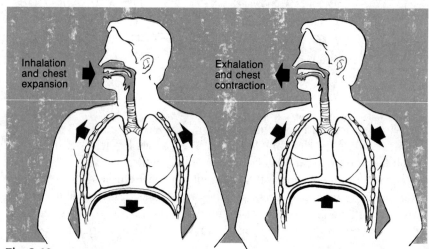

Inhalation and chest expansion

Exhalation and chest contraction

Fig. 2.13

blood by *decreasing* the depth and rate of breathing. Normally, breathing is automatic. It is possible to hold one's breath voluntarily or to breathe very rapidly and deeply for a short time only. When the normal amounts of oxygen or carbon dioxide in the blood are sufficiently altered, the respiratory center will automatically override the strongest voluntary efforts.

Fig. 2.14 *Digestive Tract*

THE DIGESTIVE SYSTEM

The digestive system consists of the **digestive tract**, a tube that conducts food through the body from mouth to anus, and associated organs that produce substances to aid digestion. This system ingests, digests, and absorbs food and fluid, and eliminates wastes. **Ingestion** means to take into the body. **Digestion** is the breakdown of food into simpler substances that can be more easily absorbed into the bloodstream. **Absorption** is the transfer of digested substances through the intestinal wall into the blood. **Elimination** is the expulsion of indigestible residues through the feces.

Starting from above, the digestive tract (Fig. 2.14) includes the **mouth, oropharynx, esophagus, stomach, small intestine, large intestine, appendix, rectum**, and **anus**. Associated organs include the **salivary glands, liver, gallbladder**, and **pancreas**.

Food enters the **mouth**, where it is chewed into small pieces by the **teeth** and mixed with **saliva**. Saliva moistens the food and starts the digestive process with an enzyme that breaks down starch. The **tongue** helps move the food and contains **taste buds** which provide the perception of bitter, salty, sweet and sour **tastes**. The different **flavors** of food are perceived by the **olfactory organ** in the nose; people actually smell the flavor of food rather than taste it.

The chewed and moistened food then passes through the **oropharynx** and **esophagus** into the **stomach**, where it is mixed with gastric juice containing hydrochloric acid and a protein-digesting enzyme. Next, the partly

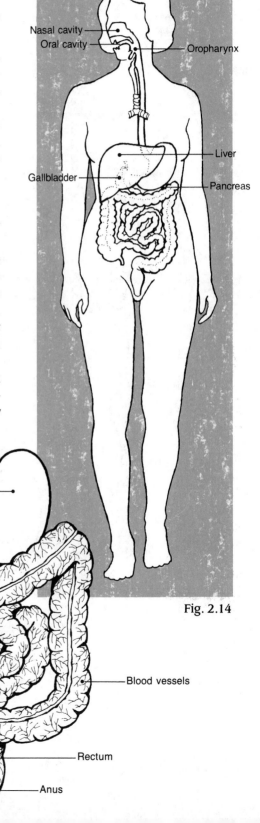

Fig. 2.14

Fig. 2.15a *Urinary System*

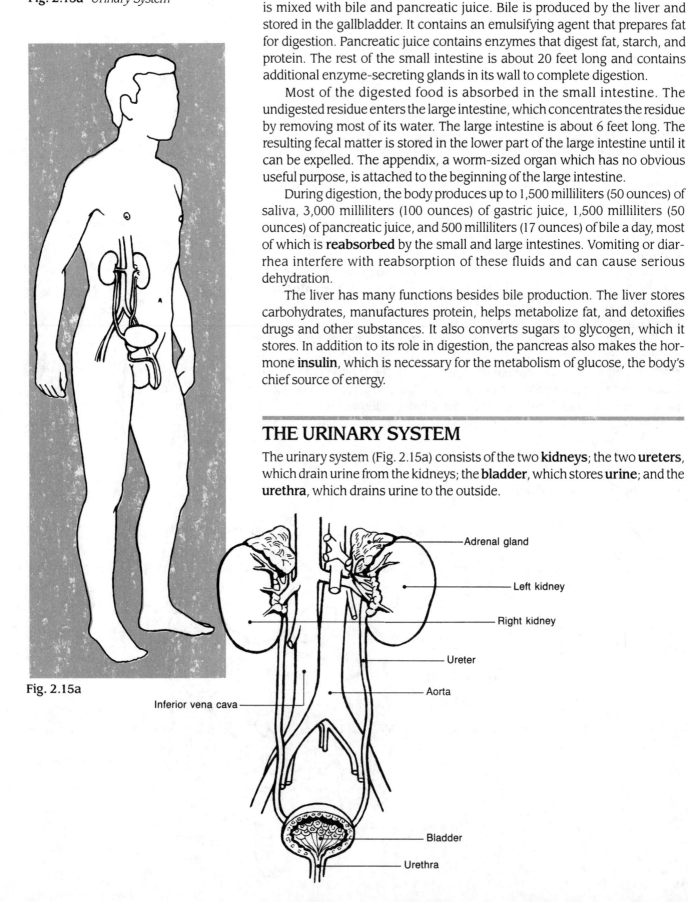

Fig. 2.15a

digested food enters the first part of the small bowel, the **duodenum**, where it is mixed with bile and pancreatic juice. Bile is produced by the liver and stored in the gallbladder. It contains an emulsifying agent that prepares fat for digestion. Pancreatic juice contains enzymes that digest fat, starch, and protein. The rest of the small intestine is about 20 feet long and contains additional enzyme-secreting glands in its wall to complete digestion.

Most of the digested food is absorbed in the small intestine. The undigested residue enters the large intestine, which concentrates the residue by removing most of its water. The large intestine is about 6 feet long. The resulting fecal matter is stored in the lower part of the large intestine until it can be expelled. The appendix, a worm-sized organ which has no obvious useful purpose, is attached to the beginning of the large intestine.

During digestion, the body produces up to 1,500 milliliters (50 ounces) of saliva, 3,000 milliliters (100 ounces) of gastric juice, 1,500 milliliters (50 ounces) of pancreatic juice, and 500 milliliters (17 ounces) of bile a day, most of which is **reabsorbed** by the small and large intestines. Vomiting or diarrhea interfere with reabsorption of these fluids and can cause serious dehydration.

The liver has many functions besides bile production. The liver stores carbohydrates, manufactures protein, helps metabolize fat, and detoxifies drugs and other substances. It also converts sugars to glycogen, which it stores. In addition to its role in digestion, the pancreas also makes the hormone **insulin**, which is necessary for the metabolism of glucose, the body's chief source of energy.

THE URINARY SYSTEM

The urinary system (Fig. 2.15a) consists of the two **kidneys**; the two **ureters**, which drain urine from the kidneys; the **bladder**, which stores **urine**; and the **urethra**, which drains urine to the outside.

Adrenal gland

Left kidney

Right kidney

Ureter

Aorta

Inferior vena cava

Bladder

Urethra

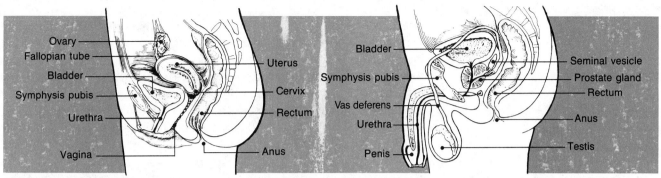

Fig. 2.15b

Fig. 2.15b *Female and Male Genitourinary Systems*

Fig. 2.16 *Components of the Skin*

The kidneys lie on either side of the spine against the upper part of the posterior abdominal wall and contain a complicated system of filters and collecting tubes. They are supplied by the renal arteries, large blood vessels that branch directly from the aorta and bring 25 percent of the heart's output to the kidneys. The kidneys filter about 75 liters (19.8 gallons) of blood per hour, removing many waste products of cellular metabolism. During this process, about 7,500 milliliters (2 gallons) of fluid per hour is removed from the blood along with the wastes. As this fluid travels through the kidneys, essential minerals and most of the water are reabsorbed and the water is concentrated to form urine. The kidneys conserve the body's content of water and essential minerals, producing only about 60 milliliters (2 ounces) of urine per hour and returning the remainder of the filtrate to the blood.

A young adult male's body is about 60 percent water, which amounts to 42 liters (11 gallons) for a 70-kilogram (150 pound) male. Of this, 28 liters (7.4 gallons) are within the cells and 14 liters (3.7 gallons) outside the cells, including about 5.5 liters (1.5 gallons) in the blood.

The kidneys carefully guard the body's water and mineral content by regulating the excretion of water and minerals such as sodium and potassium. If the diet contains enough fluid, an average adult excretes about 1,200 milliliters (41 ounces) of light-yellow urine daily. Any excess fluid is excreted, producing a large amount of pale urine. Insufficient fluid intake, or fluid loss caused by vomiting or sweating, for example, triggers conservation of fluid, with as little as 300 to 400 milliliters (10 to 13.5 ounces) of concentrated, dark urine produced each day. If the diet contains too much or too little sodium or potassium, the kidneys will vary the excretion of these minerals.

Urine drains from each kidney into the funnel-shaped **renal pelvis** at the upper end of the ureters, which are muscular tubes that run down along the back of the abdominal cavity and empty into the bladder. The bladder, a hollow organ with muscular walls, lies in the pelvic cavity behind the pubic bones (Fig. 2.15b). The bladder is drained by a tube, the urethra. In males, the urethra passes through the penis and is about 8 inches long. In females, the urethra is about 1 inch long and exits just above the vaginal opening.

THE CUTANEOUS SYSTEM

The cutaneous system consists of the skin and the underlying subcutaneous tissues. The skin (Fig. 2.16), the largest organ in the body, is made up of an outer layer, the **epidermis,** and an inner layer, the **dermis.** The epidermis is composed of many layers of flat, closely adhering cells and forms a water-

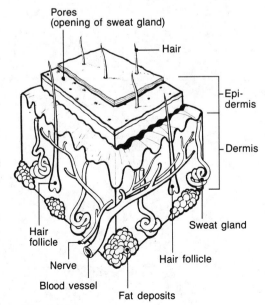

Fig. 2.16

Fig. 2.17 *Human Skeleton*

tight covering for the body. The outermost layer consists of dead cells that are constantly being rubbed off. The cells of the innermost (germinative or basal) layer multiply to continually renew the outer layers. The dermis contains hair follicles, oil glands, sweat glands, blood vessels, nerves, and the sensory organs that perceive pain, touch, and temperature.

The cutaneous system keeps the body from drying out and protects it from invasion by bacteria and other infectious organisms. It is the major

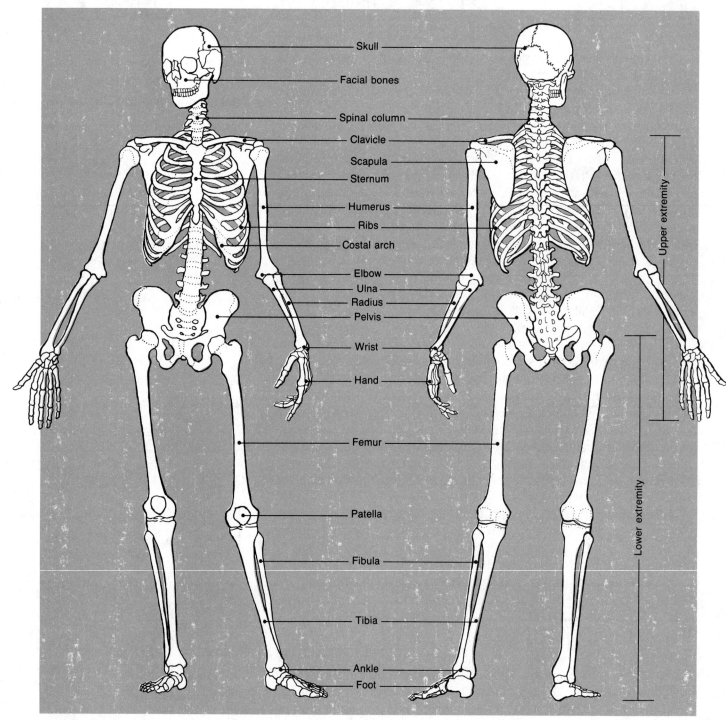

Fig. 2.17

organ system that regulates body temperature, which it controls by producing sweat and adjusting the blood flow in surface vessels.

Fig. 2.18 *Three Major Types of Bones*

THE SKELETAL SYSTEM

The skeletal system, made up of 206 **bones** and their associated **ligaments** (Fig. 2.17), provides a rigid framework to protect and support the soft tissues, gives form to the body and, together with the muscular system, allows body movement. The inner part of bone (the marrow) produces blood cells.

Looking at a dry, dead bone, it is hard to appreciate that bone is living tissue composed of a protein matrix containing deposits of a complex salt made of the important minerals calcium and phosphorus. Bones have many small cavities that contain living cells responsible for bone growth. Because bones are richly supplied with blood vessels and nerves, injury to bone can lead to severe pain and bleeding. All bones have an outer casing of hard, compact, bony tissue and an interior cavity of spongy bone and marrow. There are three major types of bones (Fig. 2.18): **long bones**, found in the limbs; **flat bones**, found in the skull and pelvis; and **irregular bones**, such as the vertebrae.

The bones of young children are less brittle than the bones of adults and, when injured, a child's bone will occasionally bend (greenstick fracture) rather than break completely through. As the body ages, calcium is gradually lost so that bones become weaker and more brittle. Even minor falls can cause fractures in the elderly.

Muscles are attached to bones by tough, fibrous structures called **tendons**. Tendons usually attach to the bone at a prominent point or ridge.

The area of contact between two bones is called a **joint**. Joints may be **freely movable**, **slightly movable**, or **immovable** (Fig. 2.19). The joints of the limbs are freely movable, while the joints between the vertebrae are only slightly movable. The joints between the skull bones and the pelvic bones are examples of immovable joints. In general, the more complex, freely movable joints are more prone to damage from trauma than the simpler, less movable joints. At immovable joints, bones are bound directly together by tough fibrous tissue.

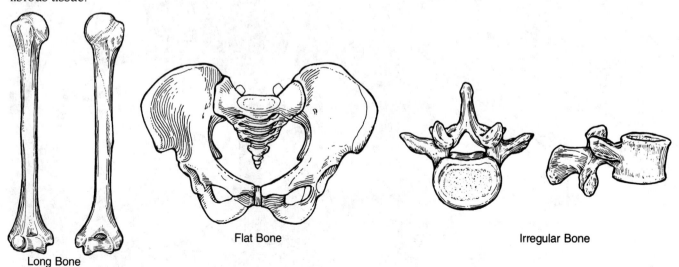

Long Bone   Flat Bone   Irregular Bone

Fig. 2.18

In movable joints, the opposing surfaces of bone are covered by cartilage, which provides a smooth riding surface. The joint is surrounded by a sac of fibrous tissue, the **joint capsule**, which is tight in some areas and loose in others to permit joint motion. Parts of the capsule that are thicker and stronger are called **ligaments**. The inner part of the capsule is lined by the **synovial membrane**, which produces the fluid that lubricates and nourishes joint tissues.

Fig. 2.19 *Three Major Types of Joints*

Fig. 2.20 *Two Major Types of Movable Joints*

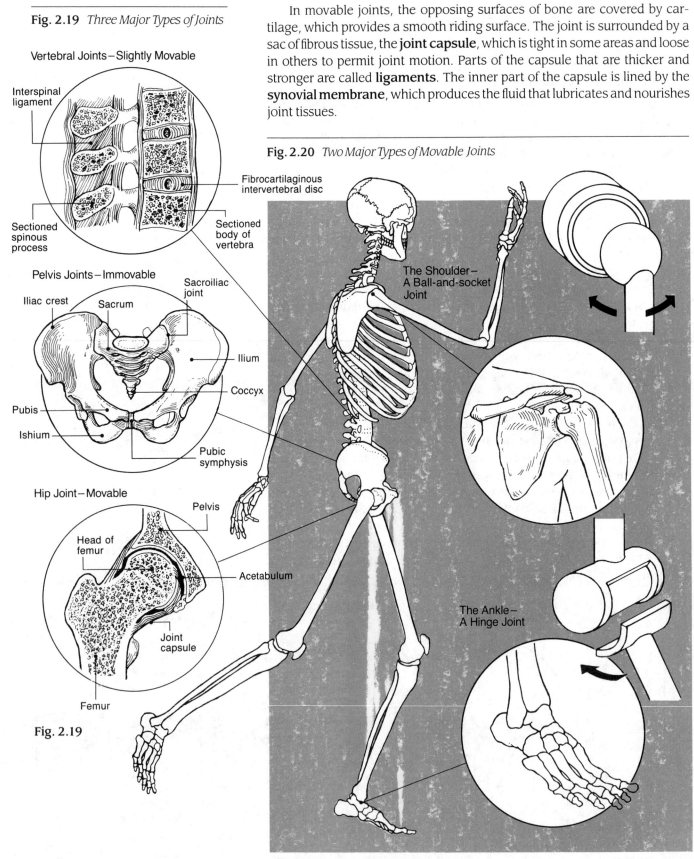

Vertebral Joints – Slightly Movable

Interspinal ligament

Sectioned spinous process

Fibrocartilaginous intervertebral disc

Sectioned body of vertebra

Pelvis Joints – Immovable

Iliac crest

Sacrum

Sacroiliac joint

Ilium

Coccyx

Pubis

Ishium

Pubic symphysis

Hip Joint – Movable

Pelvis

Head of femur

Acetabulum

Joint capsule

Femur

The Shoulder – A Ball-and-socket Joint

The Ankle – A Hinge Joint

Fig. 2.19

Fig. 2.20

The two major types of movable joints are the **ball-and-socket joint** and the **hinge joint** (Fig. 2.20). Ball-and-socket joints can both bend and rotate: examples are the hip and shoulder joints. Hinge joints usually move in only one plane: examples are the elbow and ankle joints. The knee joint, which is discussed in Chapter 12, is a special type of hinge joint that allows both bending and a small amount of rotation.

The skeleton is divided into the **axial skeleton**, which consists of the skull, spine, ribs and sternum, and the **appendicular skeleton**, composed of the upper and lower limbs and the pelvis (Fig. 2.17).

Fig. 2.21 *Bones of the Skull*

Fig. 2.22 *Spine or Vertebral Column*

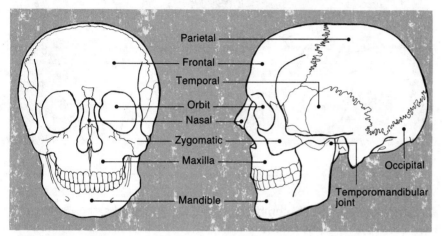

Fig. 2.21

The Skull

The **skull** (Fig. 2.21) is made up of the **cranium** and the **face**. The cranium is composed of several flat bones tightly fused together to form a rounded container for the brain. The face consists of a number of irregularly shaped bones that support the nose and other facial features. The **maxilla**, or upper jaw, contains the upper teeth. The **mandible**, or lower jaw, contains the lower teeth and is attached at the two **temporomandibular (TM) joints**.

The Spine

The **spine**, or **vertebral column** (Fig. 2.22), which is composed of 33 **vertebrae** (Fig. 2.23), forms the main support for the body and protects the spinal cord. Between each pair of vertebrae is a doughnut-shaped ring of fibrous cartilage with a soft center, the **intervertebral disc**. The vertebrae are connected by ligaments which permit some spinal movement.

Each vertebra has three parts: the **body**, the **arch**, and the **posterior and lateral processes** (processes are projections of bone or tissue). The posterior processes also are called spinous processes. When posture is erect, the vertebral bodies are *anterior* and the arches *posterior*. The processes form attachment points for the ligaments and tendons.

The vertebral arches form the **spinal canal** (Fig. 2.24), which runs like a tunnel from the top to the bottom of the spine and contains the **spinal cord**. At regular intervals, pairs of **spinal nerves** branch off and exit through notches between the vertebrae.

The spine is divided into five regions (see Fig. 2.22): **cervical**, **thoracic**, **lumbar**, **sacral**, and **coccygeal**. The cervical spine consists of the seven

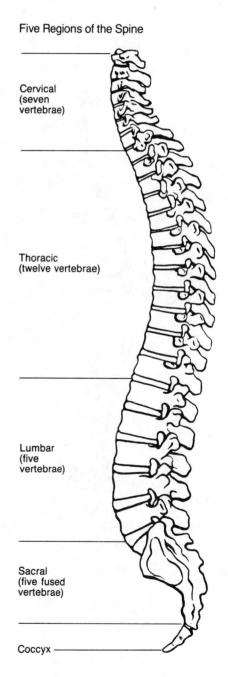

Five Regions of the Spine

Cervical
(seven
vertebrae)

Thoracic
(twelve vertebrae)

Lumbar
(five
vertebrae)

Sacral
(five fused
vertebrae)

Coccyx

Fig. 2.22

Fig. 2.23 *Parts of a Typical Vertebra*

Fig. 2.24 *The spinal cord lies in the spinal canal.*

Fig. 2.25 *Important Parts of the Thorax*

cervical vertebrae, the thoracic spine of the 12 thoracic vertebrae, and the lumbar spine of the five lumbar vertebrae. The five sacral vertebrae are fused together to form a single bone, the **sacrum**, and the last four vertebrae are fused to form the vestigial tail-like **coccyx.**

The skull rests on the first cervical vertebra. The spinal cord passes through a large hole (the **foramen magnum**) at the base of the skull and attaches to the base of the brain.

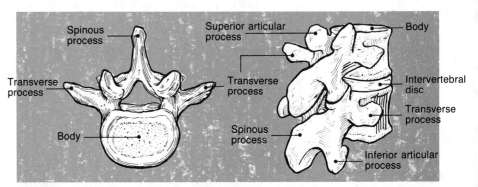

Fig. 2.23

The Thorax

The **thorax** (Fig. 2.25) is composed of the 12 pairs of **ribs**, the 12 **thoracic vertebrae**, and the **sternum** (breastbone). The thorax was discussed to some extent in the section on the respiratory system (see Fig. 2.11). Each pair of ribs is attached in back to one of the thoracic vertebrae. The upper 10 pairs of ribs also have attachments in front. The two lower pairs lack frontal attachments and are known as the floating ribs.

The front end of each rib is composed of cartilage. The junction between the bony rear portion and the cartilage is weak and easily sprained. Such sprains are a frequent cause of minor chest pain.

The first through fifth ribs connect directly to the sternum, while the sixth

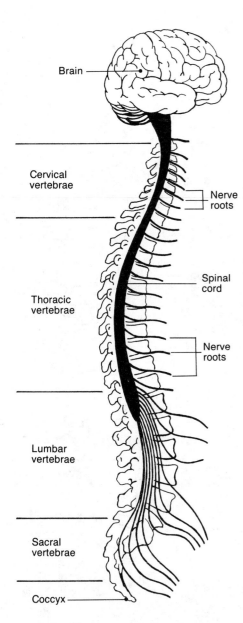

Fig. 2.24

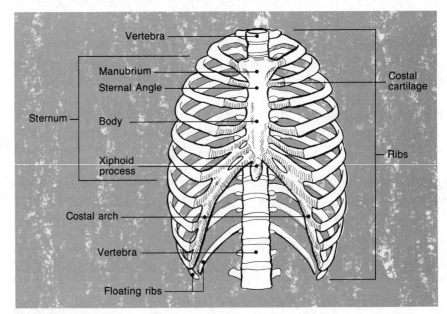

Fig. 2.25

through tenth ribs are connected by cartilage to form the **costal arch**, which is attached to the base of the sternum. Important features of the sternum include the **sternal angle**, a bony ridge at the junction of the upper and lower parts of the sternum where the second ribs attach, and the **xiphoid process**, a tail of cartilage that hangs from the base of the sternum.

The Upper Extremity

Each **upper extremity** is composed of the **shoulder, arm** (upper arm), **forearm, wrist,** and **hand** (Fig. 2.26). The upper part **(shoulder girdle)** contains three bones (Fig. 2.27): the **clavicle** (collarbone), the **scapula** (shoulder blade), and the **humerus** (upper arm bone). Each shoulder girdle also con-

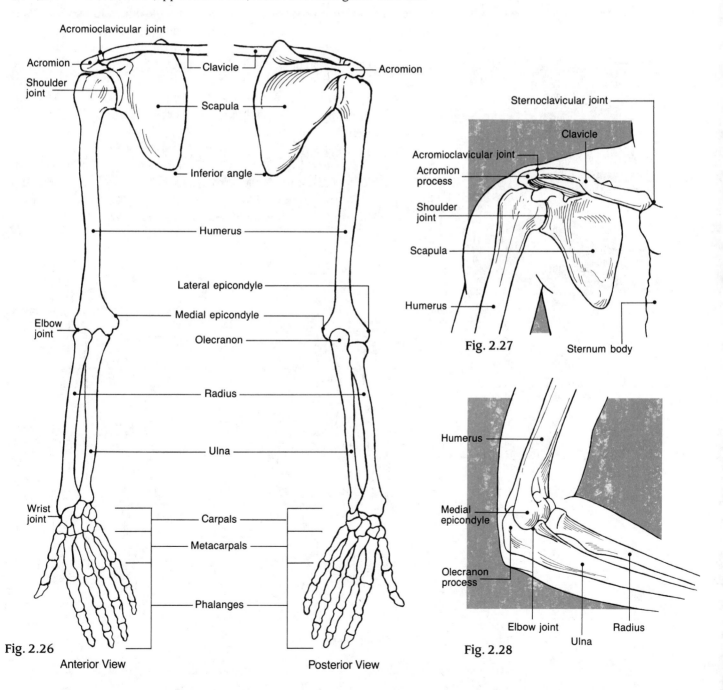

Fig. 2.26

Anterior View   Posterior View

Fig. 2.27

Fig. 2.28

Fig. 2.29 *Forearm Movements*

Fig. 2.30 *Detail of the Wrist and Hand*

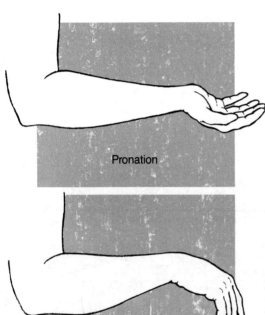

Pronation

Supination

Fig. 2.29

tains three joints: the **sternoclavicular joint,** the **acromioclavicular (AC) joint,** and the **shoulder joint.** Because the upper extremity is directly attached to the rest of the skeleton only by the sternoclavicular joint and because the shoulder joint is a ball-and-socket joint, the upper extremity has a wide range of motion. The cup of the shoulder joint is very shallow (Fig. 2.27), making it unstable and easy to dislocate.

The **clavicle** is a long, thin bone that attaches medially to the sternum and laterally to the acromion of the scapula. The **scapula,** a large, flat, triangular bone, is held by large muscles against the posterior chest wall. At its outer angle, the head of the humerus fits into the shoulder joint socket.

The lower end of the humerus is connected to the two forearm bones at the elbow joint. When a person stands with palms facing forward, the **radius** is lateral and the **ulna** is medial. The main part of the **elbow joint** (Fig. 2.28) is a simple hinge joint formed by a spool-like **condyle** on the medial part of the distal end of the humerus that fits into a notch in the proximal end of the ulna. The second part is a shallow ball and socket joint where the proximal end of the radius fits against a round knob on the lateral aspect of the distal end of the humerus. This arrangement allows the forearm to rotate (Fig. 2.29) so that the palm of the hand can face either forward or backward, and the forearm can be bent and straightened.

The distal ends of the radius and ulna are connected to the wrist, or carpal, bones at the **wrist joint** (Fig. 2.30). The eight carpal bones connect with the five **metacarpal bones,** which are found in the palm of the hand and form a base for the fingers and thumb. Each finger contains three small bones, called **phalanges**; the thumb has only two phalanges. The phalanges

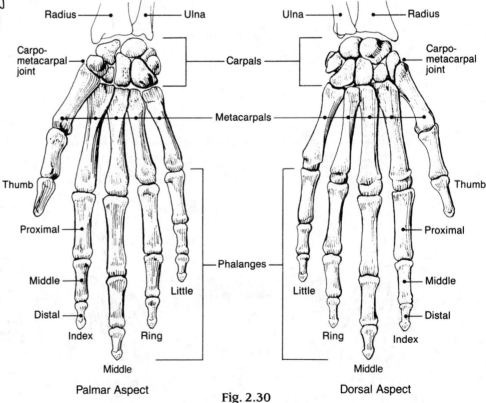

Palmar Aspect   Dorsal Aspect

Fig. 2.30

of the fingers are connected to their metacarpals and to each other by simple hinge joints. The metacarpal joint of the thumb is a modified ball-and-socket joint that allows some rotation as well as flexion and extension.

The Pelvis

The **pelvis** (Fig. 2.31) is a cone-shaped, bony ring made up of the right and left **pelvic bones**, which are joined together in front at the **pubis**. In back, the pelvis and the sacrum join at the **sacroiliac joints**. Each pelvic bone consists of three separate bones – the **ilium**, **ischium** and **pubis** – fused together to form a wing-like structure. The ilium lies superior, the pubis lies anterior, and the ischium is posterior. The main feature of the ilium is the long, curving **iliac crest.** The medial part of the pubic bone is easily felt just above the genitals. The **ischial tuberosities** are the large bony knobs in each lower buttock. The pelvis is a rigid structure that encloses and protects the organs in the pelvic cavity–the **bladder, rectum** and **female reproductive organs**– (Fig. 2.32) and adds support to the body. There is a cup-shaped depression, the **acetabulum** (Fig. 2.33), where the three pelvic bones join laterally. The

Fig. 2.31 *Pelvic Bones*

Fig. 2.32 *Pelvic Cavity*

Fig. 2.33 *The three pelvic bones form a ball-and-socket joint.*

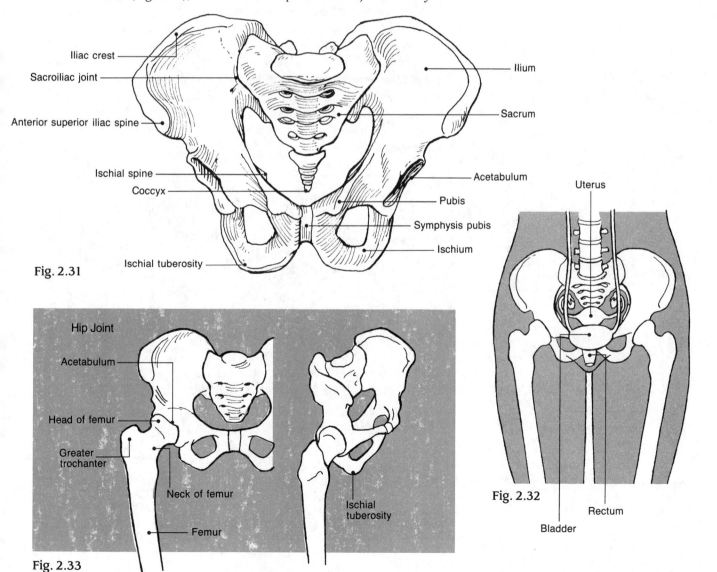

Fig. 2.31

Fig. 2.32

Fig. 2.33

Fig. 2.34 *Lower Extremity Bones*

Fig. 2.35 *Foot and Ankle Bones*

head of the femur fits into the acetabulum to form the hip joint. This joint is a ball-and-socket joint that allows both bending and rotation. Because this socket is much deeper than the shoulder joint socket, the hip is much harder to dislocate.

The Lower Extremity

Each **lower extremity** (Fig. 2.34) consists of the **thigh**, **leg**, and **foot**. The thighbone, or **femur**, is quite strong and is the longest bone in the body. It joins with the two lower leg bones at the **knee joint**. The knee joint, a complex joint important in skiing and other outdoor activities, is discussed in Chapter 12. The **patella**, or kneecap, lies in the tendon of the quadriceps muscle which extends the knee. It increases the efficiency of the knee joint.

The two lower leg bones are the **tibia** and **fibula**. The main weight-bearing bone is the tibia, which lies medially. Its edge can be felt beneath the skin and its distal end, the **medial malleolus**, can be felt where it forms the *inside* part of the ankle joint. The fibula lies laterally; its head can be felt on the outside of the knee joint and its distal end, the **lateral malleolus**, can be felt where it forms the *outside* part of the ankle joint (Fig. 2.35).

The **ankle joint** is a hinge joint formed by the lower ends of the tibia and fibula proximally and one of the foot bones, the **talus**, distally. Another important foot bone is the **calcaneus**, or heel bone, to which the large, rope-like **Achilles tendon** is attached. The other bones of the foot are similar to their counterparts in the hand; they include the five small **tarsals**, the five long, slender **metatarsals** which form the arch of the foot, and the **phalanges**, or toe bones. The great toe has two phalanges, and each of the smaller toes has three.

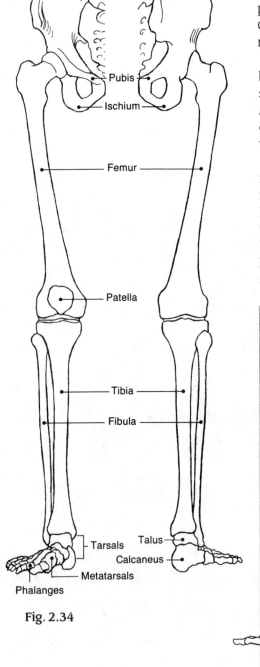

Fig. 2.34

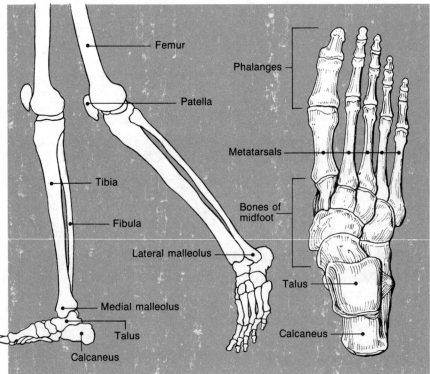

Fig. 2.35

THE BODY CAVITIES

There are three major body cavities: the **chest, abdominal, and pelvic cavities.**

The Chest Cavity

The walls of the chest cavity (Fig. 2.36a) are formed by the thoracic spine and adjacent muscles posteriorly, the sternum anteriorly, and the sweeping curve of the ribs and their muscles laterally. The chest cavity blends with the structures of the neck above and is separated from the abdominal cavity below by the diaphragm. It contains the right and left thoracic (pleural) cavities, which are separated by a central area, the mediastinum (Fig. 2.36b).

The right and left thoracic cavities contain the lungs and pleural spaces.

The mediastinum contains the heart, its enclosing sac (the pericardium), the main pulmonary artery and its two branches, the arch of the aorta, the thoracic aorta, and the roots of the large arteries supplying the upper body. It

Fig. 2.36a *Three Major Body Cavities*

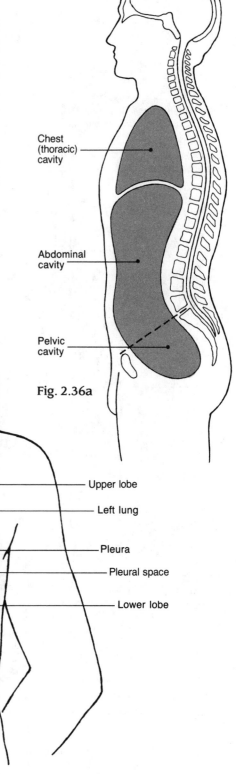

Chest (thoracic) cavity

Abdominal cavity

Pelvic cavity

Fig. 2.36a

Fig. 2.36b *Detail of the Chest Cavity*

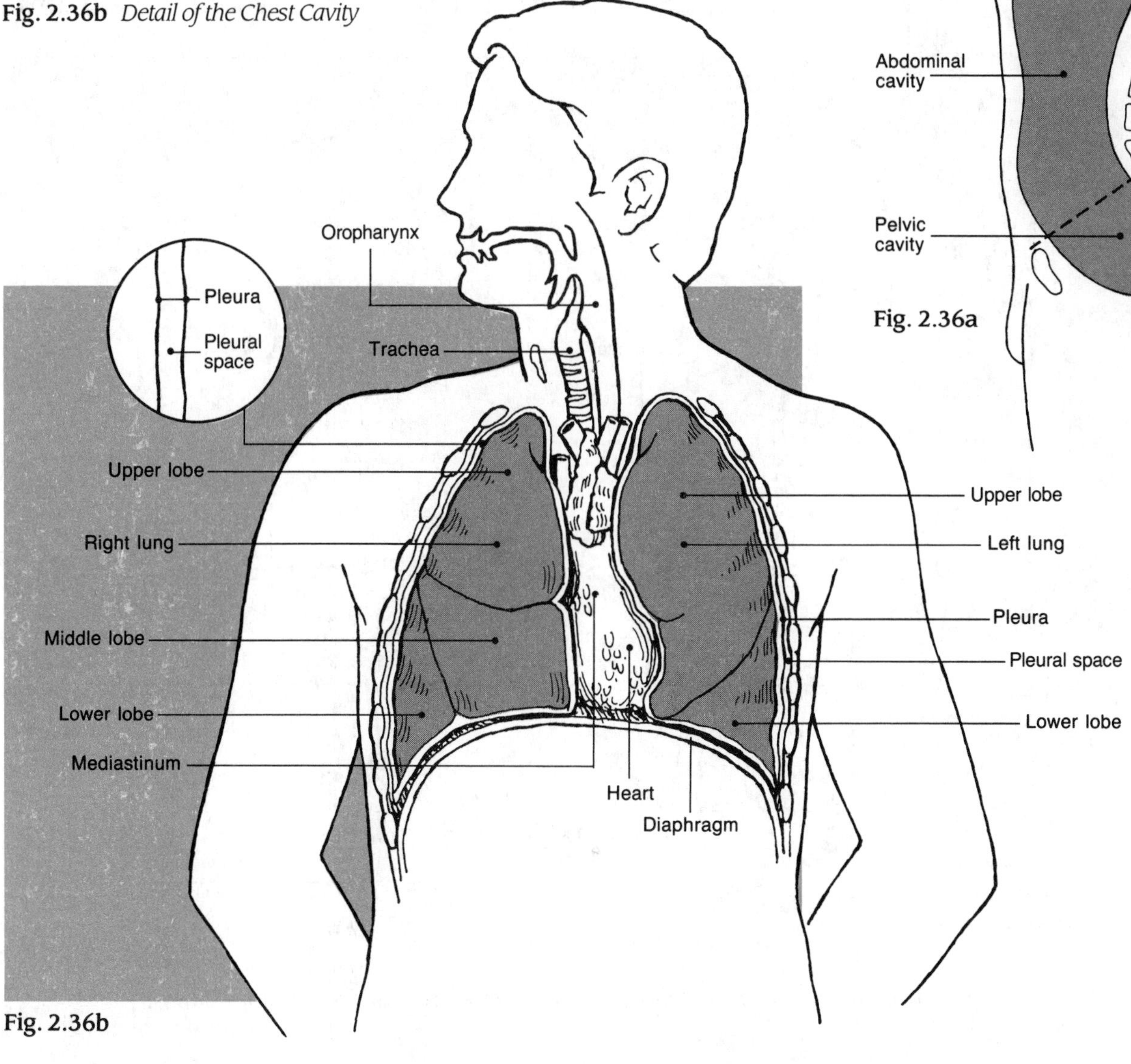

Oropharynx

Pleura

Pleural space

Trachea

Upper lobe

Right lung

Middle lobe

Lower lobe

Mediastinum

Upper lobe

Left lung

Pleura

Pleural space

Lower lobe

Heart

Diaphragm

Fig. 2.36b

Fig. 2.37 *Abdominal Cavity*

also contains the superior and inferior venae cavae, which return blood to the heart from the upper and lower parts of the body. The mediastinum contains the trachea, the two main bronchi, the esophagus, the **vagus nerves**, which help regulate the heart rate and digestive tract function, the **phrenic nerves**, which supply the diaphragm, and other major nerves.

The Abdominal Cavity

The abdominal cavity (Figs. 2.36a, 2.37) walls are formed by the lumbar spine and its associated muscles posteriorly, the abdominal muscles anteriorly, and the flank muscles and upper ilium bones laterally. The abdominal cavity is separated from the chest cavity above by the diaphragm. Below, the abdominal cavity is continuous with the pelvic cavity at the **pelvic brim**, located at the level of the pubis and upper sacrum. The abdominal aorta and inferior vena cava run through the abdominal cavity posteriorly; the cavity also contains major arteries and veins that supply the abdominal organs. Major parts of the digestive and urinary systems lie within the abdominal cavity. The cavity is lined with a thin membrane, the **peritoneum**, which is continuous with the outer coverings of the organs within the cavity, forming a closed sac similar to the pleural cavity. The peritoneum contains nerves

Fig. 2.38 *Contents of the Abdominal Cavity*

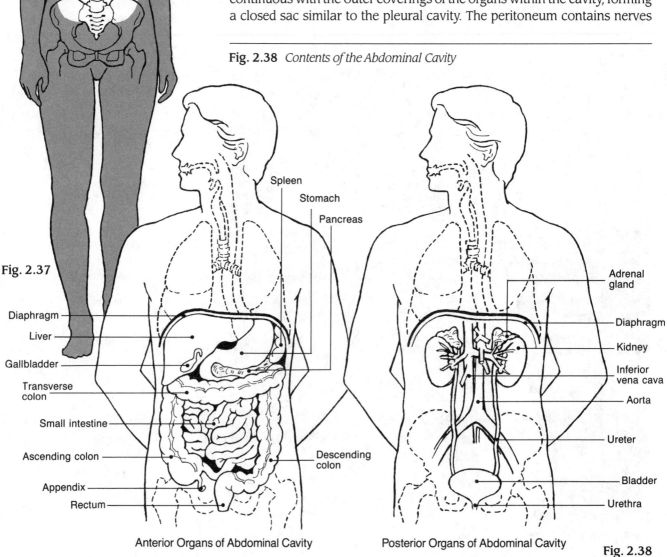

Fig. 2.37

Diaphragm
Liver
Gallbladder
Transverse colon
Small intestine
Ascending colon
Appendix
Rectum

Spleen
Stomach
Pancreas

Descending colon

Adrenal gland
Diaphragm
Kidney
Inferior vena cava
Aorta
Ureter
Bladder
Urethra

Anterior Organs of Abdominal Cavity

Posterior Organs of Abdominal Cavity

Fig. 2.38

and, when infected or irritated, causes pain. Because the nerves and nerve endings are different from those in the skin, intra-abdominal pain is harder to localize than pain in the skin.

Organs of the digestive system (Fig. 2.38) that lie *within* the abdominal cavity are the stomach, duodenum, small intestine, colon, liver, and gallbladder. The pancreas, kidneys, and ureters lie *behind* the abdominal cavity against the muscles of the back. The spleen, an organ that filters the blood, lies in the upper-left part of the abdominal cavity. The exact locations of these organs are discussed in Chapter 3.

Most of the organs within the abdominal cavity are suspended by thin sheets of connective tissue called **mesentery**. This arrangement allows the movement necessary for the normal peristaltic activity of the small and large intestines. The intestines have muscular walls that contract to mix and propel their contents forward.

The Pelvic Cavity

The **pelvic cavity** (Figs. 2.36a, 2.39) is continuous with the abdominal cavity. Its sides and floor are formed by the pelvic bones and muscles, and it is lined with a continuation of the peritoneum. The pelvic cavity contains the bladder, rectum and, in females, the reproductive organs.

In general, abdominal and pelvic organs are either **hollow** or **solid** (Fig. 2.40). Hollow organs are shaped like tubes or sacs and contain liquid or semisolid material; examples include the stomach, intestines, gallbladder, urinary bladder, ureters, and uterus. Solid organs include the liver, spleen, pancreas, and kidneys. Peritonitis (infection or irritation of the peritoneal cavity) develops when the contents of hollow organs spill into the peritoneal cavity. Injury to solid organs can cause serious bleeding.

Fig. 2.39 *Pelvic Cavity and its Contents*

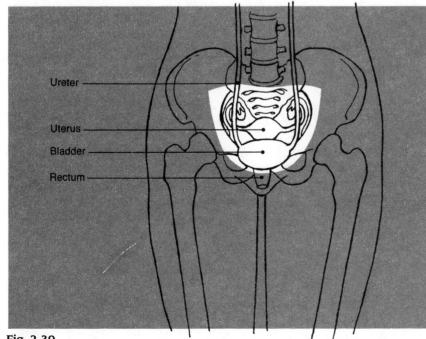

Ureter

Uterus

Bladder

Rectum

Fig. 2.39

Fig. 2.40 *Organs of the Abdominal and Pelvic Cavities*

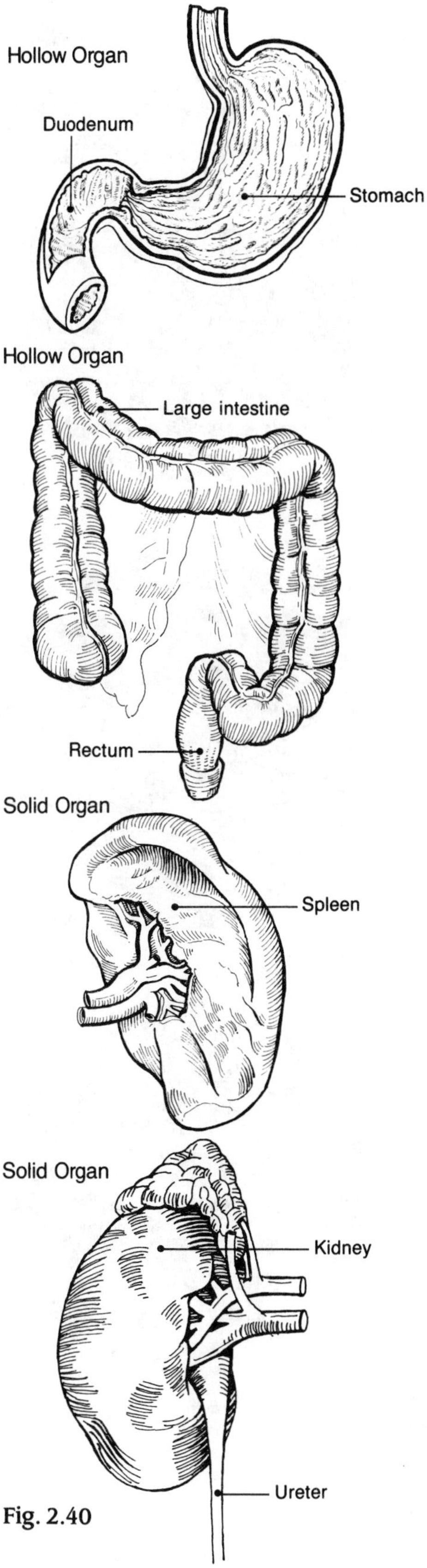

Hollow Organ

Duodenum

Stomach

Hollow Organ

Large intestine

Rectum

Solid Organ

Spleen

Solid Organ

Kidney

Ureter

Fig. 2.40

Fig. 2.41 *The Three Types of Muscle Tissue and their Microscopic Appearance*

Skeletal Muscle Tissue

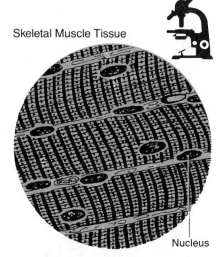

Nucleus

Smooth Muscle Tissue

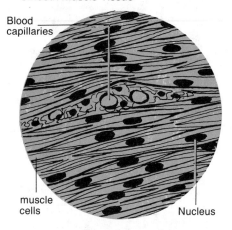

Blood capillaries

muscle cells

Nucleus

Cardiac Muscle Tissue

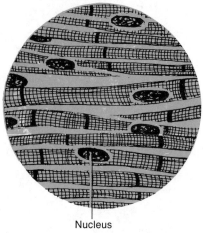

Nucleus

Fig. 2.41

THE MUSCULAR SYSTEM

Muscle is a special tissue composed of cells that can shorten, or **contract**, and lengthen, or **relax**. Muscle contraction is an active, energy-requiring process; relaxation is a passive process requiring little energy. There are three types of muscles: **skeletal**, **smooth**, and **cardiac** (Fig. 2.41).

The **skeletal muscles**, which allow body movement, generally are arranged in opposing sets extending across the joints and attached at points proximal and distal to the joints. Various types of joint movement are produced when opposing sets of muscles are alternately contracted and relaxed.

Skeletal muscles are called **voluntary muscles** because they are under conscious control and can be contracted or relaxed at will. The **motor area** of the brain's **cerebral cortex** controls this function. Nerve fibers travel from this area through the brain and spinal cord to reach the muscles via the **peripheral nerves.**

Muscles are covered by a sheath of tough, fibrous tissue called **fascia**. At the ends of the muscle, the fascia extends into strong cords called **tendons** that attach directly to bone at points close to the joints (Fig. 2.42).

Smooth muscle gets its name because when viewed under a microscope it lacks the striations, or cross-hatches, seen in skeletal and cardiac muscle. Smooth muscle usually forms in sheets rather than fibers and is under automatic rather than voluntary control. It is found in many important organs of the body, particularly the hollow organs of the respiratory, circulatory, digestive, urinary, and reproductive systems. Smooth muscle helps carry out much of the body's automatic internal work.

Cardiac muscle is a special type of striated muscle also under automatic control. Unlike other striated muscles, it never stops working and rests only between heartbeats. To meet these special demands, the heart requires a constant supply of oxygen and glucose furnished by an uninterrupted blood flow. The coronary arteries (Fig. 2.43), which are the first branches of the

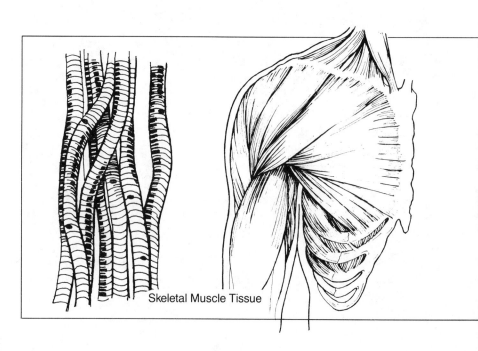

Skeletal Muscle Tissue

aorta, provide blood to the heart. The heart, an organ about the size of a fist that represents less than 1 percent of the body's weight, is nourished by 5 percent of the blood pumped each minute.

To some extent, the diaphragm also is a specialized striated muscle. Although breathing can be voluntarily controlled for short periods, it is mostly under automatic control.

Of the hundreds of voluntary muscles in the human body, only a few will be described here (Fig. 2.44). First, several new words that describe joint motions must be defined. The term **flex** is used when a joint is bent, the term **extend** is used when it is straightened. **Adduct** means to pull an extremity *toward* the midline, or medially, and **abduct** means to pull it *away* from the midline, or laterally. When referring to the feet, which normally are positioned at right angles to the legs, the term **dorsiflex** is used when the foot is bent upward, or dorsally; the term **plantarflex** is used when the foot is bent downward, or in the direction of the sole of the foot. (In Latin, *planta* means sole of the foot.)

The head is almost completely covered with muscles which open and close the eyes and mouth, and govern facial expression. The large, powerful **masseter** and **temporalis muscles** close the jaws. The **trapezius muscles** are attached to the shoulder girdles laterally and to the spine and base of the skull medially. They strengthen the shoulder girdles and lift the shoulders. The strap-like **sternomastoid muscles** on either side in front of the neck help turn the head. Back movement is provided by a complicated series of long, powerful muscles that run on either side of the spine from the base of the skull to the sacrum. For simplicity, the groups can be called **paraspinous** or **paravertebral muscles.** The **latissimus dorsi muscles**, extending like wings from the shoulder girdles to the spine, adduct the upper extremities.

The **intercostal muscles** between the ribs already have been described. Deep muscles in the neck are attached to the first ribs and clavicles, and lift them during deep breathing. The **pectoralis muscles** beneath the breasts help adduct the upper extremities. The muscles covering the front of the

Fig. 2.42 *Skeletal muscles attach directly to bones at points close to the joints.*

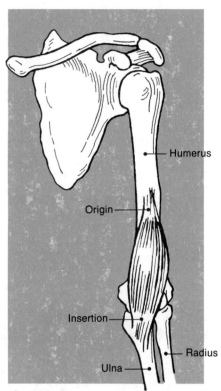

Fig. 2.42

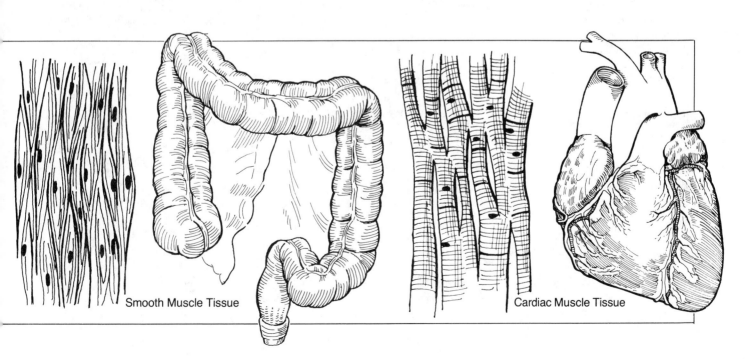

Smooth Muscle Tissue

Cardiac Muscle Tissue

Fig. 2.43 *Coronary Arteries*

abdomen include the strap-like **rectus muscles** which support the abdomen and flex the lumbar spine. The **iliopsoas muscles**, which flex the hip joints, lie at the back of the abdominal and pelvic cavities on either side of the spine.

The **gluteus muscles** form the buttocks and allow extension and abduction of the hips. The major muscles of the thighs are the **quadriceps** anteriorly, which extend the knee, and the **hamstrings** posteriorly, which flex the knee. Other muscles located on the inside of the upper thigh adduct the hips. In the lower leg, the anterior muscles flex the ankle and toes, and the calf muscles extend them.

In the upper extremity, the **deltoids** form the rounded outer part of the shoulders and are the main muscles that lift the extremities up and outward. Beneath each deltoid muscle, three small muscles form the rotator cuff, a strong, curved band of tendon and muscle that holds the head of the humerus firmly in the shoulder joint socket. These muscles and tendons can become irritated by overuse, causing painful shoulder motion, a condition known as bursitis.

The major muscles of the upper arm are the **biceps** anteriorly, which flexes the elbow, and the **triceps** posteriorly, which extends the elbow. The forearm muscles are similar to those in the lower leg, and consist of anterior muscles which flex the wrist and fingers, and posterior muscles which extend them.

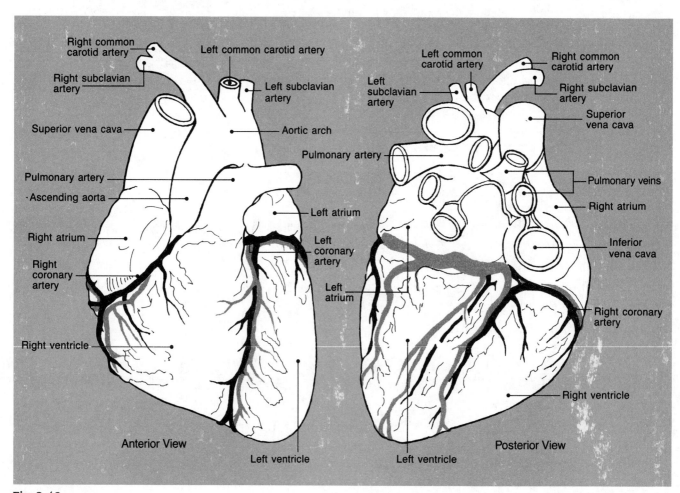

Fig. 2.43

Fig. 2.44 *Major Muscles*

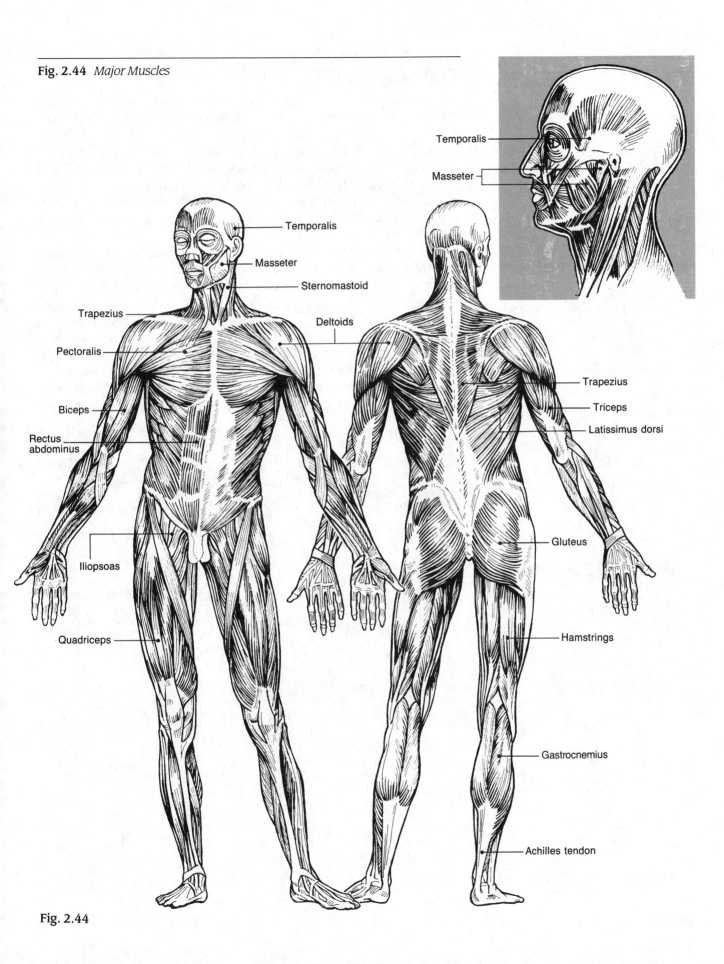

Temporalis

Masseter

Temporalis

Masseter

Sternomastoid

Trapezius

Deltoids

Pectoralis

Biceps

Rectus abdominus

Iliopsoas

Quadriceps

Trapezius

Triceps

Latissimus dorsi

Gluteus

Hamstrings

Gastrocnemius

Achilles tendon

Fig. 2.44

Fig. 2.45 *Neurons*

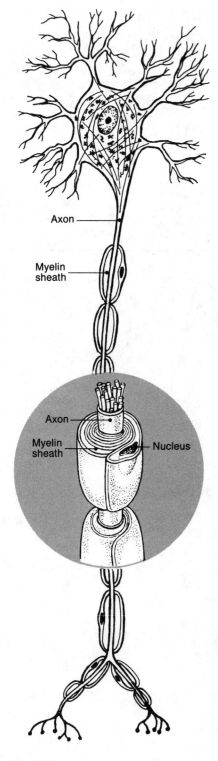

Axon

Myelin
sheath

Axon

Myelin
sheath

Nucleus

Fig. 2.45

THE NERVOUS SYSTEM

The **nervous system** contains special cells called **neurons** (Fig. 2.45) that react to stimuli and conduct impulses rapidly. Each neuron has a **body**, several short processes called **dendrites**, and a long process called an **axon**. The processes connect at **synapses**, allowing nerve impulses to be transmitted from one neuron to another. Brain cell axons that run into the spinal cord may be more than 2 feet long. Axons are enclosed in a fatty substance called **myelin**, which acts much like the insulation that prevents short circuits in electric wires. Chains of neurons linked by synapses form complicated, computer-like circuits.

Because of their gray color, groups of nerve cells are called the **gray matter** of the brain and spinal cord, while groups of myelin-covered axons, which are yellowish-white, are called **white matter**. The brain and spinal cord are covered by three layers of protective membranes called **meninges** (Fig. 2.46); inflammation of the meninges is called **meningitis**. The outermost of these protective membranes is a tough, fibrous layer, the **dura mater**, that lines the inside of the skull. The other meninges are the **arachnoid** and the **pia mater**. The **cerebrospinal fluid** circulates in the spaces between these membranes. Because the arteries that supply blood to the brain and spinal cord lack cross-connections, if one is blocked by an injury or blood clot, the area it supplies will die.

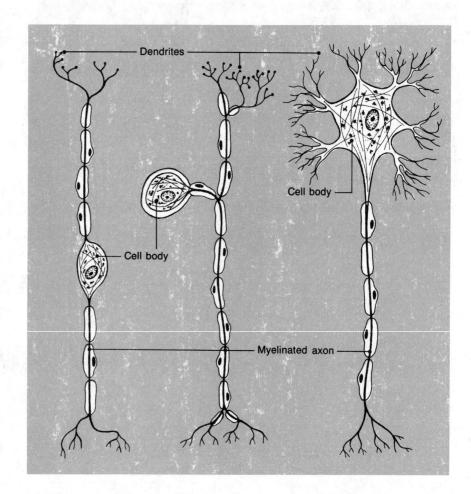

Dendrites

Cell body

Cell body

Cell body

Myelinated axon

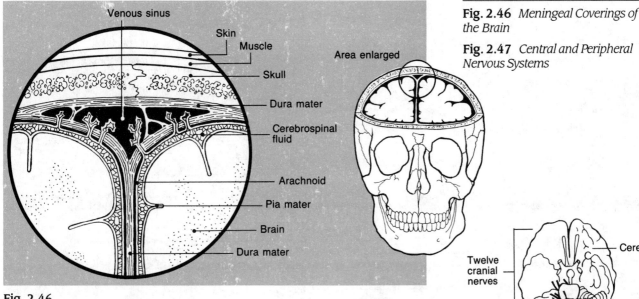

Fig. 2.46

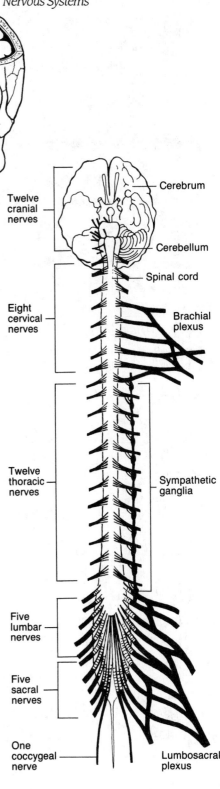

The nervous system is divided into the **central nervous system**, which includes the brain and spinal cord; the **peripheral nervous system**, which includes the nerves and their branches (Fig. 2.47); and the special sensory organs. The nervous system also can be divided into the **somatic** and the **autonomic (involuntary or automatic) nervous systems**. The somatic nervous system controls voluntary activities such as eating, walking, and talking. The autonomic nervous system controls all bodily activities not under conscious control, such as the functions of the heart and blood vessels, digestion, sweating, and shivering.

The brain (Fig. 2.48) is divided into three major parts: the **cerebrum**, **cerebellum**, and **brain stem**. The cerebrum consists of the outer right and left **cerebral hemispheres** and the inner **thalamus** and **hypothalamus**. The thalamus contains centers for temperature, pain, and emotion. The hypothalamus controls automatic functions such as regulation of the heart, circulation, digestion and blood pressure, and regulates water balance, sexual function, sleep, appetite, and body temperature.

The cerebral hemispheres, which are the largest part of the brain, control conscious functions, including voluntary movement, and the perception of sensations transmitted by the sensory organs for sight, hearing, touch, taste, and smell.

The cerebellum, which lies below and to the rear of the cerebrum, regulates posture, balance and muscle tone, and coordinates body movement.

The brain stem lies at the base of the brain and contains centers in the brain stem that help regulate breathing, heart function, and blood pressure. Long nerve fibers from upper parts of the brain pass through the brain stem into the spinal cord.

Cranial nerves supply sensory and motor fibers to the head and are responsible for sight, hearing, taste, and smell. These nerves originate in the base of the brain and leave the skull through openings called **foramina.**

Voluntary movement is controlled by special cells in the frontal lobe of each cerebral hemisphere. A series of fibers, called **motor fibers**, passes from these nerve cells through the midbrain, brain stem, spinal cord, and

Fig. 2.47

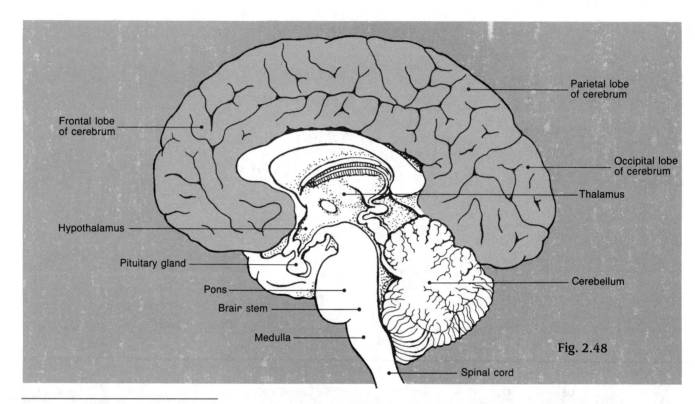

Frontal lobe
of cerebrum

Parietal lobe
of cerebrum

Occipital lobe
of cerebrum

Thalamus

Hypothalamus

Pituitary gland

Pons

Brain stem

Medulla

Cerebellum

Spinal cord

Fig. 2.48

Fig. 2.48 *Brain*

Fig. 2.49 *Nerve Pathways from the Brain to the Spinal Cord*

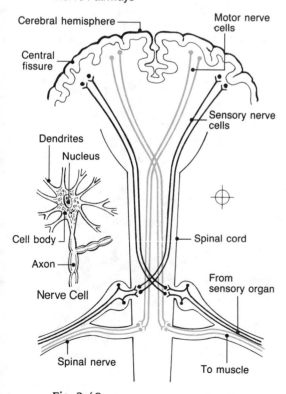

Nerve Pathways

Cerebral hemisphere

Motor nerve
cells

Central
fissure

Sensory nerve
cells

Dendrites

Nucleus

Cell body

Spinal cord

Axon

From
sensory organ

Nerve Cell

Spinal nerve

To muscle

Fig. 2.49

spinal nerves, ending in the muscles (Fig. 2.49). Injury at any point in this long pathway can cause weakness or paralysis of the corresponding muscle or muscles.

Sensory fibers carry sensation to the brain. They originate in the organs of touch, pain, and temperature in the skin and muscles, and pass through the spinal nerves, the spinal cord, the brain stem, and the midbrain to the cerebral cortex. Injury to these nerve fibers causes loss of sensation.

Both motor and sensory fibers **cross over** to the opposite side so that sensation from the right side of the body is received by the left side of the brain, and vice versa. Similarly, the muscles of the right side of the body are controlled by the left side of the brain, and vice versa. In right-handed persons, the left side of the brain is **dominant**, while in left-handed persons, the right side of the brain is dominant. The centers for speech, reading, and writing are located in the dominant cerebral hemisphere. Consciousness, thought, memory, intelligence, and other mental functions are not localized and depend upon the integrated activity of large areas of the brain.

The peripheral nervous system (see Fig. 2.47) consists of 31 pairs of spinal nerves and 12 pairs of cranial nerves. The spinal nerves exit the spinal cord between the vertebrae, and the cranial nerves leave the brain through foramina in the skull. Most peripheral nerves contain both motor and sensory fibers.

Motor fibers transmit impulses from nerve cells in the cerebral cortex to the individual muscles. The more complex sensory fibers transmit impulses to the brain from the sensory organs governing sight, hearing, taste, smell, touch, pressure, pain, and temperature. These organs include eyes, ears, taste buds, the olfactory organ in the nose, and special organs in the muscles, joints, blood vessels, pleura, peritoneum, and dermis of the skin. Sensory nerves constantly supply the brain with information about the relation of the body to its external and internal environments.

Peripheral nervous system nerve cells differ from those of the central nervous system in their reaction to injury. If a spinal nerve or its branch is cut, the cut axons will regenerate and eventually restore nerve function. A similar injury to the brain or spinal cord will not heal because these axons cannot regenerate, which is why brain and spinal cord injuries are generally permanent.

The spinal cord has many short connections between motor and sensory nerve fibers, called **reflex arcs**, that bypass the brain. They generate an immediate reaction to noxious stimuli. For example, a person who touches a hot stove will immediately withdraw his or her finger before thinking about it (Fig. 2.50).

The **autonomic nervous system** controls the automatic functions of the body and consists of two parts with opposing functions: the **sympathetic** and **parasympathetic nervous systems**. Many of the neurons of the autonomic nervous system lie outside the spinal cord in small clusters called **ganglia** (see Fig. 2.47). The sympathetic nervous system prepares the body for action in response to stress; its fibers cause the pupils of the eyes to dilate, hairs to stand erect, the heart rate to increase, sweating to occur, and body sphincters to tighten. The parasympathetic nervous system causes the pupils to constrict, the heart rate to slow, and sphincters to relax.

Some of the body's important nerves (Fig. 2.51) should be discussed briefly. The cranial nerves were described earlier in this chapter. The major nerves in the upper extremity originate in the **brachial plexus**, which lies in the neck behind the clavicle. The most important ones are the **radial, ulnar, and median nerves.**

Fig. 2.50 *Reflex Arc*

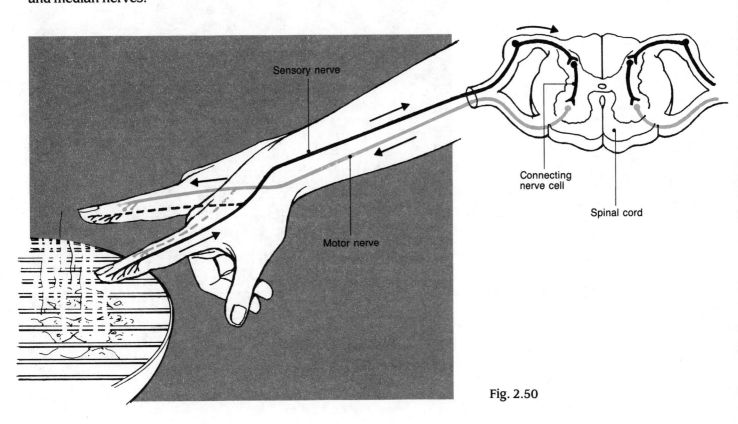

Fig. 2.50

Fig. 2.51 *Important Nerves*

The **radial nerve** supplies the muscles that extend the wrist, fingers and thumb, and runs from the plexus into the armpit and around the back of the humerus into the forearm. Its location exposes it to damage when the humerus is fractured, causing a condition called wrist drop. The **ulnar nerve** runs through the upper arm, entering the forearm behind a bony knob on the medial end of the humerus. It supplies sensation to the little finger and the medial side of the ring finger. The lateral side of the ring finger and most of the thumb and first two fingers are supplied with sensation by the **median nerve**. (Medial and lateral in this example refer to the hand held with the palm facing forward.) The median and ulnar nerves allow flexion of the wrist, gripping with the hand, and most fine movements of the fingers and thumb.

The major nerves of the lower extremity, the **sciatic** and **femoral nerves**, originate in deep-lying plexuses in the pelvis. The sciatic nerve provides sensation to the lateral leg and foot and supplies the muscles that extend the hip, flex the knee, and move the ankle and foot. The sciatic nerve is the largest nerve in the body. It runs from the plexus into the buttock and down the back of the thigh, where it divides into the **tibial** and **peroneal nerves**. The peroneal nerve winds around the head of the fibula before entering the lower leg, where it divides into superficial and deep branches. The peroneal nerve at the head of the fibula and the superficial branch near the lateral surface of the leg are vulnerable to damage from trauma or a tight splint. The femoral nerve enters the front of the thigh just lateral to the femoral artery and provides sensation to part of the front of the thigh and the inner leg. It also supplies the muscles that flex the hip and extend the knee.

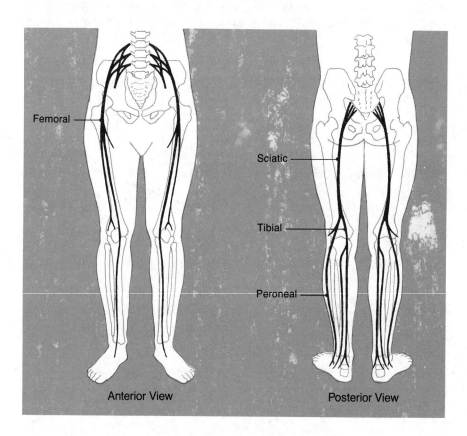

Femoral

Sciatic

Tibial

Peroneal

Anterior View

Posterior View

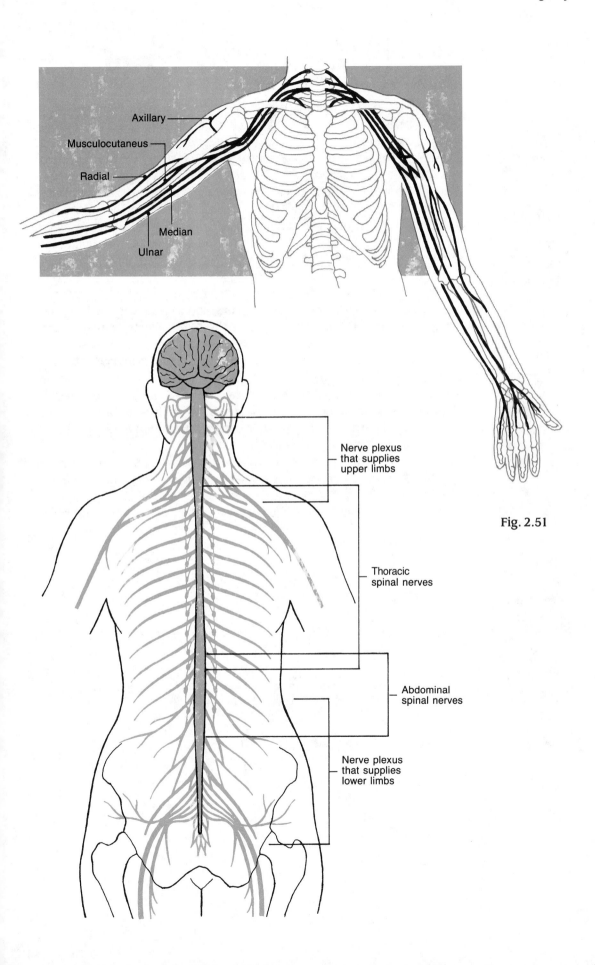

Axillary

Musculocutaneus

Radial

Median

Ulnar

Nerve plexus that supplies upper limbs

Thoracic spinal nerves

Abdominal spinal nerves

Nerve plexus that supplies lower limbs

Fig. 2.51

Fig. 2.52 *Female Reproductive System*

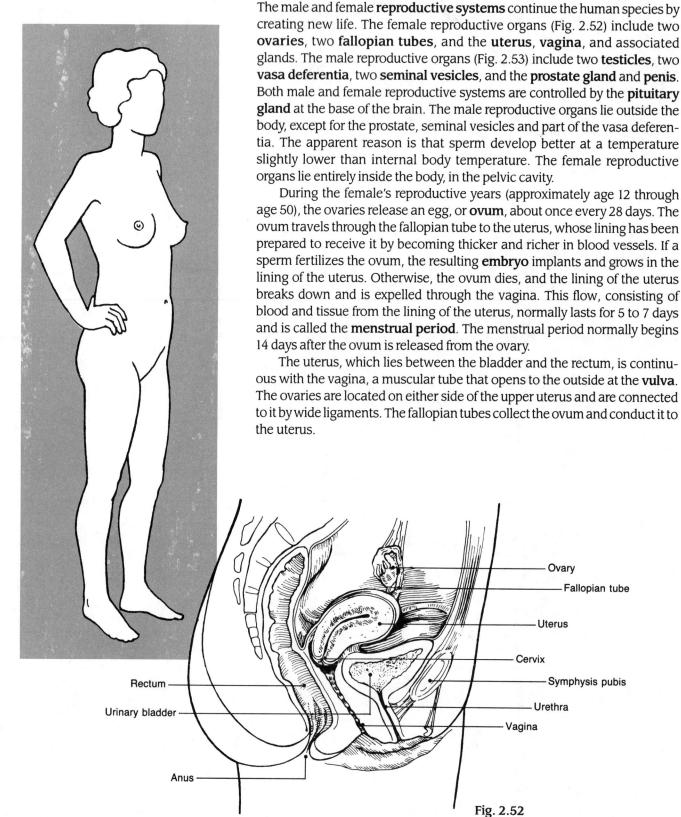

THE REPRODUCTIVE SYSTEM

The male and female **reproductive systems** continue the human species by creating new life. The female reproductive organs (Fig. 2.52) include two **ovaries**, two **fallopian tubes**, and the **uterus**, **vagina**, and associated glands. The male reproductive organs (Fig. 2.53) include two **testicles**, two **vasa deferentia**, two **seminal vesicles**, and the **prostate gland** and **penis**. Both male and female reproductive systems are controlled by the **pituitary gland** at the base of the brain. The male reproductive organs lie outside the body, except for the prostate, seminal vesicles and part of the vasa deferentia. The apparent reason is that sperm develop better at a temperature slightly lower than internal body temperature. The female reproductive organs lie entirely inside the body, in the pelvic cavity.

During the female's reproductive years (approximately age 12 through age 50), the ovaries release an egg, or **ovum**, about once every 28 days. The ovum travels through the fallopian tube to the uterus, whose lining has been prepared to receive it by becoming thicker and richer in blood vessels. If a sperm fertilizes the ovum, the resulting **embryo** implants and grows in the lining of the uterus. Otherwise, the ovum dies, and the lining of the uterus breaks down and is expelled through the vagina. This flow, consisting of blood and tissue from the lining of the uterus, normally lasts for 5 to 7 days and is called the **menstrual period**. The menstrual period normally begins 14 days after the ovum is released from the ovary.

The uterus, which lies between the bladder and the rectum, is continuous with the vagina, a muscular tube that opens to the outside at the **vulva**. The ovaries are located on either side of the upper uterus and are connected to it by wide ligaments. The fallopian tubes collect the ovum and conduct it to the uterus.

Ovary

Fallopian tube

Uterus

Cervix

Symphysis pubis

Urethra

Vagina

Rectum

Urinary bladder

Anus

Fig. 2.52

During the nine months of a normal pregnancy, the fetus grows and develops inside a fluid-filled sac, the **amniotic sac**. The fetus is attached to the wall of the uterus by the **umbilical cord** and the **placenta** (afterbirth), which provide it with oxygen and nourishment from the mother. During birth, the fetus is expelled from the uterus through the vagina to the outside by strong contractions of the uterine muscles.

In the male, the testicles are formed inside the body cavity during embryonic life and pass through canals in the body wall before birth into the sac-like **scrotum**, where they normally lie. The canals sometimes remain after birth, forming a weak spot in the body wall where an **inguinal hernia** may develop. The testicles produce both sperm and male hormones. The mature sperm travel through the vasa deferentia to be stored in the seminal vesicles, which lie within the pelvic cavity at the base of the bladder. The first part of the urethra passes through the prostate gland, which lies just below the opening of the bladder. The prostate and seminal vesicles together produce the **seminal fluid**, which nourishes and helps transport the sperm. In elderly men, the prostate gland may enlarge and partly block the urethra, causing difficulty in urinating.

The penis is called an **erectile organ** because it contains sinuses that are normally collapsed but can fill with blood to enlarge and stiffen the penis. Erection occurs so that during sexual intercourse the normally soft penis will be able to enter the vagina. At ejaculation, the muscular walls of the prostate and seminal vesicles expel the sperm, mixed with seminal fluid, out through the urethra. When sperm enter the vagina they travel up into the uterus to fertilize the ovum.

Certain diseases and injuries can cause **priapism**, a long-lasting and painful type of erection. Priapism in a patient with a back or neck injury almost always is a sign of severe damage to the spinal cord.

Fig. 2.53 *Male Reproductive System*

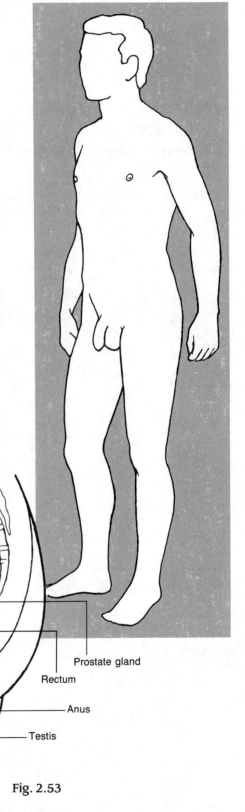

Urinary bladder

Seminal vesicle

Vas deferens

Symphysis pubis

Urethra

Penis

Prostate gland

Rectum

Anus

Testis

Fig. 2.53

3

Surface Anatomy

I profess both to learn and to teach anatomy,
not from books but from dissections;
not from positions of philosophers but from the fabric of nature.

—*William Harvey*

Fig. 3.1 *Surface Anatomy of the Head*

The surface of the human body has many characteristic features that most people have been aware of all their lives yet usually take for granted. When studied in a systematic manner, these surface features provide clues to understanding the normal body and the changes produced by disease and injury.

The human body is **bilaterally symmetrical**. This means that each half is a mirror image of the opposite half. During patient examination, one half of the body can be compared with the other to detect differences that suggest disease or injury. While reading this chapter, consult the illustrations and locate each landmark on your own body or on a companion's body. Later in this text, you will learn about the part of **assessment** called the **secondary survey**, a careful examination of each part of the body, always *in the same order* to avoid missing anything important. In general, the order of examination is from top to bottom and from front to back. This order will be followed in presenting the surface features of the head, neck, chest, abdomen, pelvis, lower extremity, upper extremity, and back.

THE HEAD

The head (Fig. 3.1) is divided into the cranium and the face. With the exception of the **forehead**, the skin over the cranium (the **scalp**) is covered by hair. From anterior to posterior, the **temporal**, **parietal**, and **occipital** parts of the scalp cover the corresponding parts of the cranium. The face contains the **eyes**, **ears**, **nose**, **mouth**, and **cheeks**. The **orbits** are the bony sockets that contain and protect the eyes; the **eyebrows** lie over the prominent upper part of the orbits. The proximal one-third of the nose is bone; the distal two-thirds are flexible cartilage. The **cheekbone** is the bony ridge of the maxilla below the orbit and above the soft part of the cheek. The ear, or **pinna**, is made of cartilage covered by skin; it surrounds the **ear canal**, which leads to the **middle** and **inner ear**. The pulse of the **temporal artery** can be felt just anterior to and above the opening of the ear canal.

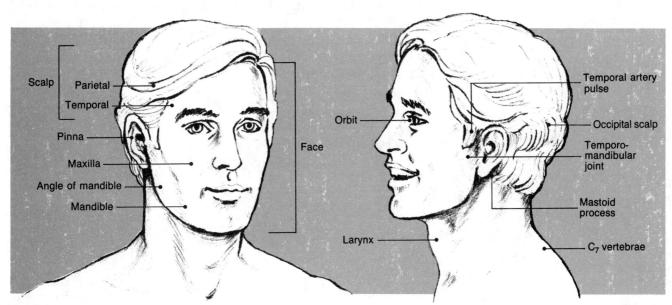

Fig. 3.1

Fig. 3.2 *Major Features of the Anterior Neck*

The **upper teeth** lie in the maxilla and are covered by the **upper lip**, which is just below the **nostrils**. The **lower teeth** lie in the **mandible**, or jawbone, which is attached to the base of the skull at the **temporomandibular (TM) joints**. You can feel the TM joints move as you open and close your mouth by placing your fingers just in front of and slightly below the ear canal on either side. Just below and behind the outer ear is the bony **mastoid process**. The **angle of the jaw** can be felt below the ear where the long lower border of the mandible bends sharply upward toward the TM joint.

THE NECK

The **neck** (Fig. 3.2) contains many important structures, some of which can be seen or felt. Posteriorly, some of the **spinous processes** of the seven cervical vertebrae can be felt in the midline just under the skin. The most prominent of these is the seventh cervical spinous process at the base of the neck. Moving anteriorly, the wide **trapezius muscles** form the upper shoulders. The **sternomastoid muscles** are attached to the mastoid processes above and run medially to the sternoclavicular joints below. The pulsations of the large **carotid arteries** can be felt between the sternomastoid muscles and the larynx.

In the anterior midline of the neck, portions of the larynx and trachea can be seen and felt. The prominent upper part of the larynx, the **thyroid cartilage**, or "Adam's apple," is more prominent in males than in females. With the neck extended, move your finger downward over the larynx until you reach a soft spot, the **cricothyroid ligament**; just below this ligament is a curved, horizontal, bony ridge, the **cricoid cartilage**.

The **trachea** is attached to the cricoid cartilage and can be felt below it in the midline of the neck. Place a fingertip on either side of the trachea and push gently. The width of the soft space between the trachea and the sternomastoid muscle should be the same on both sides. If the space is unequal, the trachea is said to be deviated. Deviation of the trachea usually is a sign that disease or injury to one of the thoracic cavities has caused a shift in the mediastinum away from the midline. The esophagus runs directly behind the trachea.

The two lobes of the **thyroid gland** are found on either side of the lower larynx and upper trachea. The thyroid gland cannot be felt unless it is enlarged, forming a goiter.

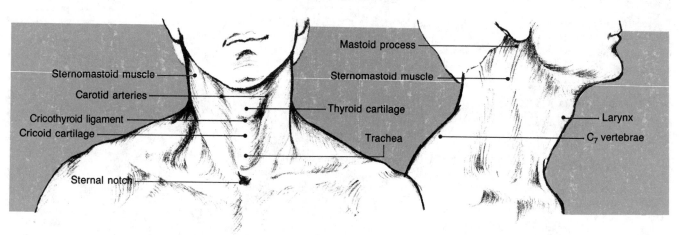

Sternomastoid muscle —
Carotid arteries —
Cricothyroid ligament —
Cricoid cartilage —
Sternal notch —
Mastoid process —
Sternomastoid muscle —
— Thyroid cartilage
Trachea
— Larynx
— C₇ vertebrae

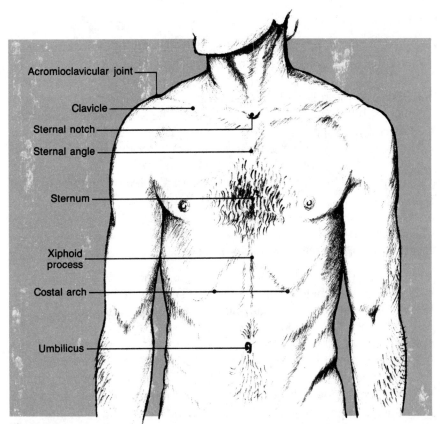

Fig. 3.3

Fig. 3.3 *Anterior Chest*

THE CHEST

The chest (Fig. 3.3) has many bony landmarks. From above downward, the **clavicles** lie just beneath the skin and can be felt from their junction medially with the **sternum** at the **sternoclavicular joint** to their lateral connection with the **acromion** of the **scapula** at the **acromioclavicular (AC) joint**. The top of the sternum forms a notch, the **sternal notch**. In the midline of the chest, the flat surface of the sternum can be felt just beneath the skin and, in many persons, the cartilaginous tail of the sternum, the **xiphoid process**, also can be felt. At the junction of the upper one-third and lower two-thirds of the sternum is a prominent horizontal ridge, the **sternal angle** (Angle of Louis), that lies where the second ribs attach to the sternum. The sternal angle serves as a useful landmark to number the ribs, which can be located one after another downward from the second ribs in slender people. The first ribs cannot be felt because they lie behind the clavicles.

The spaces between the ribs, the **intercostal spaces** or **interspaces**, are numbered according to the rib *above*, i.e., the *second* interspace lies *below* the *second* rib. The lower chest forms an inverted V where the two **costal arches** join the sternum medially. The ends of the floating ribs occasionally can be felt in slender people.

The nipples of the male breast lie at the level of the fourth interspaces. The centers of the female breasts also lie at this level but, because a woman's breasts are larger, the nipples usually lie somewhat lower.

The interior of the chest contains many important organs, including the heart, great vessels, esophagus, trachea, lungs, diaphragm, nerves, and

Fig. 3.4 *Surface Anatomy of the Abdomen with Quadrants and Landmarks*

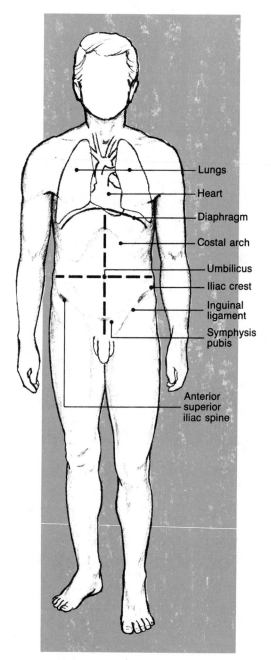

Fig. 3.4

lymph nodes. Only the **heart** and **aortic arch** can be located from surface signs. The heart lies behind and to the left of the sternum, at the level of the second to sixth ribs. In slender people, the heartbeat can be felt in the fifth interspace at the **midclavicular line**, an imaginary line running perpendicular to the midpoint of the left clavicle. The aorta arches to the left beneath the upper part of the sternum and, as it descends, lies just to the left of the spine in the posterior chest. In many people, the pulsations of the aorta can be felt in the sternal notch, especially after exercise. Both sides of the chest expand and contract equally during normal breathing. In some types of chest injuries, one side will expand less than the other.

THE ABDOMEN AND PELVIS

Visible landmarks on the anterior abdominal wall (Fig. 3.4) include the **costal arches, umbilicus** (navel), **iliac crests,** and **pubis**. The prominent knob at the anterior end of each iliac crest is the **anterior superior iliac spine**. The **inguinal ligaments** lie between the **anterior superior iliac spines** and the pubis. The pulses of the **femoral arteries** can be felt just below the midpoint of the inguinal ligaments.

The **abdomen** contains the major parts of the digestive and urinary systems. The organs of these systems are customarily located by using two imaginary lines–the midline and a line crossing the midline at the umbilicus (navel)–to divide the abdomen into four quadrants: the **right** and **left upper quadrants** and the **right** and **left lower quadrants**. (see Fig. 3.4). When pain or other symptoms arise in one of these quadrants, disease or injury of the underlying organs should be suspected.

Figure 3.5 illustrates the important organs in all four quadrants. The **right upper quadrant** contains the liver, gallbladder, and the upper right side of the colon. The liver normally lies above and behind the right costal arch, but when the liver is enlarged it can be felt below and parallel to the arch. The gallbladder is located just below the costal arch at its midpoint; tenderness in this area suggests gallbladder disease. Part of the right colon lies just below the gallbladder. Gaseous distention and certain diseases of the colon can cause tenderness at that location. Injuries to the right upper quadrant frequently involve the liver; tenderness there following trauma suggests a **ruptured liver**.

The **left upper quadrant** contains the spleen, stomach, and the upper left side of the colon. Following trauma, tenderness above and behind the left costal arch suggests a **ruptured spleen**, particularly if ribs are broken. Gaseous distention of the hairpin bend of the left side of the colon is a frequent cause of pain in the left upper quadrant and in the lower left chest under the ribs.

The **right lower quadrant** contains the lower right side of the colon and the appendix. **Appendicitis** is a frequent cause of nontraumatic pain in this quadrant. The **left lower quadrant** contains the lower left part of the colon.

A number of important organs lie in more than one quadrant. The colon begins in the right lower quadrant, travels up into the right upper quadrant, across the midline into the left upper quadrant, and then turns down into the left lower quadrant. The small intestine also occupies parts of all four quad-

Figure labels: Lungs, Heart, Diaphragm, Costal arch, Umbilicus, Iliac crest, Inguinal ligament, Symphysis pubis, Anterior superior iliac spine

rants. The pancreas is a horizontal organ that lies in both upper quadrants against the posterior abdominal wall. The urinary bladder and uterus normally lie in the pelvis, but, when the bladder is distended and the uterus is enlarged, they may extend into the midline of the lower quadrants of the abdomen.

The kidneys lie in the upper quadrants against the posterior abdominal wall and are drained by the ureters, which run through the lower quadrants into the pelvis where they enter the bladder. (The kidneys are discussed in more detail as part of the external anatomy of the back.)

The **pelvis** is separated from the abdomen by an imaginary plane running from the top of the pubis in front to a ridge on the upper sacrum in back. The main landmarks of the pelvis are the pubis and the anterior superior iliac spines. The pelvis contains the bladder, urethra, lower ureters, lower colon, rectum, the female reproductive organs (vagina, uterus, fallopian tubes, and ovaries), and the internal parts of the male reproductive system (part of the vasa deferentia, the prostate and the seminal vesicles).

Fig. 3.5 *Important Abdominal Organs in the Four Quadrants*

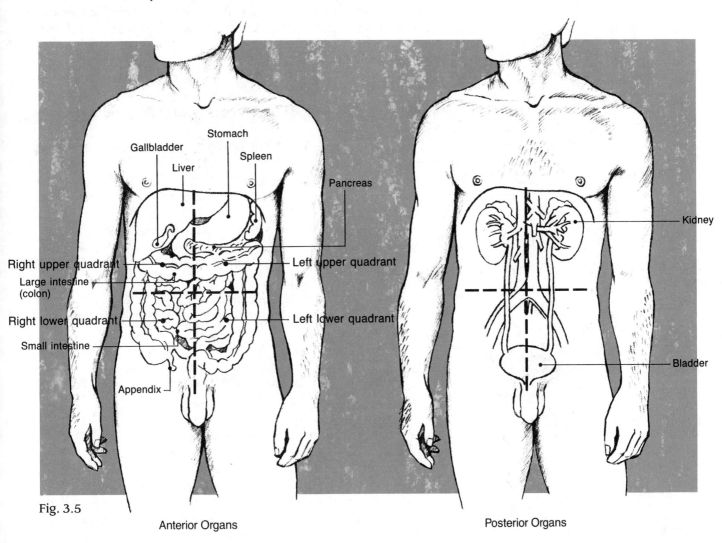

Fig. 3.5

Anterior Organs

Posterior Organs

Fig. 3.6 *Easily Felt Features of the Lower Extremity*

THE LOWER EXTREMITY (Fig. 3.6)

The bony prominence on the outside of the upper thigh is the **greater trochanter** of the femur. Many people mistake the greater trochanter for the hip joint, which is located below the midpoint of the inguinal ligament just behind the femoral artery. Trauma can cause the **bursa** that separates the greater trochanter from its overlying muscles to become inflamed and tender. Trochanteric bursitis is common in beginning skiers who hit their trochanters when they fall sideways in the snow. The shaft of the femur is buried within the thigh muscles and cannot be felt.

Many of the components of the knee joint can be felt just beneath the skin. The major landmark is the **patella**, or kneecap, in front of the joint. A broad, strong tendon attached to the major muscle of the anterior thigh, the **quadriceps femoris**, surrounds the patella. The continuation of this tendon, the **patellar ligament**, extends from the patella to the **tibial tuberosity**. As the knee joint moves, the patella glides up and down in a groove between the two rounded projections of the distal femur called the **femoral condyles**. The joint line of the knee is about an inch below the lower border of the patella and can be felt when the knee joint is flexed at a right angle. The **medial** and **lateral femoral condyles** can be felt above the joint line on either side. The **medial** and **lateral hamstring tendons** can be felt on either side of the depression behind the knee where they attach to the head of the fibula just below the joint line of the knee laterally and the upper tibia medially.

The **peroneal nerve** is a sensitive, cord-like structure that can be felt in the indentation below the head of the fibula. Because of its exposed position, the peroneal nerve is susceptible to damage from a blow to the side of the knee or from too tight a splint. Damage to the peroneal nerve can cause foot drop (inability to flex the foot).

The tibia is triangular in cross-section; its anteromedial side lies just beneath the skin and can be felt throughout its length to the point where it forms the inner part of the ankle joint at the **medial malleolus** (Fig. 3.7). The pulse of the **posterior tibial artery** can be felt just below and behind the medial malleolus. Most of the fibula is buried in the leg muscles, but the lower quarter can be felt to the point where it forms the outer portion of the ankle joint at the **lateral malleolus**.

The subcutaneous tissues of the ankle and foot are so thin that their underlying structures can be easily felt through the skin. The tendons of the muscles that bend the foot upward (flex or dorsiflex) can be felt when the muscles on the front of the leg are tightened. Easily felt features (see Fig. 3.7) include the posterior part of the calcaneus, which forms the **heel**; the **Achilles tendon**, which allows the calf muscles to extend (plantarflex) the foot; the **arch** of the foot, made up of the calcaneus, talus, and tarsal bones; the five slender **metatarsals**; and the five toes, or **digits**, with their respective **phalanges** and **joints**. The pulse of the **dorsalis pedis artery** can be felt on the top of the foot, between the first and second metatarsals. Because of their prominence and thin skin covering, the medial and lateral malleoli should be well-padded during splinting to avoid excessive pressure and skin damage.

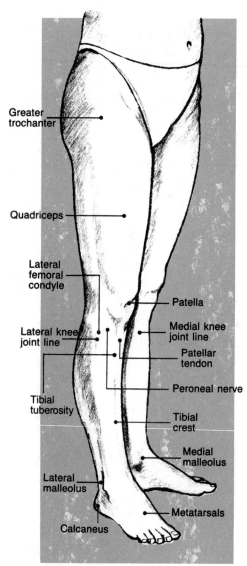

Greater trochanter

Quadriceps

Lateral femoral condyle

Lateral knee joint line

Tibial tuberosity

Lateral malleolus

Calcaneus

Patella

Medial knee joint line

Patellar tendon

Peroneal nerve

Tibial crest

Medial malleolus

Metatarsals

Fig. 3.6

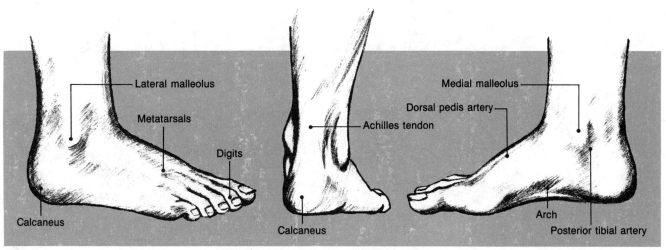

Fig. 3.7

Fig. 3.7 *Major Surface Features of the Foot*

THE UPPER EXTREMITY (Fig. 3.8)

In the upper chest and shoulder, the entire **clavicle** can be felt from the **sternoclavicular joint** to where it articulates with the acromion of the scapula to form the **acromioclavicular (AC) joint** at the point of the shoulder. The head of the humerus, which lies just below the AC joint, is covered by the **deltoid muscle** to form the rounded part of the shoulder. The medial margin and part of the spine of the **scapula** can be felt in back of the shoulder.

Most of the humerus is covered by muscles, principally the **biceps** and **triceps**, but its lower end can be felt at the elbow, where it forms two rounded points, the **medial** and **lateral epicondyles**. An important nerve, the **ulnar nerve**, can be felt in the groove behind the medial epicondyle. This nerve is called the "crazy bone" because bumping it causes a tingling sensation in the medial forearm and hand. Another important nerve, the **radial nerve**, winds around the humerus at its midpoint. Because of its location, the radial nerve can be injured when the humerus is fractured. The pulse of the brachial artery can be felt beating against the humerus on the medial side of the upper arm, midway between the shoulder and elbow.

The **olecranon**, the large process of the **ulna**, is found between the medial and lateral epicondyles posteriorly. The **triceps tendon**, which is attached to the olecranon, can be felt when the triceps muscle is tightened. The main tendon on the front of the elbow is the **biceps tendon**, which attaches to the **radius**. If the biceps muscle is tightened, the tendon can be easily felt just medial to the soft hollow at the front of the elbow.

In the forearm, the entire posterior border of the ulna can be felt just below the skin. The lower ends of the **radius** and **ulna**—the two bones of the forearm—form the upper part of the wrist joint. The prominent bony projections called the **radial** and **ulnar styloid processes** at the lower ends of the forearm bones form the lateral and medial sides of the wrist joint. The pulse of the **radial artery** can be felt anterior to the radial styloid process above the base of the thumb. Many of the muscles, bones and tendons of the wrist and hand can be seen as well as felt. The more obvious features include the long, slender **metacarpal bones**, which are easy to feel on the back of the hands, and details of the **digits** and their **phalanges** and **joints**. Tendons of the muscles that extend the wrist can be seen and felt, especially over the knuckles. On the palmar surface, the tendons of the muscles that flex the wrist can be seen in the middle of the wrist.

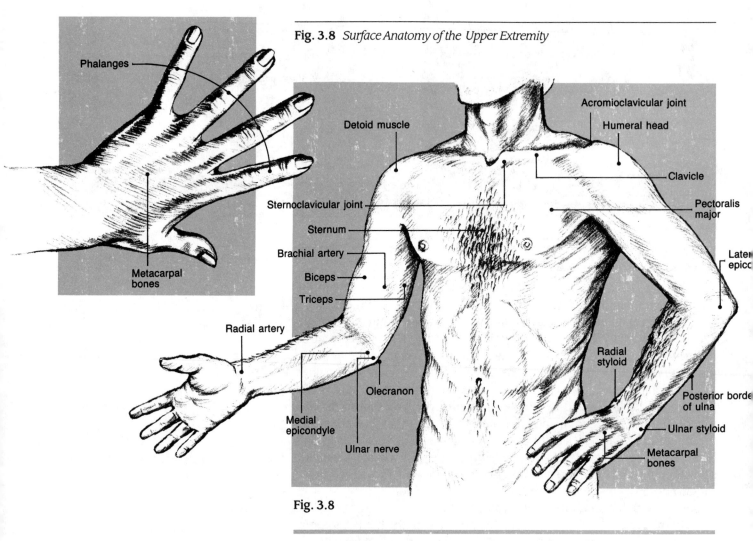

Fig. 3.8 *Surface Anatomy of the Upper Extremity*

Phalanges

Metacarpal bones

Radial artery

Medial epicondyle

Ulnar nerve

Olecranon

Detoid muscle

Sternoclavicular joint

Sternum

Brachial artery

Biceps

Triceps

Acromioclavicular joint

Humeral head

Clavicle

Pectoralis major

Later epicc

Radial styloid

Posterior borde of ulna

Ulnar styloid

Metacarpal bones

Fig. 3.8

THE BACK

The major features of the **back** (Fig. 3.9) will be covered starting from the large **trapezius muscles** that form the "web" of the neck on either side and are used to raise the shoulders. The trapezius muscles are attached to the spinous processes of the cervical and upper thoracic vertebrae medially and the scapula laterally. The spinous processes of the **cervical**, **thoracic**, and **lumbar vertebrae** can be felt beneath the skin in the midline. The flat, triangular surface of the **sacrum** lies below the lowest lumbar vertebra. The sharp **coccyx**, which hangs like a short tail from the lower end of the sacrum, can sometimes be felt. The sacrum is joined to the iliac bones at the two **sacroiliac joints**, which can be felt just beneath the skin on either side. From these joints, the **iliac crests** curve up and around toward the front. The **ischial tuberosities**, on which we sit, are the rounded knobs that can be felt on either side below the buttocks. The two **sciatic nerves** descend from the buttocks into the thighs just lateral to these tuberosities. Sitting in certain positions puts pressure on these nerves, causing the foot to "fall asleep."

The two wing-like **latissimus dorsi muscles**, which are used to adduct the upper arms, can be felt as they extend downward from the armpits on the sides of the chest. These muscles are attached to the humerus laterally and the spinous processes medially. The large, prominent, strap-like **paraspinous (paravertebral) muscles** that lie on either side of the spine are used to flex, extend, and bend the spine sideways. The triangular space formed between the lowest rib and the spine on each side is called the costovertebral angle. The kidneys lie anterior to the costovertebral angles at the back of the peritoneal cavity. Tenderness produced by tapping the muscles of the **costovertebral angle** may indicate disease or injury of the underlying kidney.

Fig. 3.9 *Major Features of the Back*

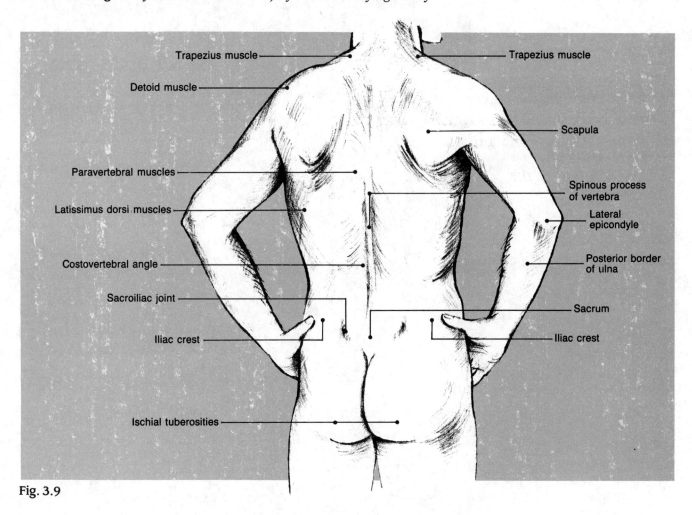

Fig. 3.9

4

Patient Assessment

Better to be despised for too anxious apprehensions,
than ruined by too confident a security.

—*Edmund Burke*

Before giving emergency care, a rescuer must know what is wrong with the patient. This may seem obvious, but many mistakes in emergency care are caused by lack of thoroughness rather than lack of knowledge. Perhaps because of the excitement of the moment, patient examination is not always systematic and thorough enough to find the true nature of the problem.

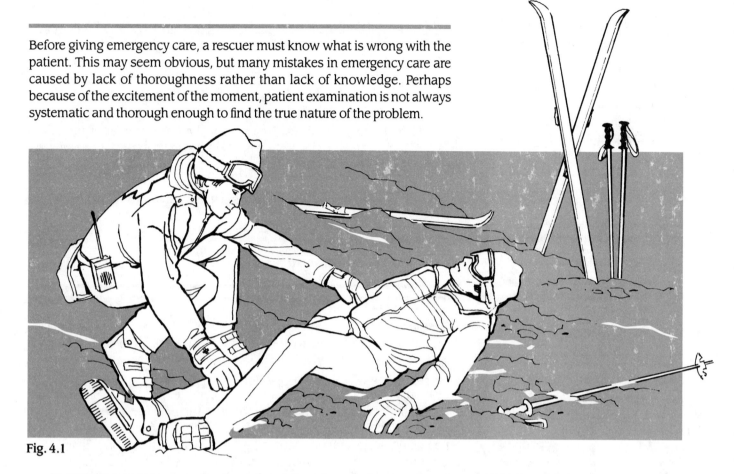

Fig. 4.1

In emergency care, examination of a patient is called **assessment** (Fig. 4.1). However, assessment means more than examination alone. In addition to using the eyes, ears, nose and hands, the rescuer must also use the brain so that appropriate questions are asked and the information gathered is evaluated and understood. Although assessment is relatively easy to learn and to perform under classroom conditions, it may be very difficult under adverse environmental conditions. Cold and wind, in particular, numb the examiner's fingers and prevent undressing the patient.

The objectives of assessment are to immediately detect and treat such urgent problems as **absence of breathing, absence of heart action,** and **severe bleeding**; to find out if anything else is wrong; and to miss nothing. Assessment is divided into three major parts: the first impression, the primary survey, and the secondary survey.

The first impression is entirely automatic and almost instantaneous. It includes recognizing the probable mechanism of injury and the presence or absence of possible hazards to the patient or the rescuer. The primary survey is conducted semi-automatically; the secondary survey is conducted more slowly and methodically.

The primary survey includes a rapid, but not hasty, evaluation of the status of the respiratory and circulatory systems. A rigid protocol is followed so that all life-threatening problems will be checked for in the proper order and treated immediately.

The secondary survey is a systematic evaluation of the remaining six organ systems always in the same order so that nothing important will be overlooked.

Fig. 4.1 *Thorough patient assessment is the foundation of emergency care.*

Table 4.1

FIVE VITAL SIGNS

Pulse
Respiration
Blood pressure
Temperature
Level of consciousness

Fig. 4.2 *Locations of the Important Pulses*

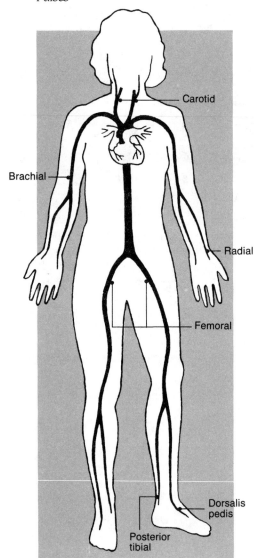

Fig. 4.2

The examiner arrives at the patient's side with a number of important intrinsic "tools": the brain, eyes, ears, hands, and nose. The examiner also should carry a watch with a second hand and a small flashlight. A stethoscope and a blood pressure cuff are also useful, but training and experience are required to use them well. The examiner should *think*, *look*, *listen*, *feel*, and occasionally even *smell*. He or she must be familiar with the normal appearance and function of the components of the organ systems and search for signs and symptoms that indicate deviations from the normal state.

A **sign** is an important characteristic of illness or injury that the *observer* notes by looking, feeling, listening, or smelling. A **symptom** is an important characteristic that the *patient* notes and discusses with the observer. The most important signs are the five **vital signs**: **pulse**, **respiration**, **temperature**, **blood pressure**, and **level of consciousness.**

THE PULSE

The **pulse** is the rhythmic, expanding tap felt when the fingers are placed over an artery lying close to the body surface. The pulse represents the pressure wave propagated in the arteries each time the heart beats. The presence of a pulse means the heart is beating, that it is beating strongly enough for the beat to be transmitted to the examiner's fingers, and that the arterial channel is open between the heart and the examiner's fingers. The absence of a pulse means either the heart is not beating, the arterial channel is blocked, or, too frequently, the examiner is searching for the pulse in the wrong place!

The normal resting pulse is 60 to 90 beats per minute in an adult and 90 to 110 beats per minute in a child. Although the pulse normally has a regular rhythm, young people may exhibit sinus arrhythmia, a pulse rate that increases slightly on inhaling and decreases slightly on exhaling.

The important features of the pulse are its **rate**, **rhythm**, and **strength**. There is a relationship between the rate and strength. The pulse is usually strong when the rate is slow (unless the heart muscle is weakened by disease), because more blood is pumped by the heart per beat; it is usually weak when the rate is very fast, because less blood is pumped per beat.

The pulse rate is controlled by two sets of nerves that have opposing effects: the **vagus nerves**, which slow the heart, and the **sympathetic nerves**, which speed it. During physical activity and in response to pain or emotions such as excitement or fright, the increased activity of the sympathetic nerves and the action of adrenalin increase the pulse rate. With fever, the pulse rate increases five to 10 beats per minute for each degree (Fahrenheit) the body temperature rises. Shock, serious illnesses such as peritonitis, and many types of heart disease can cause a fast, weak pulse.

The pulse is *slow* during sleep. It also is slow in patients with hypothermia, because of the effect of cold, and in those who have fainted or have certain head injuries. Slowing of the pulse occurs mainly because of increased activity of the vagus nerves. Certain types of heart disease also can slow the pulse. A slow pulse is normal in well-conditioned athletes. The normal heart rate is as low as 45 to 50 beats per minute in marathon runners and nordic ski racers.

An *irregular* pulse can be caused by heart disease with atrial fibrillation, or frequent extra beats. The strength of the pulse is related to the strength of each contraction of the heart. A *strong* pulse is found in many conditions that produce a fast or slow pulse, including fever, high blood pressure, hyperthermia (heatstroke), increased intracranial pressure, and the early stages of hemorrhage and other causes of shock. A *weak* (thready) pulse is common in cases of advanced shock.

In an emergency, the best places to find the pulse are the large, easily located vessels such as the **carotid artery** in the neck, or the **femoral artery** in the groin. When extremities are injured, the pulses can be used to determine whether circulation *distal* to the injury is present.

The easiest pulse to find in the upper extremity is the **radial pulse**, located just *proximal* to the base of the thumb at the wrist. The **brachial pulse** can be felt at the midpoint of the inside of the upper arm. In the lower extremity, the **dorsalis pedis pulse** is on the *dorsum* (top) of the foot between the first and second metatarsals, and the **posterior tibial pulse** is *posterior* to the medial malleolus. These pulses usually are easy to find on young, previously healthy people, but may be very difficult to find in those who are elderly, ill, severely injured, or who have arteriosclerosis or other blood-vessel disease.

Important pulse points are shown in Figure 4.2 and also are described in Chapter 3. Practice locating the six important pulses listed above on yourself and fellow students until you can find them within a few seconds (Fig. 4.3). Use the first three fingers to feel the pulse. Never use the thumb, which has a strong pulse of its own that can be mistaken for the patient's pulse. The pulse is counted for 30 seconds and multiplied by two to calculate the rate in beats per minute.

The **pulse rate** and **characteristics** should be recorded at regular intervals when attending to a seriously ill or injured patient. In a patient with a severely injured extremity, record the presence or absence of a pulse distal to the injury initially and again before and after alignment or splinting.

Fig. 4.3 *Technique of Feeling the Radial Pulse*

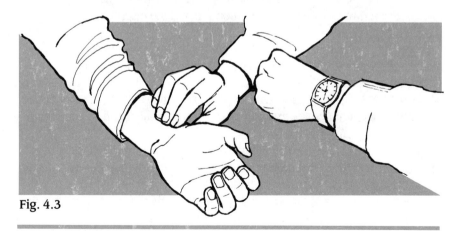

Fig. 4.3

RESPIRATION

Normal breathing is noiseless, effortless, and regular. The normal respiratory rate is 12 to 20 breaths per minute for adults and somewhat higher for children and infants. Respiration may be changed by disease or injury, becoming slower or faster, deeper or shallower, or noisier than normal.

Fig. 4.4 *Standard rectal and oral thermometers are shown on the left. The Zeal is a brand of special low-reading thermometer used for detecting hypothermia.*

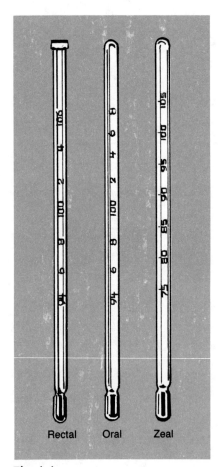

Rectal   Oral   Zeal

Fig. 4.4

Abnormal respiration may reflect changes in the upper or lower respiratory tract, the thoracic cage, the blood, the breathing control center in the brain, or the body as a whole as interpreted by special sense organs that send impulses to the breathing control center.

For example, a patient with fractured ribs or inflammation of the pleura (pleurisy) will have shallow, rapid respirations because it is painful to breathe deeply. A rise in either blood **temperature** (fever) or blood **acidity** (acidosis) increases the rate and depth of breathing. A fall in blood temperature (hypothermia) slows the breathing rate. A head injury that damages the respiratory control center may lead to either rapid, shallow breathing or slow, deep breathing. However, think first of an *obstruction of the upper airway* when an unconscious patient has an altered breathing pattern.

When the oxygen content of the blood falls, there is a compensatory increase in the rate (**tachypnea**) or depth (**hyperpnea**) of breathing. Common causes include pneumonia, pulmonary edema, heart failure, shock, and high altitude. In an unconscious patient, noisy breathing may be caused by relaxation of the tissues of the pharynx or partial obstruction of the upper airway by the tongue. Bronchitis, pneumonia, asthma, and other lung diseases cause characteristic coughs, wheezes, and rattles in the lungs and upper airway.

Abnormal breath odors may be caused by poor oral hygiene, recent ingestion of alcohol or pungent foods, or indigestion. The breath may have a fruity odor in patients with diabetic acidosis and a urinous odor in patients with kidney failure.

TEMPERATURE

Normal body temperature is approximately 98.6°F (37°C), when measured by a thermometer placed under the tongue. Body core temperature, measured rectally, is a degree higher, and the temperature measured in the armpit is a degree lower. Body temperature varies slightly during the day, with the lowest temperature occurring after midnight and the highest temperature in the evening.

Despite normal variations, a reading more than 1°F above normal signifies **fever**. Fever usually is caused by infection or, occasionally, by an injury. A temperature below 98°F (36.7°C) is subnormal; hypothermia occurs at and below 95°F (35°C). Temperatures of 104 to 105°F (40 to 40.6°C) or higher can be seen in cases of fever, especially in children, but also can indicate heatstroke (hyperthermia).

Body temperature usually is taken by placing the bulb of an oral thermometer under the tongue and leaving it in place, with the lips closed around it, for three minutes. If the patient is a child or a disoriented adult, the temperature can be read more reliably and safely by placing a thermometer in the armpit (axilla), and leaving it in place for 10 minutes.

Rectal temperatures, though quite accurate, often are inconvenient or difficult to obtain. In general, rectal thermometers can be distinguished from oral thermometers by differences in their bulbs: the bulb of a rectal thermometer is shorter, wider, and rounder, while the bulb of an oral thermometer is longer and thinner. Frequently, the top end of a rectal thermometer is flat (Fig. 4.4).

An ordinary clinical thermometer contains mercury and is graded from 94°F to 106 or 108°F. Thermometers that read in Centigrade also are available. If an oral temperature reading is 94 to 95°F (34.4 to 35°C), a rectal temperature reading should be taken with a special thermometer capable of documenting the lower body temperatures that occur with hypothermia.

BLOOD PRESSURE

Blood pressure is the pressure transmitted to the walls of the arteries by the blood as it is propelled by the rhythmic contractions of the heart. Thus, blood pressure is closely related to blood flow. Because blood circulates in a **closed system**, a change in one component of the system affects the other components. The body has a complicated feedback system to monitor the pressure within the blood vessels so that the brain can vary heart contractions and blood vessel tone as necessary to ensure adequate blood pressure for maintaining circulation.

Blood pressure is determined by the interaction of the **pulse rate**, **cardiac output**, **blood volume**, and the **tone** of the **blood vessel walls**. An increase in any of these tends to raise blood pressure; a decrease tends to lower blood pressure. For example, an injury that causes blood loss tends to lower blood pressure because less blood is expelled with each beat of the heart. Pressure monitors in the circulatory system respond to a fall in blood pressure by signalling the control center in the brain to increase the heart rate and narrow the blood vessels. If bleeding stops, these adjustments usually will restore adequate blood pressure. If bleeding continues, the blood pressure will drop despite these compensatory adjustments. A marked fall in blood pressure is one of the characteristics of **shock** (discussed in Chapter 7).

Abnormally high blood pressure also is dangerous, because it can strain the heart and damage or even rupture blood vessels. When blood pressure is high, the control center in the brain tends to slow the heart rate. It is important to diagnose and treat the causes of both high and low blood pressure.

The pressure in the aorta and arteries rises when the heart muscle contracts and falls when the heart muscle relaxes. This produces a wave-like pressure curve (Fig. 4.5); the highest point of the curve corresponds to the **systolic pressure** and the lowest point to the **diastolic pressure**. A blood pressure cuff (sphygmomanometer) and a stethoscope (Fig. 4.6) are used to measure blood pressure. Because the cuff should be at least 20 percent wider than the diameter of the arm, different-sized cuffs are needed for adults, children, and obese individuals. Cuffs that are too small may give false high readings; cuffs that are too large, false low readings. Because blood pressure readings can vary depending on the patient's emotional state, readings usually are more accurate when taken *early* in the assessment *before* painful or anxiety-producing procedures are carried out.

To measure blood pressure, wrap the cuff snugly around the arm (Fig. 4.7) so that its lower edge is 1 inch above the bend of the elbow. Place the center of the cuff (marked with an arrow) over the brachial artery. Blood pressure can be taken either by **feeling (palpation)**, or by **listening (auscultation)**. Traditionally, the blood pressure is measured in millimeters of mercury (mm Hg), corresponding to the height a column of mercury is raised within a glass tube. Many sphygmomanometers use a mercury tube.

Fig. 4.5 *Relation of the Systolic and Diastolic Pressures to the Pulse Curve*

Fig. 4.6 *Blood Pressure Cuff and Stethoscope*

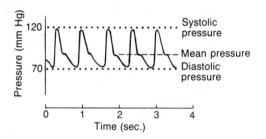

Fig. 4.5

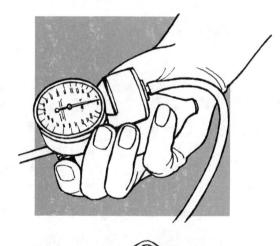

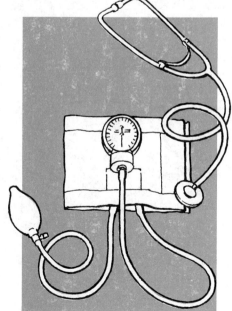

Fig. 4.6

Fig. 4.7 *Technique of Taking Blood Pressure by Palpation*

Fig. 4.8 *Technique of Taking Blood Pressure by Auscultation*

Aneroid sphygmomanometers use a dial to record the cuff pressure directly. Digital sphygmomanometers also are available, but they are more expensive, less durable, and less reliable than the mercury or aneroid types.

It is difficult to read blood pressure by auscultation in noisy places and in moving vehicles; under these circumstances, palpation may have to be used. If the radial pulse can be felt, the patient's systolic blood pressure is at least 80 mm Hg; if the femoral pulse can be felt, at least 70 mm Hg; and if the carotid pulse can be felt, at least 60 mm Hg.

To take blood pressure by **palpation**, locate the patient's radial pulse (for technique, see **THE PULSE**, above). Inflate the cuff for an additional 30 mm Hg after the pulse disappears, then slowly deflate the cuff until the pulse reappears. The reading on the gauge at the point the pulse reappears is the **systolic pressure**. Because the palpation method is less accurate than auscultation, follow the systolic pressure reading obtained by palpation with a P, i.e., 120/P.

To take blood pressure by **auscultation** (Fig. 4.8), locate the brachial artery pulse at the bend of the elbow by palpation. Place the end piece of the stethoscope over the brachial pulse so that, when the rubber-tipped earpieces are placed in the ears, the earpieces will point anteriorly (i.e., forward, toward the nose). Inflate the cuff while listening with the stethoscope. You can begin to hear the pulse when the pressure in the cuff reaches about 80 mm Hg.

Continue to inflate the cuff until the audible pulse disappears and for about 30 mm Hg above that point. Then, slowly deflate the cuff until the audible pulse reappears. The recorded pressure at this point is the **systolic blood pressure**. Continue to slowly deflate the cuff until the audible pulse disappears. The reading at this point is the **diastolic pressure**. Record the systolic and diastolic pressure readings obtained by auscultation separated by a slash, e.g., 120/80, and indicate the patient's position as the reading was taken, i.e., lying, sitting or standing.

The blood pressure of a healthy, young adult usually is about 120/80; pressures from 90/50 to 140/90 are within the normal range. Blood pressure tends to rise slowly with age and can vary widely in the same individual in

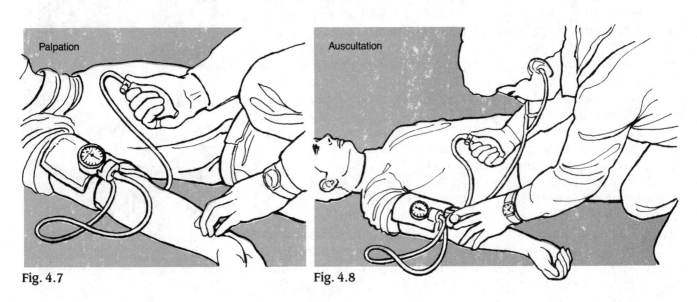

Fig. 4.7   Fig. 4.8

response to pain, emotion, or even the minor stress of having the blood pressure taken. An isolated abnormal blood pressure reading means little, but repeated resting values over 140/90 or below 90/50 are abnormal at any age and should be investigated by a physician.

LEVEL OF CONSCIOUSNESS

An individual with *a normal* level of consciousness is alert, oriented, and talks coherently to the examiner and can easily answer questions about identity, location, day, date, and time of day. Consciousness can range from this normal state to a completely unconscious state where only the activity of the circulatory and respiratory systems can be detected.

Impaired consciousness can be caused by head injury, shock, poisoning, drug use, stroke, hypothermia, hyperthermia, or damage to the circulatory or respiratory systems. When attending to an injured patient, it is important to record the level of consciousness initially and at regular intervals. This is done by repeatedly asking the patient simple questions, such as "How do you feel now?" "Are you doing all right?" and "Can you remember your name and where you are?"

The level of consciousness is usually recorded with the aid of the AVPU scale, which grades the patient's neurologic status from normalcy to complete unconsciousness.

Table 4.2

AVPU SCALE

Alert: The patient appears normal, talks coherently to the examiner, knows his or her own identity, location, address, telephone number, day, and date.

Responds to Verbal Stimuli: The patient is not alert, the eyes do not open spontaneously, but the patient responds in some way when spoken to.

Responds to Pain: The patient does not respond to verbal stimuli, but moves or cries out in response to pain, i.e., a gentle pinch. This response is not valid if the stimulated extremity is numb or paralyzed.

Unresponsive: The patient does not respond to either verbal stimuli or to pain.

The Glasgow Coma Scale (Table 4.3) is another useful but more complicated scale. It is based on three types of response (eye, motor, and verbal) and catalogs what happens to each as a patient's condition deteriorates or improves.

In addition to the five vital signs, five other important signs and symptoms must be described: **skin temperature, moisture** and **color; capillary refill time; appearance of the pupils of the eyes, ability or inability to move on command,** and **reaction to touch and pain.**

Table 4.3

GLASGOW COMA SCALE

		Scale:
Eyes:	Opens eyes **spontaneously**.	4
	Opens eyes to **examiner's speech**.	3
	Opens eyes to **painful stimuli**.	2
	Does not open eyes.	1
Motor:	Follows **simple commands** to move hand or foot.	6
	Pulls **examiner's hand** away when pinched.	5
	Pulls **body part** away when pinched.	4
	Flexes body or body part when pinched.	3
	Extends body or body part when pinched.	2
	No motor response to pinching.	1
Verbal:	Talks **appropriately,** knows name, date, location.	5
	Speech, intelligible, but **confused** and **disoriented**.	4
	Talks, but makes **no sense** at all.	3
	Makes **sounds** but no words.	2
	Makes **no sounds** at all.	1

Table 4.4

FIVE OTHER IMPORTANT SIGNS AND SYMPTOMS

Skin temperature, moisture
and color
Capillary refill
Reaction of the pupils
Ability to move
Reaction to pain

SKIN TEMPERATURE, MOISTURE, AND COLOR

Skin temperature is the net result of the difference between the temperature of the environment and the temperature of the blood. Skin wetness depends on the activity of the sweat glands. Skin color depends on the state of the surface blood vessels and the blood within them. However, in dark-skinned people, skin pigment may mask color changes, and examination of the whites of the eyes or the nailbeds may be more reliable.

As the blood flows through the capillaries in the skin, oxygen is extracted and the blood changes from bright red to a more bluish red. If the blood vessels are **widened (dilated)**, there is an increase in the volume and speed of blood flow to the skin, less oxygen is removed from each unit of blood, and the blood (and skin) become redder and warmer. If the blood vessels are **narrowed (constricted)**, there is a decrease in the volume and speed of blood flow to the skin, more oxygen is removed from each unit of blood, and the blood (and skin) become bluer and cooler. If blood vessels are markedly narrowed, very little blood reaches the surface capillaries and the skin appears pale, ashen or grey, and cool or cold.

In patients with anemia, a condition characterized by too few red blood cells, the skin appears pale. The skin is pale, clammy, and cold in patients with an illness or injury that stimulates a stress response from the sympathetic nervous system, leading to increased heart rate, narrowing of surface blood vessels, and increased sweating.

Redder, warmer skin typically is seen in association with fever or heatstroke (hyperthermia) and in warm environments. Red skin can be a sign of too many red blood cells (polycythemia) because of high altitude or blood disease, too high blood pressure, or carbon monoxide poisoning. In patients who are severely ill or injured, sympathetic nervous system stimulation or shock can result in skin that is pale (white or grayish), cold, and clammy. Cold exposure and hypothermia produce pale or bluish, cold, dry skin. When there is inadequate oxygen in the blood because of high altitude or disease of the heart or lungs, the skin is a bluish color (a condition called **cyanosis**). Hepatitis and other types of liver disease can lead to an accumulation of bilirubin that turns the skin and the whites of the eyes yellow. This condition, called **jaundice**, should not be confused with the yellowing of the skin caused by eating large quantities of foods, such as tomatoes and carrots, that contain high levels of the vitamin A precursor carotene.

Even though examination of the skin does not reveal everything the rescuer needs to know, it does furnish important clues regarding oxygenation, general body stress, and the status of circulation to the skin.

CAPILLARY REFILL

Capillary refill is the ability of the circulatory system to refill small vessels after blood has been squeezed out of them (Fig. 4.9). Using the thumb and forefinger, squeeze a finger or toe tip until the nail blanches; then release the pressure. The tissues under the nail should return to their normal pink color within two seconds (count "one-and-two-and" or say "capillary refill").

This test is a rough measure of blood flow through the blood vessels; capillary refill is prolonged or absent in cases of serious illness or injury, particularly shock. Unfortunately, the test is unreliable in the cold, when circulation in the skin and extremities is normally slowed.

REACTION OF THE PUPILS

The pupils are normally round and equal to each other in diameter. Ten percent of normal individuals have unequal pupils. An artificial eye, changes caused by prescription drugs or eye drops, or eye surgery (e.g., for a cataract), also can cause differences in pupil size. Conditions causing pupillary change can be divided into those that change both pupils and those that change only one pupil.

Shining a bright light into one eye normally causes both pupils to **constrict** (become smaller). Both pupils will constrict in response to strong glare or opiates. **Dilation** (enlargement) of both pupils occurs normally in response to dim light. Abnormal dilation occurs in response to certain drugs (e.g., marijuana and barbiturates), and in individuals who are frightened or unconscious. Patients who are in cardiac arrest generally have dilated pupils that do not constrict in response to a bright light. The pupillary response to light also is lost after death.

Unequal pupils, which usually means one pupil is normal and the other dilated, frequently indicate a serious injury involving the brain on the same side as the dilated pupil. When a patient has a brain injury or is unconscious, it is important to *recheck* and *record* the pupil size and equality at regular intervals. Figure 4.10 illustrates common pupillary changes.

Fig. 4.9 *Technique of Testing Capillary Refill Time*

Fig. 4.10 *Normal Pupils and Pupillary Changes*

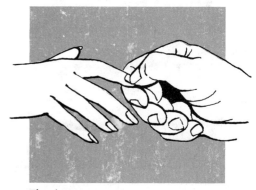

Fig. 4.9

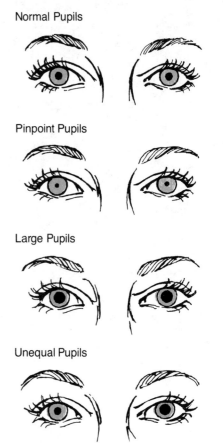

Normal Pupils

Pinpoint Pupils

Large Pupils

Unequal Pupils

Fig. 4.10

Fig. 4.11 *Testing for Pain and Sensation*

Fig. 4.12 *Testing for Impaired Movement*

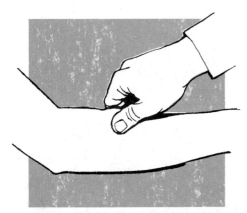

Fig. 4.11

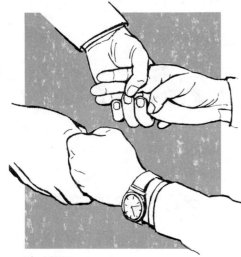

Fig. 4.12

REACTION TO PAIN

The normal reaction to pain is to cry out or withdraw the body part being hurt. Test for a normal pain reaction by gently pinching the skin or scratching it with a fingernail (Fig. 4.11) while asking "Can you feel this?" An inability to feel pain usually means damage to the nerve pathways running from that body part to the brain. This can occur because of damage to the spinal cord or damage to the peripheral nerves. Lack of sensation is frequently, but not always, accompanied by impaired ability to move the affected body part.

ABILITY TO MOVE

To test for impaired movement, ask the patient to move his or her fingers and toes and to squeeze your hands (Fig. 4.12). A conscious patient who is unable to comply is said to be **paralyzed**. Paralysis can involve a single extremity, one side of the body, or both sides of the body. Record exactly what the patient can or cannot do.

Paralysis of a single extremity most often is caused by nerve damage resulting from injury to that extremity. Paralysis can be caused by severe injury without nerve damage if motion is so painful that the patient refuses to try to move. Test motion in an injured extremity initially and again before and after any attempt to align or splint the extremity. Paralysis of one side of the body usually is caused by a stroke, but unilateral paralysis can follow a head injury involving the *opposite* side of the head. Injury to the spinal cord in the neck may result in paralysis of all four extremities and the body below the neck; spinal cord injury below the neck may paralyze only the legs.

PSYCHOLOGY OF DEALING WITH THE ILL OR INJURED

Two things should be firmly in mind when approaching a patient: your initial reaction to the patient and the patient's initial reaction to you as the rescuer. Everyone responds to outside events in two ways: emotionally and intellectually. The emotional reaction to a patient who is hysterical, in pain, or horribly injured is to do something, e.g., provide emergency care, tell a hysterical patient to calm down, summon assistance, or even to vomit or run away. All of these reactions are normal and will differ among people in both type and degree. Fortunately, with training and experience, the initial reaction to an emergency can be managed so that the intellect rather than the emotions predominates (Fig. 4.13).

Most, though not all patients, will be reasonable and cooperative. Any severe stress tends to cause a regression to a more infantile, more dependent state. Take advantage of this reaction by assuming a calm air of trustworthiness, competence, kindness, and authority. The patient's concerns should be taken seriously. Avoid making jokes and uttering banalities such as "Don't worry, we'll take care of it," or "There is nothing to worry about."

As a rescuer, make eye contact with the patient, introduce yourself as a trained rescuer and emergency care provider, and ask "May I be of help?" or "May I help you?"

In some cases, help will be refused. A refusal always should be documented and witnessed, even if the patient has a normal level of consciousness and appears to have trivial injuries. The patient must be told what may happen if care is refused, and this also must be documented for a refusal to be valid. Members of the National Ski Patrol and other rescue organizations carry special forms for the patient to sign that signify care has been offered and refused. If help is refused, stay with the patient until you are satisfied that everything is under control. The patient may have a change of heart or a change of condition. If an irrational patient refuses help, necessary care may have to be given; this also should be documented and witnessed.

Giving care to a seriously ill or injured child may be difficult and emotionally taxing, especially for rescuers who have children of their own. The child often will be frightened and may be hysterical, but children usually respond to an adult who behaves in a kind and parental manner. Children often are more modest than adults, and assessment may be difficult. The rescuer should move slowly, use simple terms, make eye-level contact, and explain procedures – especially painful ones – before they are carried out. When parents or siblings are present they may be helpful in calming the child and explaining what is happening.

When assessing a child, begin at the feet and move toward the head. Painful procedures and examination of obvious injuries are best left until after a trusting relationship has been established.

Always think before speaking, since statements are easily misinterpreted by patients and their friends and relatives at the scene. Explain each action to the patient *before* it takes place. Do not lie to the patient, particularly about a procedure that will obviously be painful. Rescuers should *never* argue or criticize each others' actions within the hearing of the patient or bystanders (Fig. 4.14). Discuss plans for emergency care and evacuation privately; inform the patient after the arrangements are complete.

Remember, rescuers are not physicians. It is inappropriate for rescuers to offer detailed information on possible further treatment or outcome. In particular, avoid guessing how soon the patient will be well again. First aid and emergency care is an inexact science. Even the best assessment is imperfect, diagnostic facilities outside of a medical center are primitive, and a serious injury or illness may not be obvious in the field. Remember that more than one condition can be present, and avoid the tendency to attribute all signs and symptoms to the most obvious injury.

People who are under the influence of alcohol or other drugs are more prone to injury; it is important not to overlook these injuries or attribute signs and symptoms solely to the effects of the drug. People under the influence of drugs or alcohol and those who are senile or psychotic must sometimes be protected from injuring themselves or others. They may behave erratically. Their normal judgment and usual protective reflexes and instincts may not be functioning. They may fall and injure themselves, wreck their vehicles, wander into danger, promote fights, and become belligerent and obnoxious. They may occasionally become violent and dangerous.

Remain calm, patient, nonjudgmental, and reassuring. Refrain from arguing and, except in an emergency and preferably with witnesses present, do not attempt forceful restraint. Do not leave any patient alone until he or she has been turned over to the EMS system or another responsible agency.

Fig. 4.13 *While approaching a patient, consider the person's emotional reaction.*

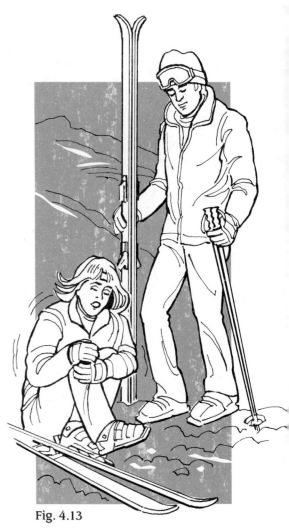

Fig. 4.13

Fig. 4.14 *Don't be guilty of this!*

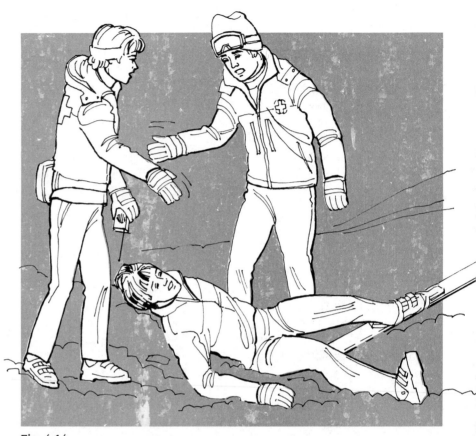

Fig. 4.14

FIRST IMPRESSION

While approaching the patient, the examiner forms an immediate **first impression** of the situation, which takes less time to do than to read about here. The first impression includes the following information, which is registered almost simultaneously (Fig. 4.15):

1. Is there any *danger* to the rescuer(s), the patient, or others at the scene (from rockfall, snow avalanche, other skiers, etc.)
2. What has most likely occurred, as indicated by the patient's location, position, probable *mechanism of injury,* etc.?
3. Is the patient *responsive* or unresponsive?
4. Is the patient *breathing*?
5. Does the patient have *severe bleeding*?

The examiner should wear disposable rubber gloves while examining a patient if there is a chance of contact with the patient's blood or other body fluids.

PRIMARY SURVEY

After forming the first impression, proceed with the **primary survey**, whose purpose is to immediately identify and treat life-threatening emergencies. The primary survey is conducted semi-automatically following a rigid protocol and consists mainly of a rapid, but not hasty, evaluation of the status of the respiratory and circulatory systems. The ABCDE sequence is useful in remembering what to do and in what order (Fig. 4.16-19):

A: Airway, including stabilization of the cervical spine, if indicated.
B: Breathing.
C: Circulation (including severe bleeding).
D: Disability.
E: Exposure (undress the patient only enough to identify all injuries in preparation for the thorough secondary survey examination).

Shortly after reaching the patient, the rescuer should have a good idea whether the patient is responsive or unresponsive. If not, ask, ''Are you okay?'' If there is no answer, immediately determine the presence or absence of breathing and circulation and, if indicated, begin rescue breathing or cardiopulmonary resuscitation (CPR), described in Chapter 5.

Assess breathing by opening the airway, listening for breath sounds by placing your ear next to the patient's mouth and nose, and watching for chest movements. The airway can be opened by either the chin-lift or jaw-thrust methods described in Chapter 5; however, if there is a possibility of a neck injury or if the patient is unresponsive because of an injury or unknown cause, use only the jaw-thrust method and stabilize the cervical spine. It also may be useful to examine the skin for cyanosis. Note the presence of breathing, the rate and regularity of respirations, and whether or not the chest is moving normally. Assess circulation by checking the carotid artery pulse.

Fig. 4.15 *The first impression is formed while approaching the patient.*

Unresponsive Patient

If the patient is unresponsive but is breathing and has a carotid pulse, note the color, temperature and moisture of the skin, and check capillary refill time. At the same time, monitor the upper airway and stabilize the cervical spine manually *and* with an extrication collar (see Chapter 9). Find and control sources of major bleeding (Fig. 4.17). If a patient has suffered major trauma, it may be necessary to remove the patient's clothing and logroll the patient onto one side to find every source of bleeding. Check blood pressure by feeling for major pulses (see **THE PULSE**) or using a sphygmomanometer.

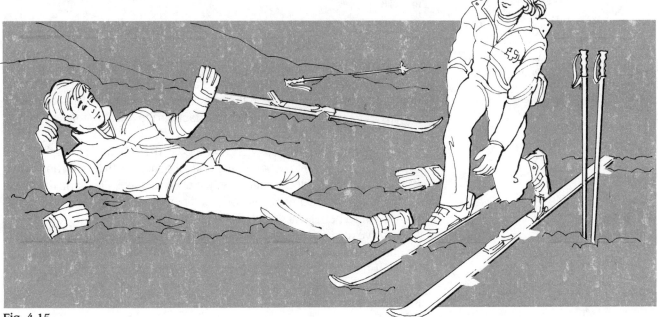

Fig. 4.15

Fig. 4.16 *Begin the primary survey by assessing breathing and the carotid pulse.*

Fig. 4.17 *Find and control major sources of bleeding.*

Fig. 4.18 *Manual stabilization is applied to the head and neck when the patient is unresponsive.*

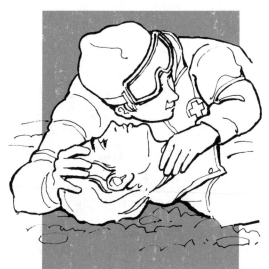

Fig. 4.16

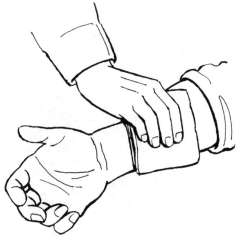

Fig. 4.17

If there is no external bleeding but changes in the pulse, skin color, blood pressure, and capillary refill time indicate blood loss, open clothing so that the chest, abdomen, pelvis, and thighs can be examined for signs of internal bleeding, discussed in Chapter 7.

Next, establish and monitor the extent of **disability**, i.e., injury to the **nervous and musculoskeletal systems**. Grade the level of consciousness with the aid of the AVPU scale or Glasgow Coma Scale, discussed previously (Tables 4.2 and 4.3).

Whenever a patient is unresponsive following trauma or from an unknown cause, the cervical spine is assumed to be injured. If not handled properly, such injuries can lead to damage of the spinal cord and possible permanent disability; therefore, the cervical spine (Fig. 4.18) *must* be stabilized immediately and maintained throughout the primary and secondary surveys (see Chapter 5).

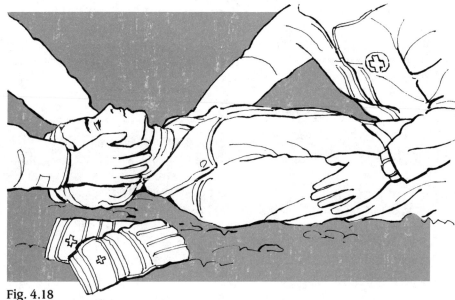

Fig. 4.18

Responsive Patient

Approach the patient, make eye contact, and introduce yourself as a person trained in emergency care. Next, ask what happened and if the patient will allow you to be of assistance. If the answer is yes, ask, ''How do you feel?'' and ''What is wrong?'' Continue eye contact during questioning and examination to detect the patient's reactions.

Next, grasp the patient's wrist and assess the rate and strength of the radial pulse (Fig. 4.19) to separate the critical patient with a rapid and weak pulse from the non-critical patient with a normal pulse. Checking the pulse also identifies you as a medically oriented person and helps establish trust, reliance, and a beneficial giver-receiver relationship.

Observe the patient's face for color changes and excessive perspiration, and check the temperature and moisture of the skin of the wrist. Test capillary refill time, and then examine the major problem sites identified by the patient. When this examination is completed, ask, ''Is there anything else wrong?''

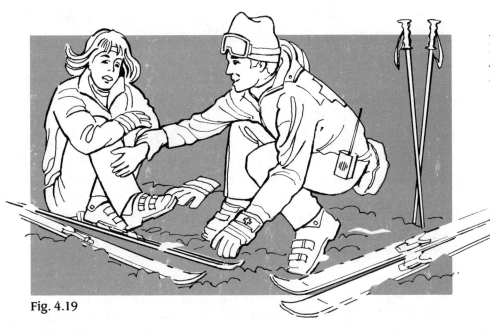

Fig. 4.19 *Check the radial pulse to separate a critical patient from a non-critical patient.*

Fig. 4.19

Table 4.5

PRIMARY SURVEY

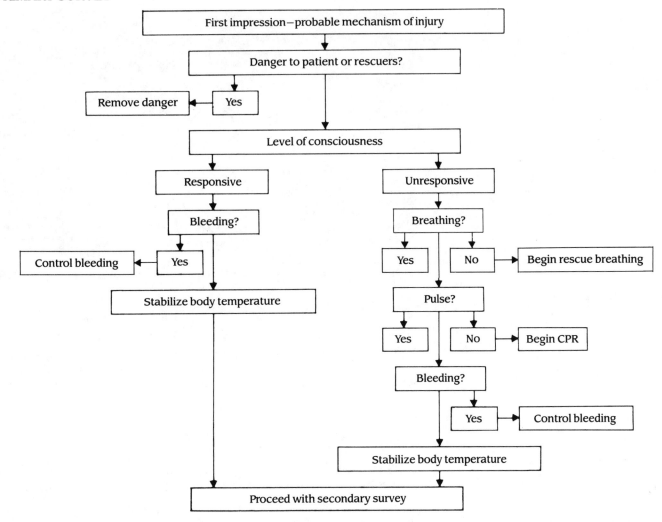

Fig. 4.20 *First things first!*

SECONDARY SURVEY

The **secondary survey** is conducted more slowly and involves evaluation of the remaining six organ systems in a systematic manner and in the same order each time so that nothing important is overlooked. Whenever possible, the secondary survey is conducted in a place and manner chosen with respect for the patient's modesty.

The extent of the secondary survey depends partly on the nature of the primary injury. The secondary survey always is carried out completely when the patient is unresponsive, has suffered serious multiple injuries, or appears to be mentally impaired or unreliable. It can be abbreviated if the injuries are trivial or solitary and the patient can *clearly* indicate that no additional problems exist.

For example, when a patient has fallen and sprained a knee at an alpine ski area and has a normal level of consciousness, it is more important to prevent hypothermia by transporting the patient by toboggan to a warm first aid room than to do a secondary survey on the ski slope (Fig. 4.20). Similarly, because it is important to maintain spinal stabilization, do not unstrap a patient from a spine board to do a secondary survey.

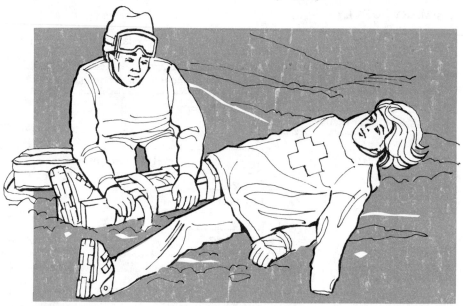

Fig. 4.20

In conducting the secondary survey, the rescuer should think, ask questions, look, listen, feel, and occasionally smell. Look for deviations from the normal state and, if in doubt, compare the area in question with the opposite, uninjured part of the body. Look for swellings, lumps, bruises, and open wounds; deformities, abnormal positions, and abnormal motion or lack of motion; abnormal skin color and moisture; and medical-alert tags or bracelets.

Avoid leading questions, listen to what the patient says, and also listen for abnormal sounds, particularly in the respiratory system. Feel the pulses, check the skin for abnormal temperature or moisture, and examine the body for deformities, lumps, indentations, abnormal hard or soft areas, and tender areas. Note abnormal odors, particularly of the breath.

The first step in the secondary survey is to record the vital signs: pulse, respiratory rate, body temperature, blood pressure, and level of consciousness (Fig. 4.21). Then interview the patient to document in detail exactly what happened and the mechanism(s) of injury, if appropriate. Make sure that all painful areas have been identified.

Next, seek important information from the patient's history. EMTs frequently use the mnemonic AMPLE to help remember the important elements of the patient history:

A: Allergies.

M: Medicines or drugs, both legal and illegal.

P: Past medical history.

L: Last meal.

E: Events prior to the incident in question.

The most important items are:

1. Preexisting illness (diabetes, heart disease, epilepsy, etc.) or injuries, especially those to the same area of the body.
2. Any medication taken regularly.
3. Any allergies, particularly to drugs.
4. Finally, ask the patient, "Is there anything else about your health that I should know?"

The answers to these questions will provide important leads to follow.

The important signs and symptoms for injured patients include general body weakness or excessive fatigue, headache, dizziness, or even momentary loss of consciousness; double vision or inability to see normally; numbness, tingling, weakness, or paralysis of an extremity; pain, pain on motion; shortness of breath, cough, blood in sputum, pain on breathing; and nausea, vomiting, abdominal pain or cramps, blood in the feces or in the urine, or difficult urination.

The description of pain should include time of onset, location at onset, change in location or severity, radiation, character (dull, achy, crushing, sharp, burning, stabbing, crampy, constant, intermittent), and severity. Also

Fig. 4.21 *The secondary survey is best conducted in a warm environment.*

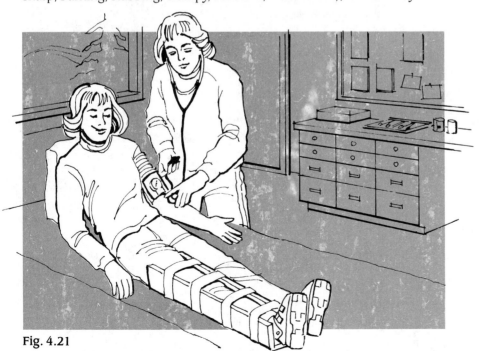

Fig. 4.21

record whether the pain changes in response to breathing, coughing, motion or change in position and whether the patient has had similar pain in the past.

Most of the above symptoms can occur with illness as well as injury. Important symptoms that usually occur only in illness include chills, the sensation of being hot or cold, insomnia, pus or blood in the sputum, pain or difficulty on swallowing, diarrhea, painful urination, and change in bowel habits.

After questioning the patient about symptoms, thoroughly examine the patient's body from the head down. Remove as much clothing as possible. In cold weather, expose one small area of the patient's body at a time. Although the patient should be shielded from the eyes of bystanders, an attempt to avoid embarrassing the patient is no excuse for missing a significant illness or injury.

The rescuer should know the meaning of two anatomical terms used to describe the patient's position when lying down. **Prone** indicates the patient is lying face down; **supine**, that the patient is lying face up. The sequence for assessment of an adult is: head, neck, chest, abdomen and pelvis, lower extremity, upper extremity, and back. For a child, it is: lower extremity, abdomen and pelvis, upper extremity, chest, neck, head, and back.

Table 4.6

SUMMARY OF SECONDARY SURVEY

1. Vital Signs
   Pulse, blood pressure, respiration, temperature, level of consciousness.
2. Interview
   a. Description of what happened.
   b. Any other current problems.
   c. Important facts from medical history.
      (1) Preexisting illnesses or injuries.
      (2) Current medications.
      (3) Allergies, particularly to drugs.
      (4) If there is anything else the rescuer needs to know about the patient's health.
3. Important Signs and Symptoms
   Weakness, fatigue, headache, dizziness, loss of consciousness, double vision, trouble seeing, numbness, tingling, weakness or paralysis, pain, pain on motion, shortness of breath, cough, blood in sputum, pain on breathing, nausea, vomiting, abdominal pain, cramps, blood in stools or urine, painful or difficult urination. Chills, fever, insomnia, pus in sputum, difficulty in swallowing, diarrhea, change in bowel habits.
4. Characteristics of Pain
   Time of onset, location, change in location or severity, radiation, character, severity, relationship to position or motion, previous episodes of similar pain.
5. Examination
   The examiner looks for open and closed wounds, bleeding, bruises, swellings, depressions, discharge, abnormal positions, deformities,

abnormal odors, asymmetry, loss of motion, changes in skin color or moisture, tenderness.

Examine the body from top to bottom in the same order each time, systematically and thoroughly checking each body area for the abnormalities listed above.

The Head

Reassess the level of responsiveness and reexamine the eyes and pupils (Fig. 4.22). It is generally safe to leave contact lenses in place, even if the patient is unresponsive, as long as the eyes are kept closed (by taping, if necessary) and the patient can be transported to a hospital within two to three hours. Alert hospital personnel by writing "Contact Lenses" on a piece of tape and affixing it to the patient's forehead. Contact lenses should never be removed if the patient has sustained an injury to the eye area.

Hard contact lenses are difficult to remove without a special suction cup made for this purpose. Individuals who travel to remote areas usually carry this equipment. If a hard lens cannot be removed, it sometimes can be slid from the clear part of the eye (cornea) onto the white of the eye.

Some soft contact lenses are designed to be left in place for weeks and will not injure the eye as long as they remain moist. This can be assured by taping the eyelids shut. If it is necessary to remove soft contact lenses, they usually can be lifted by pinching them gently between the thumb and index finger. Rescuers who wear contact lenses can be useful when lenses need to be removed.

Next, inspect the scalp and face for open wounds, bleeding, bruises, swellings, and depressions; gently feel the scalp for bumps and depressions. Inspect the ears and nose for a clear or bloody discharge, and check the mouth for dentures, foreign objects, wounds, and bleeding. Note whether the lower jaw is properly aligned under the upper jaw when the patient's mouth is closed. Smell the breath for unusual odors.

The Neck

Inspect the neck for open and closed wounds, bleeding, swellings, bruises, asymmetry, engorged neck veins, and unusual positions. Being careful not to bend or twist the neck, feel the back of the neck for tender areas, lumps, and deformities. In front, check the sternal notch to make sure that the trachea is in the midline, and feel for masses and swellings.

The Chest

Clothing must be opened for adequate assessment of the chest. Inspect the front of the chest for open and closed wounds, bleeding, bruises, asymmetry, and deformities. Note the effort required for breathing. Feel the thoracic cage, including the sternum, to detect swellings, tenderness (especially over the ribs) and the impression of "Rice Krispies" produced by air under the skin (subcutaneous emphysema). Place one hand on either side of the anterior chest to see whether both sides are expanding equally with inhalation; listen for audible wheezes and other noises (Fig. 4.23).

Fig. 4.22 *Assessment of the Head*

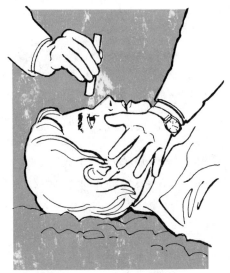

Fig. 4.22

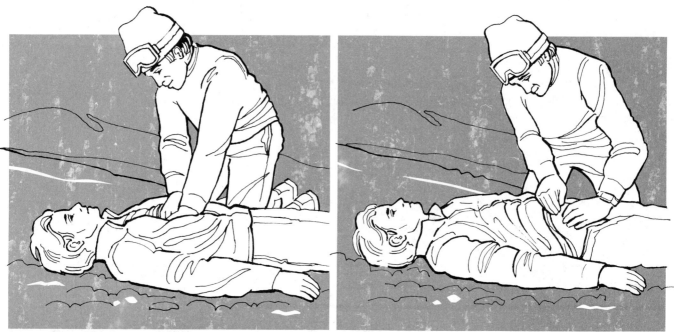

Fig. 4.23

Fig. 4.24

Fig. 4.23 *Assessment of the Chest*

Fig. 4.24 *Assessment of the Abdomen and Pelvis*

Fig. 4.25 *Assessment of the Lower Extremity*

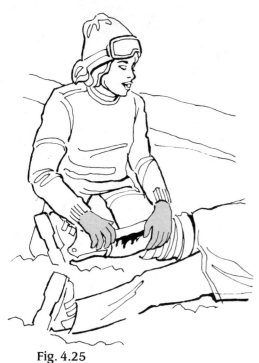

Fig. 4.25

Rescuers with experience using a stethoscope can compare the breath sounds on either side of the chest. This also can be done by placing the naked ear against the patient's chest.

Abdomen and Pelvis

Open the patient's clothing to allow adequate assessment of the abdomen and pelvis (Fig. 4.24). Inspect the abdominal skin for open and closed wounds, bleeding, bruises, and distention. Using the pads of the fingertips, palpate the abdominal wall to check for tenderness, rigidity, swellings, masses, and tightening of abdominal muscles overlying a tender area ("guarding").

Considerable experience is needed to judge how hard to press on the abdomen. Begin with a light touch and press slowly, gently, and no deeper in than 1 inch. *Never* start by examining known tender areas, because pain will cause reflex tightening of all the abdominal muscles, making further assessment difficult.

Note audible gurgling noises. If the patient has experienced trauma, gently press the sides of the pelvis backward and then toward each other to see if this causes pain.

The Lower Extremity

Inspect the thighs, legs, and feet for open and closed wounds, bleeding, bruises, deformities, abnormal shortening, and unusual positions. If in doubt, compare the injured extremity with the opposite normal extremity. Locate and palpate the femoral, dorsalis pedis, and posterior tibial pulses. Feel the skin for tender areas, swellings, and depressions. Ask if the patient's legs or feet feel numb or tingly. Check sensation in both lower extremities by gently pinching or scraping the skin with a fingernail. Next, ask if the patient can move the toes and ankles. Compare the two sides of the body throughout the examination (Fig. 4.25).

The Upper Extremity

Inspect the skin of each arm, forearm, and hand for open and closed wounds, bleeding, bruises, deformities, swellings, abnormal shortening, and unusual positions. Again, if in doubt, compare the injured extremity with the opposite normal extremity. Feel the radial pulse at the wrist, and check the skin of each extremity for abnormal swellings, tender areas, and depressions. Ask if the patient's fingers or hands feel numb or tingly, and check for sensation as described for the lower extremity. Ask if the patient can move the elbow, wrist and fingers. Instruct the patient to squeeze both your hands simultaneously to test strength and to compare the grip of each hand (Fig. 4.26).

The Back

If there is any possibility of back injury (except one involving the spinal cord), logroll the patient onto one side to examine the back (Fig. 4.27). The technique, described in Chapter 14, should be done at the time the patient is placed on a spine board to avoid unnecessary logrolling. Clothing must be opened for adequate assessment of the back. Inspect the skin of the back and buttocks for open and closed wounds, bleeding, bruises, swellings, deformities, or unusual positions. When feeling for swellings and tenderness, pay particular attention to tenderness over the spinous processes of the vertebrae.

Fig. 4.26 *Assessment of the Upper Extremity*

Fig. 4.27 *Assessment of the Back*

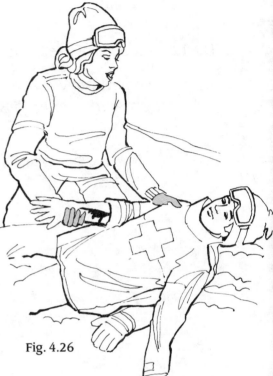

Fig. 4.26

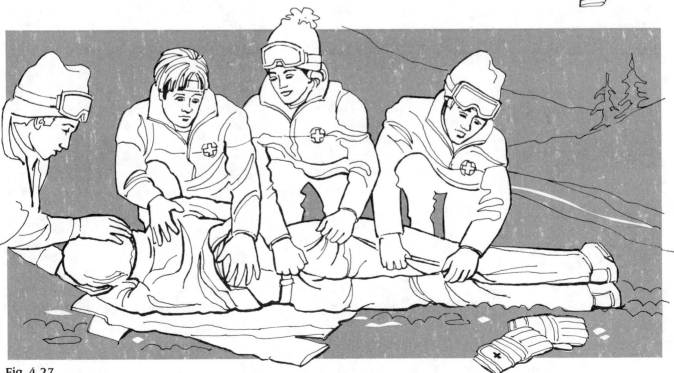

Fig. 4.27

5

Basic Life Support

The heart moves of itself and does not stop unless for ever.

–Leonardo da Vinci
  Dell' Anatomia, Fogli B.

BASIC LIFE SUPPORT

When the circulatory and respiratory systems fail to carry out their vital function of delivering oxygen to every body cell, the most frequent cause is heart disease. Heart disease is a major health problem in modern society. In 1984, coronary heart disease caused 540,000 deaths in the United States – the majority of these were sudden deaths. Currently, more than 6 million Americans are known to have coronary heart disease. Many of these individuals are at significant risk for sudden death or an acute heart attack (myocardial infarction).

About two-thirds of sudden deaths caused by heart disease take place outside a hospital, usually within two hours of the onset of symptoms. A significant proportion of these deaths are caused by abnormal heart rhythms in people whose hearts would otherwise function adequately for many years. In many cases the patient has had no warning of the impending catastrophe. Sudden death from coronary heart disease is the most common serious medical emergency in the U.S. today. It is a major concern for every emergency care giver and a major topic in every emergency care course.

Cardiac arrest is any condition where blood circulation stops because the heart malfunctions. Either the heart stops beating entirely or the heart beats too fast (ventricular tachycardia) or in an uncoordinated manner (ventricular fibrillation).

A technique called cardiopulmonary resuscitation, or CPR, was developed in the early 1960s to resuscitate victims of cardiac arrest. The rescuer restores ventilation (lung action) by breathing into the patient's lungs and restores heart action by rhythmically pressing on the patient's chest. Pressing on the chest raises the pressure inside the chest and squeezes the heart between the sternum and the thoracic spine, forcing the blood out of the heart into the circulatory system.

To be effective, cardiopulmonary resuscitation must begin within four to six minutes after cardiac arrest. Thus, the only way to save an appreciable number of cardiac arrest victims who collapse outside a medical facility would be to teach the technique to laypersons on a widespread basis. Consequently, the American Heart Association and the American Red Cross developed courses in basic life support and cardiopulmonary resuscitation. Over 50 million people have taken these courses since the early 1970s.

Basic life support saves few lives unless it is quickly followed by advanced cardiac life support (ACLS). ACLS is performed by paramedics, nurses, or physicians who may reach the patient by ambulance or helicopter. While basic life support requires only the tools that the rescuer carries at all times – the brain, eyes, ears, mouth, and hands – the ACLS team is equipped to treat the heart patient using heart monitors, electrical defibrillation equipment, and intravenous drugs. Therefore, an important part of basic life support is summoning ACLS by contacting the EMS system. It is estimated that, eventually, 100,000 to 200,000 lives per year can be saved by prompt basic life support followed rapidly by advanced cardiac life support. Everyone should memorize the phone number used locally to summon the EMS system.

An even more important public health measure is the *prevention* of coronary heart disease. Major risk factors such as age and heredity cannot be

Fig. 5.1 *Shout for help if the patient is unresponsive.*

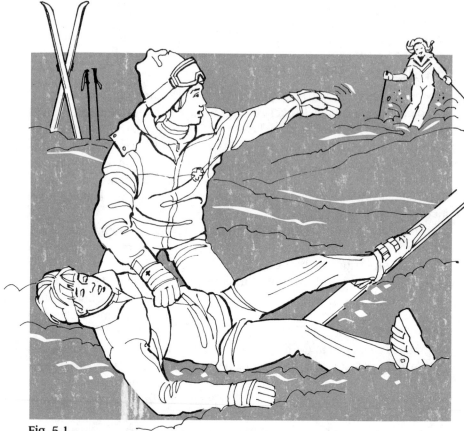

Fig. 5.1

Table 5.1

INFORMATION TO GIVE THE EMS DISPATCHER

What happened.
Where it happened:
   Location, street address, map coordinates if appropriate, nearby landmarks or prominent structures, telephone number of phone from which call is being made.
Number of patients.
Condition of patients.
Emergency care being given.

changed, but risk factors such as cigarette smoking, high blood pressure, elevated blood cholesterol, and diabetes can be eliminated or treated. Maintaining normal weight and engaging in regular aerobic exercise also appear to be important.

The techniques of basic life support described below follow the recommendations of the 1985 National Conference on Cardiopulmonary Resuscitation (CPR) and Emergency Cardiac Care (ECC) as published in the June 6, 1986 issue of the *Journal of the American Medical Association*. The section on Pediatric Basic Life Support has been modified according to the guidelines of the Pediatric Working Group of the American Red Cross, as of January 30, 1987. Remember that skills must be *refreshed* regularly if rescuers are to perform effective basic life support.

Basic life support includes techniques for **rescue breathing, cardiopulmonary resuscitation**, and **clearing upper-airway obstructions**. Not everyone who collapses needs these techniques. After an episode of simple fainting, a common cause of collapse, the patient will recover without assistance. Therefore, an important part of basic life support is patient assessment to determine which, if any, life support techniques are needed. Basic life support is more successful and easier when carried out by two rescuers. Because only one rescuer may be available, at least initially, the technique for one-rescuer basic life support will be described first.

Immediately after reaching a patient who has collapsed, perform a primary survey (Chapter 4); this should take only a few seconds. Then follow these steps:

1. **Determine the mechanism of injury or illness**. It is important to distinguish a patient who collapses because of primary cardiac arrest from one who suffers a secondary cardiac arrest as a result of a

serious injury. A spine injury must be assumed in any patient who suffers cardiac arrest accompanying trauma.

Fig. 5.2 *Positioning a Patient for Basic Life Support*

2. **Determine responsiveness** by tapping or gently shaking the patient and shouting "Are you okay?" If the patient is *truly* unresponsive, shout immediately for help (Fig. 5.1). Send someone to telephone the local emergency number (often this is 911) or otherwise **notify the EMS system.**

    The EMS dispatcher will need the following information: the location, including street address, directions, and landmarks if necessary; the telephone number from which the call is being made; what happened, i.e., auto accident, drowning, etc.; the number of patients; the condition of the patient(s); and the type of emergency care being given. The caller should not hang up before the EMS dispatcher hangs up.

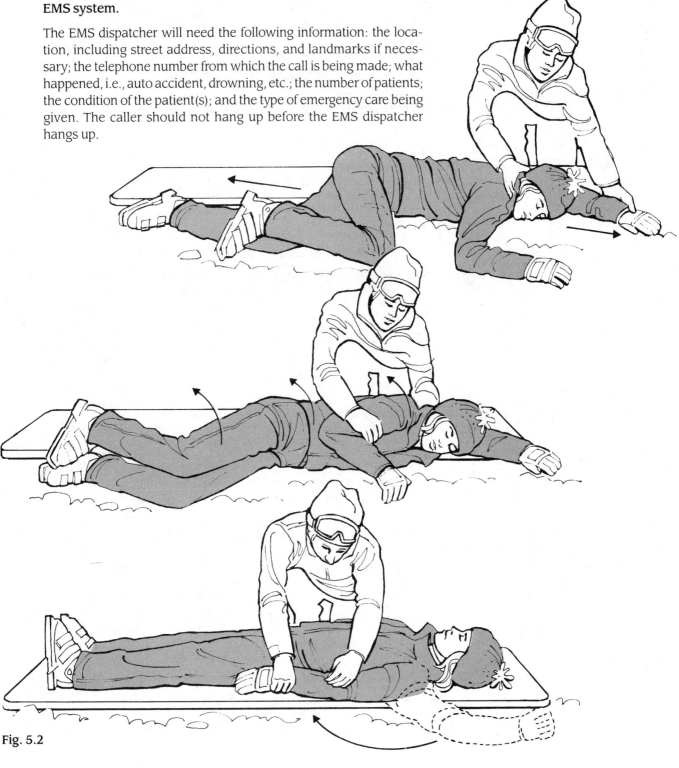

Fig. 5.2

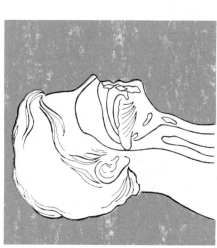
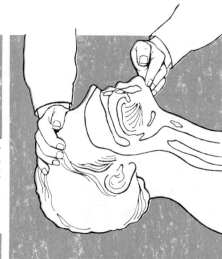
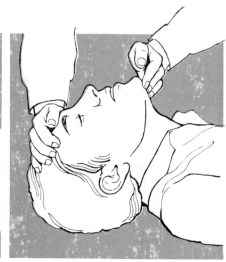

Fig. 5.3

Fig. 5.3 *Opening the Airway with the Head-tilt/Chin-lift Method*

Fig. 5.4 *Open the patient's mouth with the crossed-finger technique and remove visible foreign material with a hooked finger.*

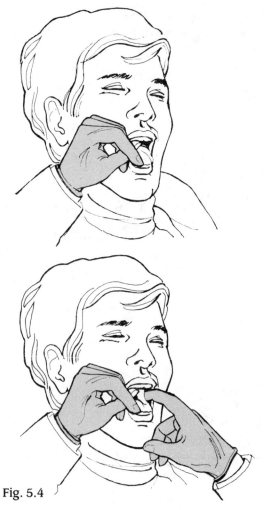

Fig. 5.4

3. **Position the patient supine** on a firm, flat surface with the head no lower than the chest (Fig. 5.2). If the patient must be moved, treat the head and body as a unit so that the back, head, and neck are not twisted or bent. Place the patient's arms alongside his or her body. Kneel by the patient's shoulder, facing the patient.

4. **Open the airway.** In the unconscious patient, the muscles of the upper airway relax, allowing the tongue to fall back and close the airway by obstructing the pharynx. Because the tongue is attached to the lower jaw, any maneuver that brings the lower jaw *forward* should open the airway. Such maneuvers should cause minimal or no bending or twisting of the neck to prevent worsening an undetected neck fracture. However, because the patient will die if the airway is not opened and breathing is not restored, it is acceptable to bend the neck slightly if necessary to open the airway. Neck injuries are unusual in patients who collapse from cardiac arrest.

The preferred method of opening the airway is the **head-tilt/chin-lift** (Fig. 5.3). Place one hand on the patient's forehead and tilt the patient's head back. At the same time, using your other hand, place several fingertips under the tip of the patient's chin just behind the point of the jawbone and lift to bring the chin forward. The patient's mouth should be partly open. If it is necessary to open the patient's mouth, use the "crossed-finger" technique (Fig. 5.4a). If the patient is wearing dentures, remove them. Also remove any visible foreign material with a hooked finger or a piece of cloth (Fig. 5.4b).

If the head-tilt/chin-lift method does not open the airway, or if a neck injury is suspected, use the **jaw-thrust method** (Fig. 5.5). This technique is very effective in opening the airway but is technically difficult and will slow the CPR process if only one rescuer is available. Place the ring and little fingers of each hand behind the angles of the patient's jawbone and thrust the jaw forward by lifting your hands while stabilizing the patient's head and neck with your thumbs and the index finger and adjacent middle finger of each hand. During this maneuver, rest your elbows on the surface on which the patient is lying.

5. **Determine breathlessness** (Fig. 5.6). Once the airway is open, determine whether the patient is breathing spontaneously by observing whether the chest rises and falls, listening for the escaping air (place your ear next to the patient's mouth and nose), and feeling for the flow of air. If the patient is breathing, continue to maintain an open airway. If the patient is not breathing, begin rescue breathing (step 6).

6. **Start rescue breathing** (Fig. 5.7). The mouth-to-mouth technique is used for rescue breathing because exhaled air retains sufficient oxygen to maintain life. Keep the patient's airway open and pinch the nostrils closed to prevent air from escaping through the nose. If the airway is maintained with the head-tilt/chin-lift method, use the thumb and index finger of the hand on the patient's forehead to pinch the nostrils closed. If the jaw-thrust method is used, you may have to press your cheek across the patient's nostrils to prevent air from escaping through the nose.

Take a deep breath, seal your lips around the patient's lips, and blow into the patient's mouth. Give two rescue breaths of one to one-and-a-half seconds each. Take a deep breath before each rescue breath. The patient's chest should rise and fall with each breath, and you should hear and feel air escaping during exhalation.

Fig. 5.5 *Opening the Airway with the Jaw-thrust Maneuver*

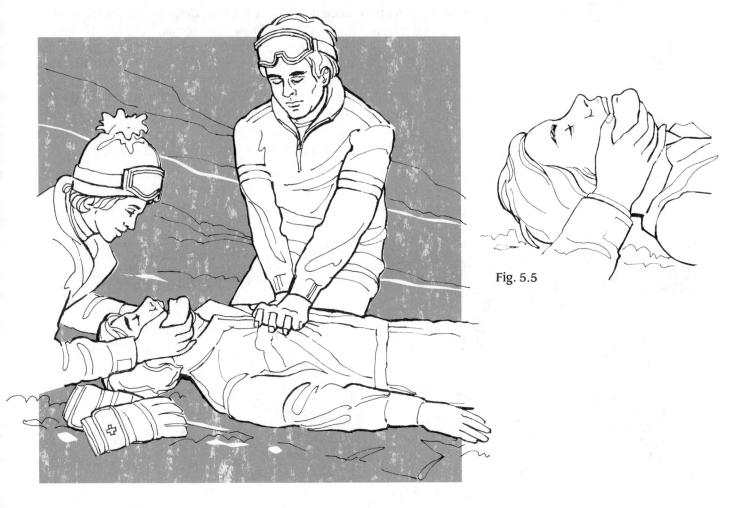

Fig. 5.5

Fig. 5.6 *Determine if the patient is breathing spontaneously.*

Fig. 5.7 *Rescue Breathing*

Fig. 5.8 *Locate the carotid artery lateral to the Adam's apple and check for a pulse.*

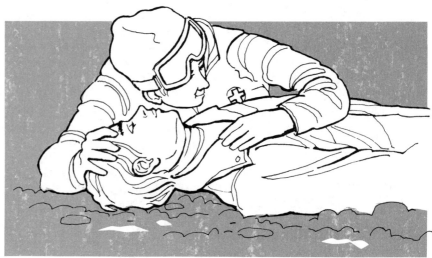

Fig. 5.6

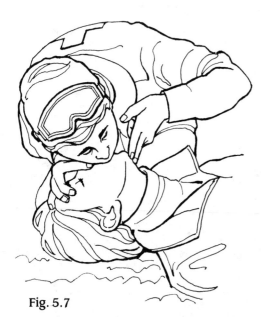

Fig. 5.7

If this is unsuccessful, the patient's airway probably is still not open. Reposition the patient's head and chin (or jaw) and repeat rescue breathing. If a second set of breaths is unsuccessful, a foreign body may be blocking the airway. The technique for relieving airway obstruction caused by a foreign body is described in the section on **Upper Airway Obstruction.**

After two successful rescue breaths, determine pulselessness by checking the carotid artery for five to 10 seconds (Fig. 5.8). This artery lies between the trachea and the sternomastoid muscle, just lateral to the Adam's apple. It is important that a weak or slow pulse is not missed because serious complications can be caused by performing external chest compressions on a patient with a pulse. If there is any question, continue checking for the pulse for several more seconds. Check for up to a minute in patients with hypothermia, because their pulses may be very slow and weak.

If the patient has a pulse but is not breathing spontaneously, continue rescue breathing at a rate of one breath every five seconds (12 breaths per minute).

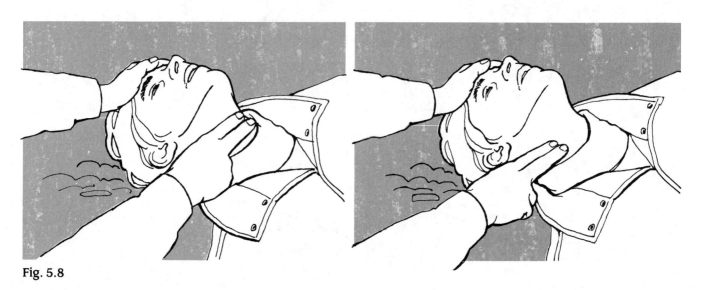

Fig. 5.8

The **mouth-to-nose technique** (Fig. 5.9) may be more effective than mouth-to-mouth in some patients, particularly in the case of facial injury, or when the rescuer cannot open the patient's mouth or achieve a tight seal around the mouth. Maintain an open airway using the head-tilt/chin-lift or jaw-thrust maneuver, except this time keep the patient's mouth tightly closed. Take a deep breath, seal your lips around the patient's nose, and blow into the nose. Excessive pressure on injured tissue should be avoided. Mouth-to-nose rescue breathing is given at the same rate as mouth-to-mouth.

The AIDS epidemic has caused concern about giving mouth-to-mouth breathing. Hepatitis and other contagious diseases also are possible dangers. Even though no case of AIDS or hepatitis is known to have been transmitted in this manner to date, the virus has been found in human saliva. It is considered prudent for rescuers to carry pocket masks to use when performing rescue breathing or CPR. These masks should be made of clear, soft plastic and have a one-way valve (Fig. 5.10). Their use is described in Chapter 6.

If there is no pulse, the patient is in cardiac arrest and external chest compressions should be started along with rescue breathing.

7. **Start external chest compressions**. Apply pressure over the lower half of the sternum in a regular, rhythmic manner. The cardiac output produced in this way, though only about 25 percent of normal, is enough to sustain life. Because blood flow to the brain is below normal, the patient's head should not be above the level of the chest. The patient should be lying supine on a firm, flat surface for chest compressions to be effective. If the patient is lying on a soft surface, such as a bed, place him or her on the floor.

The *proper hand position* (Fig. 5.11) is important. Continue to kneel facing the patient at shoulder level and, using the middle and index fingers of the hand nearer the patient's feet, locate the costal arch. Slide your fingers up the arch until your middle finger is in the notch between the two costal arches. Then place your index finger next to your middle finger on the lower end of the sternum. Place the heel of your other hand on the lower half of the sternum, next to your index finger. Place the first hand on top of and parallel to the hand on the sternum. Your fingers should be pointing across the sternum and should be kept off the patient's chest.

To achieve *proper compression*, straighten your arms, locking your elbows into an extended position. Keep your shoulders above your hands so that the thrust for each compression is directed straight down (Fig. 5.12). Depress the patient's sternum 1½ to 2 inches with each compression. Release pressure on the chest completely between compressions but do not lift your hands completely off the chest. Perform compressions at a rate of 80 to 100 per minute. To aid in timing, count "*one*-and-*two*-and-*three*-and," etc.

Fig. 5.9 *Mouth-to-nose Technique of Rescue Breathing*

Fig. 5.10 *SealEasy Pocket Mask*

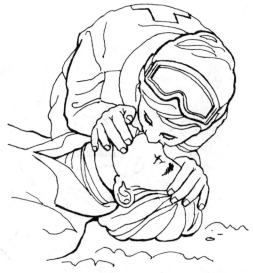

Fig. 5.9

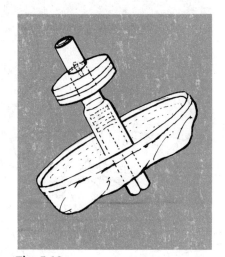

Fig. 5.10

Fig. 5.11 *Locating the Proper Hand Position for Chest Compressions*
 a. *Locate the costal arch.*
 b. *Place the middle finger in the notch with the index finger next to it.*
 c. *Put the heel of the other hand on the lower half of the sternum.*
 d. *Place the first hand on top of the second hand.*

One-rescuer Adult CPR

One-rescuer CPR (Fig. 5.13) maintains adequate circulation and ventilation but is more exhausting than two-rescuer CPR. When a second rescuer arrives, proceed with two-rescuer CPR (see page 110).

In one-rescuer CPR, maintain a ratio of 15 compressions to two breaths. After completing 15 chest compressions, move quickly to the patient's head, open the airway and deliver two rescue breaths of one to one-and-a-half seconds each. Move quickly to the patient's chest, locate the proper hand position, and give another set of 15 chest compressions. It is obvious that using a pocket mask or employing the jaw-thrust method of opening the

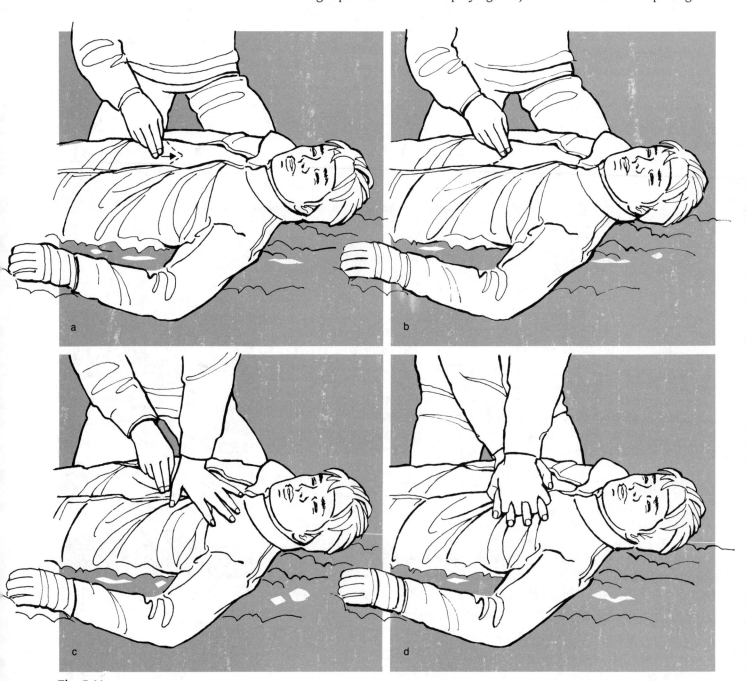

Fig. 5.11

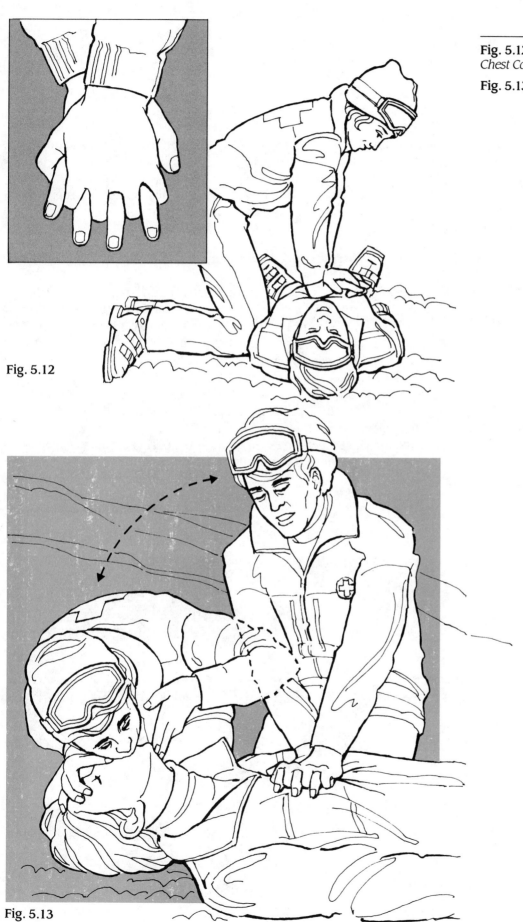

Fig. 5.12 *Proper Arm Position for Chest Compressions*

Fig. 5.13 *One-rescuer CPR*

Fig. 5.12

Fig. 5.13

Fig. 5.14 *Two-rescuer CPR*

airway would not allow the desired number of compressions and ventilations per minute. Give four complete cycles of 15 chest compressions interspersed with two rescue breaths, and then reevaluate the patient. Check the carotid pulse for five seconds and, if it is absent, resume CPR. If a pulse is present, check breathing for three to five seconds. If breathing is absent, continue rescue breathing at a rate of one breath every five seconds, and closely monitor the pulse. If breathing is present, stop CPR and monitor breathing and pulse. If CPR must be continued, check for the return of a spontaneous pulse and spontaneous breathing every few minutes. Do not interrupt CPR for more than seven seconds except in exceptional circumstances (see below).

Two-rescuer Adult CPR

One rescuer goes to the patient's head and determines responsiveness. If the second rescuer needs to notify the EMS system, the first rescuer initiates one-rescuer CPR. Otherwise, the first rescuer positions the patient, opens the airway, and checks for breathing. If breathing is absent, the first rescuer says "no breathing" and gives two ventilations; the first rescuer then checks the pulse and, if it is absent, says "no pulse." Simultaneously, the second rescuer, kneeling at the patient's other side, has been locating the proper hand position so that external chest compressions can be started when the first rescuer says "no pulse."

Two-rescuer CPR continues with the rescuer positioned at the patient's side performing external chest compressions and the rescuer on the opposite side at the patient's head maintaining an open airway, monitoring the carotid pulse for adequacy of chest compressions, and providing rescue breathing (Fig. 5.14). The ratio of compressions to ventilations is 5:1 rather

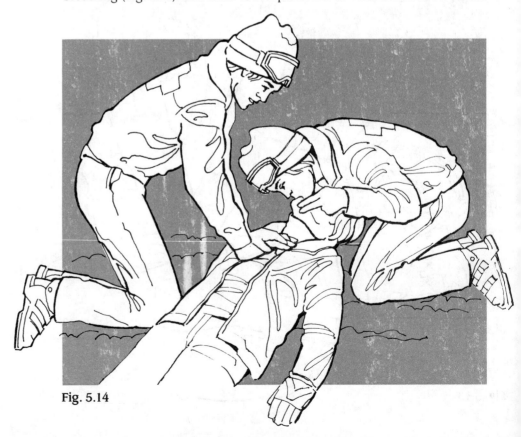

Fig. 5.14

than 15:2, with a pause of one to one-and-a-half seconds between each set of five compressions to allow for ventilation.

If the rescuer responsible for compressions becomes fatigued, the two should switch positions. The best time to switch from one-rescuer CPR to two-rescuer CPR is just after a cycle of 15 compressions and two breaths; the best time to switch positions in two-rescuer CPR is just after a cycle of five compressions and one breath.

Check the pulse during compressions to evaluate their effectiveness. Stop chest compressions for five seconds after one minute and every few minutes thereafter to see if the pulse and breathing have returned.

UPPER-AIRWAY OBSTRUCTION

The causes of upper-airway obstruction were discussed in Chapter 1. By the time the rescuer arrives, an unconscious patient may have developed an upper-airway obstruction caused by the tongue, relaxed soft throat tissues, or vomitus. Conversely, unconsciousness may be caused by lack of oxygen following upper-airway obstruction. For example, the airway can be blocked by injured tissue or blood clots in the case of a facial or head injury or by snow in the case of avalanche burial. Other types of foreign matter, such as food particles, can cause acute airway obstruction, which can mimic cardiac arrest. Because CPR is ineffective if the airway is obstructed, techniques to relieve airway obstruction are important in basic life support and, if needed, should be performed before beginning external chest compressions.

In adults, foreign-body obstruction of the airway most commonly occurs during eating – meat is a frequent culprit. Important associated factors are drinking alcohol, wearing dentures, and failing to chew food properly. In children, obstruction is most commonly caused by the accidental aspiration of peas, nuts, popcorn, beads, or other small objects.

The following precautions will decrease the incidence of foreign-body obstruction in adults and children: cut food into small pieces and chew each bite slowly and thoroughly (especially important for those who wear dentures), avoid laughing or talking while chewing and swallowing, avoid excessive alcohol intake around mealtime, prevent children from running or playing with food in their mouths or placing foreign objects in their mouths, and keep small, hard objects such as peanuts, beads, and marbles away from small children.

Recognition of Foreign-body Airway Obstruction

Foreign-body obstruction of the upper airway can cause death quickly yet is treatable if recognized early. Therefore, prompt recognition of foreign-body obstruction is the cornerstone of successful emergency care. More than 3,000 deaths occur annually from foreign-body obstruction of the airway. Obstruction of the airway must be distinguished from simple fainting, stroke, heart attack, convulsive seizure, drug overdose, and other conditions that have similar signs and symptoms but are managed differently.

Airway obstruction may be either complete or partial. With partial obstruction, the patient is still able to inhale some air into the lungs. If air exchange is good, and the patient can still cough forcefully (although there

Fig. 5.15 *Universal Distress Signal for Choking*

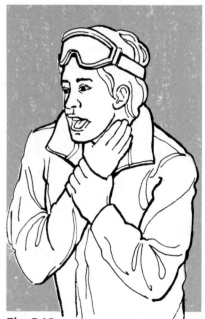

Fig. 5.15

Fig. 5.16 *Proper Way to Position the Hands for the Heimlich Maneuver*

Fig. 5.17 *Performing the Heimlich Maneuver on a Standing Patient*

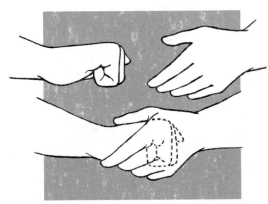

Fig. 5.16

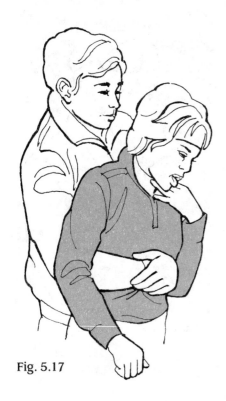

Fig. 5.17

may be some wheezing between coughs), encourage the patient to cough and attempt to expel the foreign body while being monitored by the rescuer. Either the patient will expel the foreign body, the obstruction will persist unchanged, or the condition will progress to poor air exchange or complete obstruction. If the patient does not expel the foreign body rapidly, notify the EMS system. Poor air exchange is indicated by a weak, ineffective cough and increased respiratory distress. Cyanosis may develop.

A patient with complete airway obstruction is unable to speak, breathe, or cough, and will frequently clutch the neck (Fig. 5.15). This universal distress signal to indicate choking should be taught to the public and to rescuers. Ask, "Are you choking?" If unable to reply, the patient will usually nod his or her head.

The Heimlich Maneuver

The Heimlich maneuver is recommended for relieving partial upper-airway obstruction with poor air exchange and complete upper-airway obstruction in adults and children (but not in infants). It uses the residual air in the lungs to expel a foreign object blocking the upper airway. The rescuer, or the patient, administers a sudden abdominal thrust, which increases intra-abdominal pressure, driving the diaphragm upward and expelling the residual air from the lungs. The force of the expelled air frequently is sufficient to expel the obstructing material out of the airway like a bullet fired from a gun. The maneuver may have to be repeated six to 10 times to clear the airway. The hands must be properly positioned (Fig. 5.16) to obtain maximum effectiveness and to avoid injury to the abdominal or thoracic organs. Despite the best technique, the maneuver occasionally causes organ damage or regurgitation of material from the stomach.

Patient Standing

If the patient is standing (Fig. 5.17), stand behind the patient, wrapping your arms around the patient's waist. When the patient is conscious and standing, the proper hand position (see Fig. 5.16) is to place the thumb side of one fist against the midline of the patient's abdominal wall midway between the navel and the xiphoid process (the lowermost part of the sternum). With your other hand, grasp the fist and press it into the patient's abdomen with a quick, upward thrust. Relieve the abdominal pressure completely between thrusts.

Patient Lying Down

If the patient is lying, turn the patient to the supine position (see Fig. 5.2 for technique) and kneel astride the patient's thighs, facing the patient's head. Place the heel of one hand on the patient's abdomen midway between the xiphoid process and the navel, with the second hand on top of the first. Press into the abdomen with a quick, upward thrust (Fig. 5.18).

Use the finger sweep (see Fig. 5.4) only on an unconscious adult or older child. Open the patient's mouth by grasping both the tongue and the lower jaw between your thumb and fingers and lifting the mandible. This draws the tongue forward. Insert the index finger of your other hand along the side of the cheek and deeply into the throat at the base of the tongue. Use a hooking motion to bring the foreign body up into the mouth where it can be removed. Be careful not to force the material deeper.

Fig. 5.18 *Performing the Heimlich Maneuver on a Supine Patient*

Fig. 5.19 *Self-administered Heimlich Maneuver*

Fig. 5.20 *Chest Thrusts on an Obese Patient*

Self-administered Heimlich Maneuver

The self-administered Heimlich maneuver (Fig. 5.19) allows you to dislodge a foreign body from your own throat. Position your hands as described in Figure 5.16. If you are unsuccessful after several thrusts, press the upper abdomen quickly against any firm surface, such as the back of a chair, side of a table, or porch railing.

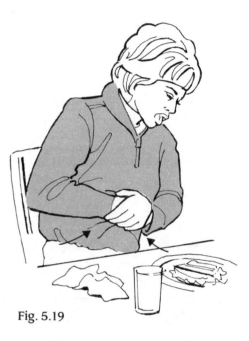

Fig. 5.19

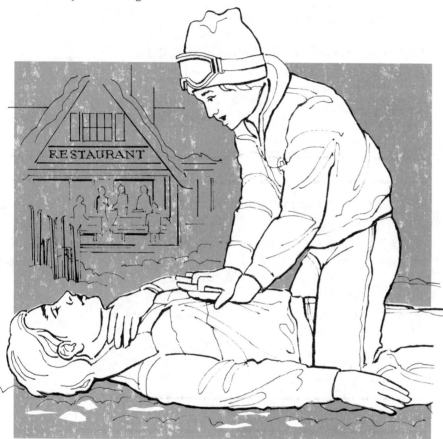

Fig. 5.18

Chest Thrust on Pregnant or Obese Patients

To perform chest thrusts on pregnant or obese patients (Fig. 5.20), stand behind the patient and wrap your arms around the patient's chest under the armpits. Place the thumb side of your fist over the *middle of the sternum*, avoiding the ribs and the xiphoid process. Grasp your fist with the other hand and press backward with quick thrusts, relieving pressure completely between thrusts as described above.

The same hand position is used for the pregnant or obese patient who is lying down. Turn the patient to the supine position and kneel astride the patient's thighs facing the patient's head.

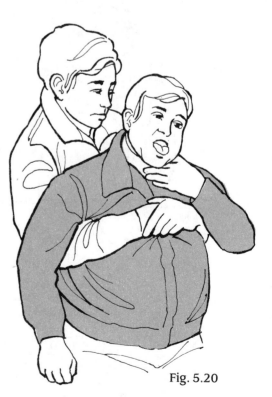

Fig. 5.20

Table 5.2

SEQUENCE FOR CONSCIOUS ADULT WITH OBSTRUCTED AIRWAY

1. When airway obstruction is suspected, ask "Are you choking?" Have someone notify the EMS system.
2. Repeat the Heimlich maneuver until the foreign body is expelled or the patient loses consciousness.
3. If the patient loses consciousness, open the patient's mouth and perform the finger sweep.
4. Open the airway and attempt rescue breathing.
5. If ventilation fails, perform additional (six to 10) subdiaphragmatic abdominal thrusts.
6. Open the mouth and repeat the finger sweep.
7. Repeat attempts to perform rescue breathing.
8. If unsuccessful, repeat the Heimlich maneuver, finger sweep, and attempts at rescue breathing.
9. Continue with these sequences until the airway is clear, or you are relieved by another responsible person, are exhausted, or the patient is pronounced dead.

Table 5.3

SEQUENCE FOR UNCONSCIOUS ADULT WITH OBSTRUCTED AIRWAY

1. If rescue breathing cannot be performed although the airway has been opened with the head-tilt/chin-lift or jaw-thrust methods, reposition the head and chin, or jaw, and repeat one attempt at rescue breathing.
2. If unsuccessful, perform subdiaphragmatic thrusts.
3. Perform the finger sweep.
4. If unsuccessful, continue to repeat 1, 2, and 3 until the airway is clear, or you are relieved by another responsible person, are exhausted, or the patient is pronounced dead.

Fig. 5.21 *Keep small objects away from small children.*

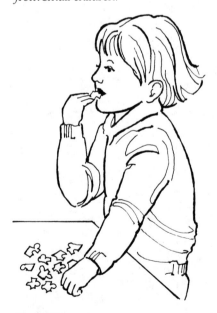

Fig. 5.21

PEDIATRIC BASIC LIFE SUPPORT

Cardiac arrest in infants and children is more commonly caused by shock or abnormal function of the respiratory system than by primary heart disease. Both shock and respiratory system abnormalities affect the heart by reducing blood oxygen levels. The long period of hypoxia that usually precedes cardiac arrest in infants and children is one reason for their low survival rate following CPR. Conversely, survival following rescue breathing for respiratory arrest alone is much higher in children than in adults.

Common causes of respiratory and cardiac arrest include injuries with shock, suffocation (as from crawling into a plastic bag), aspiration of small objects such as beads or peanuts, smoke inhalation during fires, injuries to the face or neck, respiratory infections, drowning, poisoning, and sudden infant death syndrome (SIDS).

Many of these childhood emergencies are preventable. Do not allow infants and children to play with matches, cigarette lighters, sharp objects, small objects such as beads and marbles, or toys with small, removable parts

(Fig. 5.21). Use car seats and seat belts in moving vehicles. Teach children water safety at an early age.

The sequence of CPR for infants and children is the same as for adults but the techniques for infants and small children are somewhat modified because of the smaller size of the pediatric patient. For these purposes, an infant is defined as a young child who has not yet begun to walk well, i.e., under 12 to 15 months old.

Basic life support always is given with the patient in the supine position. If the child is found prone, turn the child's body as a unit, firmly supporting the head so the neck is not bent or twisted. The child's air passages are smaller and more easily obstructed by mucus, blood, or vomitus. The head-tilt/chin-lift technique is the preferred method for opening the airway. The jaw-thrust technique is used only if the head-tilt/chin-lift technique fails or if a neck injury is likely. Avoid overextension of the neck, which may cause or aggravate airway obstruction.

In smaller children and infants, perform rescue breathing with the rescuer's mouth over *both* the mouth and nose of the child (Fig. 5.22). Rescue breaths should make the patient's chest rise and fall. The volume of air needed is less than for an adult. The rescue breathing rate is *20* times per minute for infants and young children and *15* times per minute for older children.

In infants under one year old, the brachial artery pulse usually is easier to feel than the carotid pulse, which is used in older infants and children. Give external chest compressions, if needed, as described for adults but with certain modifications:

For a child under age eight, compress the chest to a depth of 1 to 1½ inches, using *one* hand rather than two (Fig. 5.23a). The hand position is the same as for adults. Chest compressions for infants are performed with only two or three fingers rather than the entire hand (Fig. 5.23b). The finger position for chest compressions is as follows: draw an imaginary line between the infant's two nipples, and place the index finger of the hand closest to the infant's feet just under this line where it crosses the sternum. The area of compression lies under the middle and ring fingers.

Using two or three fingers, compress the breastbone to a depth of ½ to 1 inch. For infants and children, maintain a 5:1 ratio of compressions to ventilations during *either one- or two-rescuer* CPR. The compression rate is 80 to 100 per minute for children and 100 per minute or more for infants.

Fig. 5.22 *Cover both the child's mouth and nose during rescue breathing.*

Fig. 5.23 *Use the heel of one hand for chest compressions on a child and use two fingers for chest compressions on an infant.*

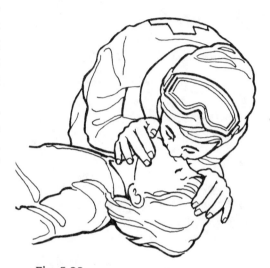

Fig. 5.22

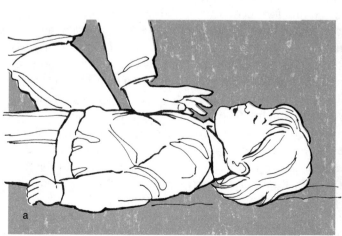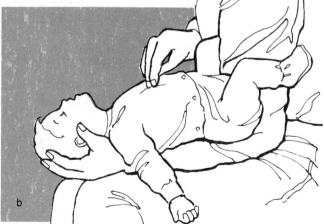

Fig. 5.23

For infants, first open the airway with the head-tilt/chin-lift. If only res-cue breathing is required, maintain the airway with this technique as well.

During one-rescuer CPR on infants, relocating the finger position for chest compression takes so long that the necessary compression rate of 100 or more per minute cannot be maintained. To achieve adequate chest com-pressions, attempt to maintain an open airway *with the head-tilt only*, without losing the finger position on the infant's chest. Watch the infant's chest to make sure it rises and falls with each rescue breath. If the head-tilt alone cannot keep the airway open, the chin-lift will also have to be performed before each rescue breath. In this case, it may be possible to administer ade-quate chest compressions by relocating the hand position *visually* rather than manually.

In children, *both the head-tilt and chin-lift* usually are needed to maintain an open airway. During chest compressions with one-rescuer CPR, maintain the head-tilt with the hand closest to the patient's head. After every fifth com-pression, use the hand doing the compressions for the chin-lift and give a rescue breath. Relocate the finger position for chest compressions visually, since finding the landmarks manually requires using both hands and takes so much time that too few chest compressions and rescue breaths can be administered.

Airway Obstruction in Infants and Children

Foreign-body airway obstruction in children can be relieved by the Heimlich maneuver; for infants, chest thrusts are used instead because abdominal thrusts are likely to cause organ damage. Foreign-body obstruction must be carefully distinguished from infections such as croup that cause airway swelling sufficient to obstruct the airway. A foreign body always should be suspected when there are *sudden* signs or symptoms of obstruction in a pre-viously well child.

Airway obstruction caused by croup usually develops slowly and is pre-ceded by a period of hoarseness and signs and symptoms of upper respira-tory infection such as runny nose, sore throat, fever, sneezing, and cough. When a child suffers from airway obstruction caused by *infection*, attempts to relieve the obstruction with rescue techniques will be futile. Take the patient to a hospital without delay.

Use the Heimlich maneuver for children in whom aspiration is witnessed or strongly suspected and for unconscious, non-breathing children whose airways remain obstructed after the usual maneuvers for opening airways have been attempted. If aspiration has been witnessed or is strongly sus-pected, encourage the child to breathe and cough spontaneously as long as the cough is forceful. Attempt to relieve the obstruction *only* after the cough becomes ineffective or if the child develops increased difficulty in breathing accompanied by stridor (a high-pitched, crowing noise on inhalation).

Perform the Heimlich maneuver on children exactly as described above for adults. In infants under one year of age, a modified technique is used to avoid injuring the liver. Lay the infant prone over your forearm so the head is lower than the body. Sit with your forearm resting on your thigh. Support the infant's head by grasping the jaw firmly with your fingers. Then, using the heel of your other hand, deliver four forceful blows to the infant's back between the shoulder blades (Fig. 5.24).

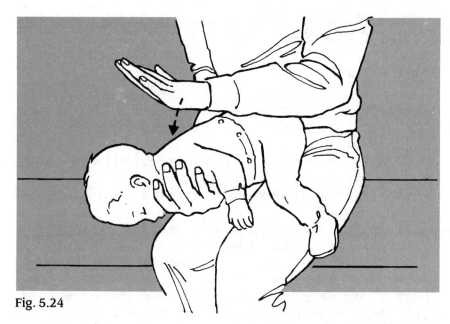

Fig. 5.24

Fig. 5.24 *Four back blows are part of the Heimlich maneuver when the patient is an infant under one year old.*

Next, place one hand on the infant's back and turn the infant's body as a unit to the supine position. Place the infant on your thigh with the head lower than the body. Deliver four chest thrusts with your fingers at the same location as for external chest compressions but at a slower rate. An alternate method is to lay the infant prone on your lap, with the head firmly supported and lower than the trunk. Give four back blows, then turn the infant over as a unit and deliver four chest thrusts (Fig. 5.23b).

Blind finger sweeps are *not* performed on infants and young children because the danger of pushing the foreign body further down into the airway is greater than for adults.

WHEN TO WITHHOLD OR DISCONTINUE CPR

Few authorities would insist that CPR be started on a person who is obviously dead or who has sustained a lethal injury. Lethal injuries include decapitation, massive evisceration, a severed trunk, or massive injuries of the head and chest. CPR should also be withheld when performing it would seriously endanger the rescuer(s), e.g., one-rescuer CPR with no shelter in very cold, windy weather.

Once started, CPR should not be discontinued except in these situations:
1. Effective spontaneous breathing and circulation are restored.
2. The patient's care is transferred to another responsible person who continues basic life support.
3. The patient's care is transferred to a physician or advanced life support team.
4. The rescuer is unable to continue because of exhaustion.
5. An authorized person certifies death. (In most states, only physicians are legally authorized to pronounce a person dead.)

These rules, while reasonable and proper in an *urban* environment, may be less applicable in a *wilderness* environment. This aspect of CPR is discussed in Appendix B.

Fig. 5.25 *Relieve gastric distention by turning the patient onto one side and pressing on the epigastric area.*

COMPLICATIONS OF CPR

Gastric Distention

During rescue breathing, air can enter the stomach instead of the lungs, causing the stomach to swell (**gastric distention**). If this swelling is severe, it may interfere with lung expansion by preventing downward motion of the diaphragm. Gastric distention frequently is associated with regurgitation of gastric contents, which may be aspirated, blocking the airway. Although some degree of gastric distention probably occurs in even the most skillfully performed CPR, it can be minimized by proper airway positioning and by limiting the amount of air blown into the patient's mouth to just enough to make the chest rise. The new method of CPR replaces several rapid breaths with two slower breaths and is less likely to force air into the stomach.

Massive gastric distention often can be relieved by turning the patient onto one side and pressing on the epigastric area with the hand (Fig. 5.25). When this is done, equipment should be available to suction the airway because the patient may regurgitate gastric contents as well as air.

Organ Damage

Rib fractures commonly occur during CPR, especially in older people whose bones are more brittle. While these fractures cannot always be avoided, their frequency can be reduced by making certain that the compressions are delivered to the center rather than the side of the sternum and that compression pressure is not excessive. Rib fractures usually heal without complications. Damage to the heart, lungs, stomach, and liver should be rare in properly performed CPR.

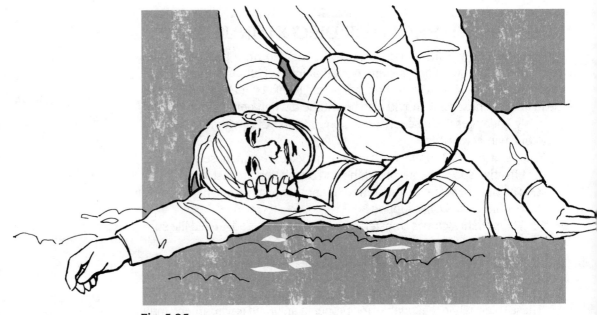

Fig. 5.25

6

Oxygen and Other Types of Respiratory System Support

I would rather dwell in the dim fog of superstition
than in the air rarefied to nothing by the air pump of unbelief;
in which the panting breast expires,
vainly and convulsively gasping for breath.

—Jean-Paul Friedrich Richter

Earlier chapters of this textbook stress that oxygen is needed for living cells to function properly. Some organs, such as the brain and heart, are so sensitive that they are irreversibly damaged if deprived of oxygen for more than a few minutes.

Delivery of oxygen to the tissues requires open respiratory passages, so air can reach the gas-exchange surfaces of the alveoli; normal alveoli, so oxygen can move from the alveolar air into the bloodstream; a normal heart and circulatory system, to transport oxygen from the lungs to the tissues; and normal ability of the tissues to absorb oxygen from the blood. The various ways in which this progression can be disrupted are listed in Chapter 1.

Aside from standard emergency care techniques such as opening the airway, closing a sucking chest wound, stabilizing a flail chest, and CPR, tissue oxygenation can be improved by adding oxygen to the inhaled air. Giving supplemental oxygen ensures that the blood carries the greatest possible amount of oxygen to the tissues; however, giving oxygen is *not* so urgent a need that it should take precedence over *standard measures* of emergency care. If the oxygen in ordinary air cannot get to the tissues, neither will added oxygen.

Inhaled air contains 21 percent oxygen, which is more than enough for normal body function. The body extracts about 25 percent of the oxygen from inhaled air, so that exhaled air contains 16 percent oxygen. Rescue breathing and CPR can be effective because, at altitudes below 9,000 to 10,000 feet (2,743 to 3,048 meters) even this amount of oxygen is enough to sustain life. However, patients who are ill or injured have increased oxygen requirements, yet their respiratory and circulatory systems may be unable to take up and transport oxygen at a normal rate. Adding oxygen to the inhaled air increases the amount of oxygen that can be taken up by the blood and transported to the cells, thereby improving chances of survival and recovery of normal function.

The ability to use supplementary oxygen and mechanical respiratory support devices is an essential component of modern emergency care. Illnesses and injuries that interfere with tissue oxygenation are not rare in the outdoors. Although supplemental oxygen is not available to the casual outdoor traveler, it is found in most ski patrol first aid rooms, wilderness search and rescue caches, and Forest Service and National Park Service emergency vehicles.

OXYGEN EQUIPMENT

Basic oxygen equipment (Fig. 6.1) includes oxygen cylinders, pressure reducing valves, pressure gauges, flowmeters, tubing, masks, nasal cannulas, oral airways, bag-mask devices, and suction equipment. In addition, ambulances, helicopters, and hospital emergency departments usually are equipped with automatic ventilators and other complicated oxygen delivery equipment.

The following are general guidelines to familiarize the student with the principles of assembling and operating basic oxygen equipment. No attempt has been made to list all available options, as these vary widely across the country. The equipment chosen should be compatible with the protocols of

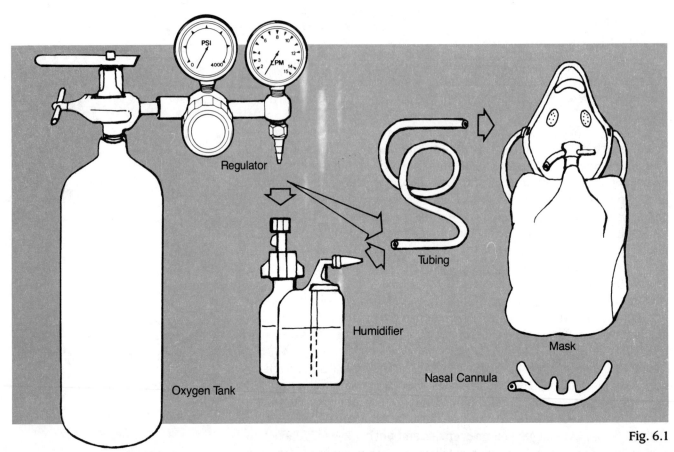

Regulator

Tubing

Humidifier

Mask

Nasal Cannula

Oxygen Tank

Fig. 6.1

Fig. 6.1 *Basic Oxygen Equipment*

Fig. 6.2 *Three sizes of Oxygen Cylinders*

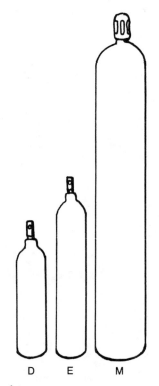

D   E   M

Fig. 6.2

local EMS units. The value of choosing equipment carefully and becoming thoroughly familiar with its use cannot be overemphasized.

Figure 6.2 illustrates three different sizes of oxygen cylinders. The most practical oxygen cylinders for field use are D cylinders (approximately 20 inches high, weighing 10¼ pounds empty, and containing 360 liters of oxygen) and E cylinders (approximately 30 inches high, weighing 15 pounds empty and containing 625 liters of oxygen). At a flow rate of 6 liters per minute, a full D cylinder will last 60 minutes and a full E cylinder will last 104 minutes. (This is calculated by dividing the tank capacity in liters by the flow rate.) The large M cylinders, which contain 3,000 liters of oxygen, are useful as stationary units in first aid facilities.

In the United States, federal regulations require that cylinders containing oxygen be painted green or have green markings to distinguish them from cylinders containing other gases. Cylinders can be purchased or rented from hospital supply companies. The pressure gauge reading provides an estimate of the oxygen remaining within a cylinder. When fully loaded, the pressure within a cylinder is 2,000 pounds per square inch (psi); if the gauge shows 1,000 psi, the cylinder is half full. When the gauge reads less than 200 psi, the cylinder should not be used since, for all practical purposes, it is empty.

Cylinders smaller than size D are impractical when patient transport times are long. Two D cylinders with their accompanying attachments can be easily mounted on a pack frame and carried to the site of an emergency (Fig. 6.3). Larger cylinders are more suitable for stationary use. Aluminum cylinders, which weigh considerably less than steel cylinders, also are available.

Each cylinder must have a pressure-reducing valve, a pressure gauge and a flowmeter, which together are commonly called a **regulator**. The regulator reduces the pressure of the oxygen from the high level within the cylinder to about 50 psi as it reaches the patient and allows the flow rate to be regulated between 1 and 15 liters per minute. Regulator systems are designed so they cannot be attached to the wrong size or type of tank by mistake. This is to prevent patients from accidentally receiving nitrous oxide, acetylene, or some other gas instead of oxygen. D and E cylinders both accept a yoke-style regulator (Fig. 6.4a) that uses a keyed pin system to ensure that the yoke will fit only the cylinder for which it is designed. The larger M, H, and K cylinders usually are equipped with DISS threaded outlet valves, which accept screw-on regulators (Fig. 6.4b).

The most practical regulator for field use is one that contains a Bourdon gauge flowmeter (Fig. 6.5a), which is unaffected by position, altitude or gravity. However, because it measures pressure rather than flow, the reading will be affected if the tubing has a kink or is obstructed. Flowmeters that use a graduated glass tube containing a steel ball (Fig. 6.5b) are more accurate, but depend on gravity to register flow rate and work correctly *only in the upright position*.

Patients who require oxygen can be divided into two general categories: those who are breathing spontaneously and those who are being resuscitated by rescue breathing or CPR. Patients breathing spontaneously are given supplemental oxygen with disposable, transparent delivery devices such as a non-rebreather mask or a nasal cannula. Patients who are being resuscitated are given oxygen by attaching the oxygen tubing to the oxygen input nipple of a pocket mask or bag-mask. In emergency care, oxygen should always be given in high concentration and at high flow rate, except to patients with chronic obstructive pulmonary disease (emphysema).

The best apparatus for delivering a high concentration of oxygen is a non-rebreather mask (Fig. 6.6a). This is a transparent mask fitted with a plastic reservoir bag and a one-way valve so that the patient can inhale oxygen from the bag but cannot exhale into the bag. A non-rebreather mask can provide 80 to 90 percent oxygen at flow rates of 10 to 15 liters per minute. The reservoir bag should be kept one-third to one-half full of oxygen so that it will not collapse completely when the patient inhales.

A nasal cannula (Fig. 6.6b) delivers lower concentrations of oxygen; it can provide 25 to 50 percent oxygen at flow rates of 2 to 6 liters per minute. A cannula may be preferred for field use because it allows the patient to talk, drink and eat, making it more acceptable to the patient. A cannula also is preferred for delivering oxygen to patients with emphysema and for patients in whom vomiting is likely.

The nasal cannula and non-rebreather mask will be sufficient for the vast majority of situations when supplemental oxygen must be administered at alpine ski areas or in the outdoors in general. Other types of masks, such as positive pressure and Venturi masks, are necessary only in special situations; their use usually is confined to ambulances, helicopters, and hospitals.

Oxygen from a tank is very dry and has an undesirable drying effect on the tissues of the respiratory tract. A humidifying device should be used during prolonged administration of supplementary oxygen. Usually, a small jar

Fig. 6.3 *Example of an Oxygen Backpack*

Fig. 6.4 *Yoke-style Regulator and DISS Threaded Outlet Valve*

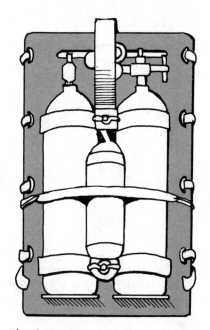

Fig. 6.3

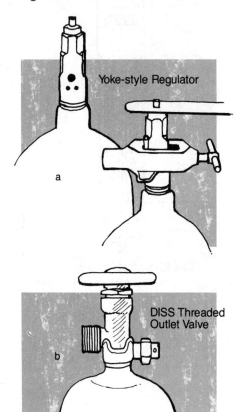

Yoke-style Regulator

DISS Threaded Outlet Valve

Fig. 6.4

Fig. 6.5 *Bourdon Gauge Flowmeter and Gravity-dependent Flowmeter*

Fig. 6.6 *Non-rebreather Mask and Nasal Cannula*

of water is attached to the tank so that the oxygen bubbles through the water before reaching the patient (Fig. 6.7). This system is difficult to use outdoors, particularly at subfreezing temperatures, and probably is unnecessary if the patient can be transferred to an ambulance or hospital within 30 minutes or so. Stationary oxygen units in first aid facilities should be equipped with humidifying devices.

Procedure For Giving Oxygen (Fig. 6.8)

1. Place the cylinder upright and position yourself to the side. Open and close the tank valve slowly with a wrench to clean debris from the outlet. This process is called "cracking" the tank.
2. Close the regulator flow valve and attach the regulator to the tank, tightening it securely in place. Don't lose the O-ring.
3. Open the tank valve slowly to one-half turn beyond the point where the regulator becomes pressurized. Note the tank pressure registered on the pressure gauge of the regulator in pounds per square inch (psi).
4. Attach the plastic delivery tubing to the regulator output nipple, and attach the mask or cannula to the other end of the tubing.
5. Open the regulator flow valve until the desired flow rate registers on the flow gauge in liters per minute.
6. Explain to the patient why oxygen is needed and what you are going to do. Test the mask or cannula on yourself to make sure the oxygen is flowing, then position it on the patient's face.
7. When you are finished administering oxygen, remove the mask or cannula from the patient. Turn the regulator flow valve until the rate on the flow gauge registers zero.
8. Shut off the main tank valve and remove the delivery tubing from the regulator output nipple.
9. Bleed the valves by opening the regulator flow valve again until the flow rate stays at zero.
10. Close the regulator flow valve.

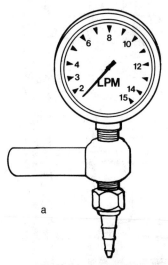

a

Bourdon Gauge Flowmeter

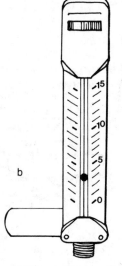

b

Gravity-dependent Flowmeter

Fig. 6.5

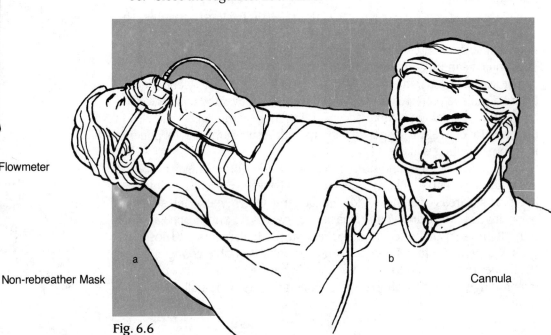

Non-rebreather Mask

a

b

Cannula

Fig. 6.6

Precautions

1. Remember that oxygen tanks contain oxygen under very high pressure and can be as lethal as bombs if mistreated. Do not position any part of a rescuer's or patient's body directly in line with the tank valve, because a loose-fitting regulator can be blown off the top of the cylinder with enough force to amputate or kill. Do not expose oxygen tanks to excessive heat, and always secure them so there is no danger that a tank can topple over and knock off the valve. *Never* drop a tank.
2. *Never* use an oxygen tank without a proper fitting regulator. *Never* use tape and other "foreign" material on oxygen equipment.
3. Close all valves when a tank is not in use, even if it is empty.
4. Oxygen will not explode when exposed to fire but *will* cause a burning object to flare up, with the danger of setting other combustibles on fire. Smoking and other sources of open flame are prohibited where oxygen is being used; combustible materials such as oil or grease should not come in contact with oxygen equipment.
5. *Never* move an oxygen cylinder by rolling it on its side or its bottom.
6. Inspect valve seat inserts and gaskets regularly.
7. Store oxygen cylinders in cool, ventilated areas. Avoid exposing cylinders to temperatures below freezing and above 125°F (52°C).
8. Have oxygen cylinders hydrostatically tested at regular intervals. The dates of previous tests are stamped on the cylinder.

Other Equipment for Oxygen Administration

A **pocket mask with oxygen inlet** (Fig. 6.9) should be made of a transparent plastic that does not become brittle or rigid in the cold. The mask must be soft enough that a good seal can be maintained and should have a one-way valve to protect the rescuer from the patient's saliva or vomitus. An oxygen inlet nipple on the mask allows the patient to be ventilated with air from the res-

Fig. 6.7 *Humidifying Device–Figure 6.1 shows how to hook up the device in the proper sequence with the rest of the oxygen apparatus.*

Fig. 6.8 *Sequence of Administering Oxygen*

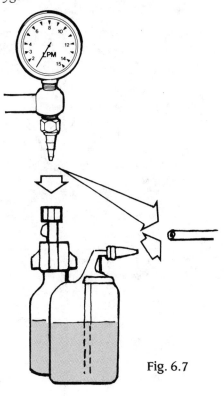

Fig. 6.7

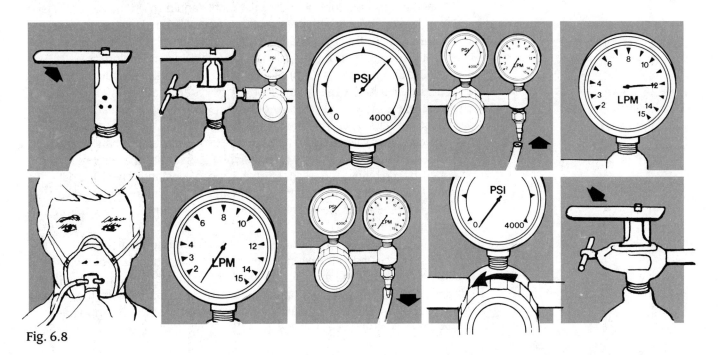

Fig. 6.8

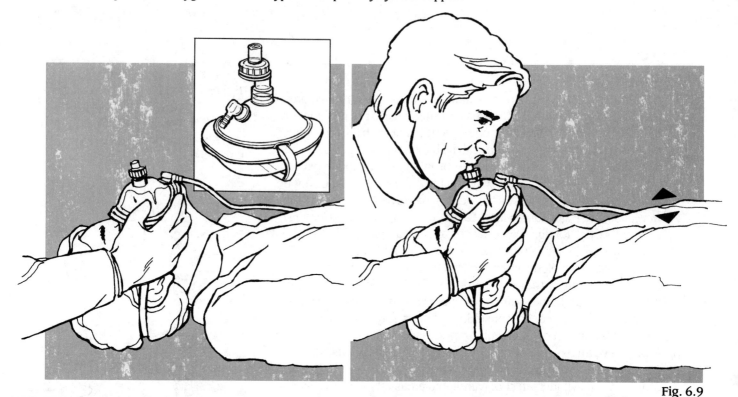

Fig. 6.9

Fig. 6.9 *Pocket Mask with Oxygen Inlet Nipple and One-way Valve*

cuer's lungs enriched by oxygen added from a tank. The mask should have an elastic cord to slip over the patient's head and hold the mask in place.

It is cumbersome to perform one-rescuer CPR with a pocket mask, but rescue breathing alone or two-rescuer CPR can be done as easily with a mask as without one. To use a mask, kneel at the patient's head and open the airway with the jaw-thrust maneuver. Place the mask over the patient's nose and mouth, with the apex over the bridge of the nose and the base in the groove between the lower lip and chin. Place your hands at the sides of the patient's head, with thumbs and index fingers pressing on the sides of the mask to maintain an airtight seal. Place the remaining fingers along the lower edge of the jaw and behind its angle to maintain the forward jaw thrust. Attach the oxygen tubing to the inlet nipple and turn on the oxygen. Place your lips on the intake valve of the mask. Perform rescue breathing at the same rate as with the standard mouth-to-mouth technique; watch between breaths to make certain the patient's chest is rising and falling.

Oral airways (Fig. 6.10) are designed to keep the tongue from falling back and occluding the upper airway. Airways are made in infant, child, and adult sizes. They are used *only* on *unconscious* patients because they will cause conscious or semiconscious patients to vomit. Oral airways should be carried in every first aid kit and used on every unconscious patient. They do not eliminate the rescuer's responsibility to see that the airway remains open, but do relieve the rescuer from having to constantly check the patient's airway, a benefit when manpower is limited. If a patient who is regaining consciousness retches, remove the oral airway immediately before the patient vomits.

To choose the proper size, hold the airway against the side of the patient's face. It should extend from the corner of the mouth to the angle of the jaw. Moisten the airway with water, open the patient's mouth with the crossed-finger technique (Chapter 5), and insert the airway with the tip *up* to avoid pushing the tongue backwards. When the airway is inserted halfway, rotate it 180 degrees so that, when fully inserted, its curve will lie along the curve of the tongue, holding the tongue forward. The flange of the airway will rest against the patient's lips or teeth. To remove the airway, simply pull it out gently.

Fig. 6.10 *Technique of Inserting an Oral Airway*

Fig. 6.11 *Mechanical Suction Devices*

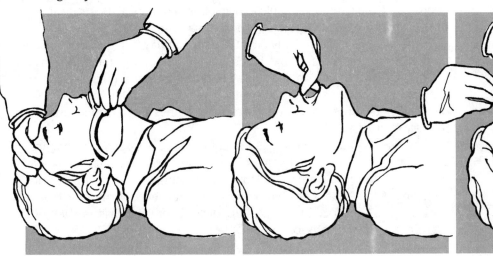

Fig. 6.10

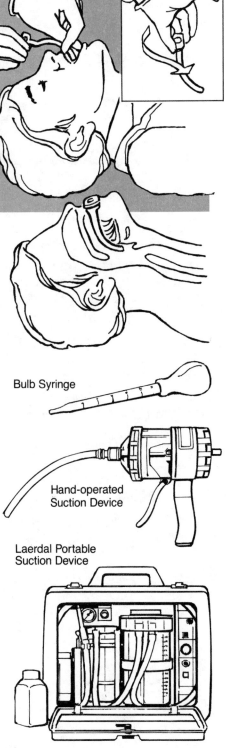

Bulb Syringe

Hand-operated Suction Device

Laerdal Portable Suction Device

Fig. 6.11

Suction apparatus include mechanical suction devices (Fig. 6.11) that can be either fixed or portable. For outdoor emergency care, a high-quality, battery-operated, rechargeable, portable device such as the Laerdal or Ohmeda is ideal. A portable suction unit can be kept on the recharge setting in a first aid room or rescue cache and used on-site or transported on a moment's notice to the site of an emergency. The unit should have a wide-bore, non-kinking rubber tube and a rigid, plastic pharyngeal suction tip called a "tonsil" or Yankauer tip. A supply of water will be needed to rinse the suction tip and tubing.

In the cold, suction tubing should be insulated during use. Do not use small-bore tubing because it freezes too easily. The active battery life of battery-operated units is reduced when they are used in the cold, so they should be insulated during transport to the accident site.

Plastic pharyngeal tips are best for suctioning both the mouth and the pharynx because their rigidity permits them to be easily inserted and controlled. Use them with caution if the patient is unconscious or semiconscious because they may induce vomiting.

To use a suction device, open the patient's mouth using the crossed-finger technique and clear out any solid debris with your fingers. Insert the tip with its convex side along the roof of the mouth, and start the suction by releasing the clamp. Suction should be intermittent and should never continue for more than 15 seconds at a time. Wear disposable rubber gloves to avoid contact with the patient's vomitus and saliva.

Foot- and hand-operated suction units are light and highly portable but are not as effective as electrical units. Hand-operated suction bulbs and bulb syringes similar to turkey basters are better than nothing.

It is a serious matter for a patient to vomit and aspirate the vomitus. The aspirated material can cause suffocation from airway blockage or a serious and hard-to-treat case of pneumonia. It is much better to prevent aspiration than to try to treat it with suction. All unconscious or semiconscious patients

Fig. 6.12 *Sequence of Turning a Patient to the NATO or Stable Side Position*

without neck or back injuries should be placed in the semiprone position, also called the NATO or stable side position (Fig. 6.12). Any patient with a serious illness or injury should be watched carefully. Remember that the rescuer assumes full responsibility for the airway of a patient strapped to a spine board, since the patient is unable to help himself or herself. Be ready at any time to tip the board to one side and apply suction.

Suctioning is indicated any time the upper airway is in danger of being blocked by sputum, edema fluid, blood, vomitus, or foreign material such as snow. Unconscious persons lose the ability to cough and may suffocate from the normal secretions produced by the nose, throat, and lungs. Listen for danger signs such as noisy rattling or crowing sounds coming from the upper respiratory tract.

The use of a **bag-mask** (Fig. 6.13) requires special training, experience, and frequent practice to maintain skills, but bag-masks are easier and more effective than rescue breathing for resuscitating patients who are not breathing. A bag-mask can deliver oxygen at a higher concentration than a pocket mask. The procedure for the bag-mask system, which is used with an oral airway in place, is as follows:

1. Inflate the mask's inflatable cushion to improve the seal.
2. Attach the oxygen tubing to the intake nipple of the bag reservoir and set the oxygen flow at 15 liters per minute.
3. Kneel at the patient's head, open the airway with the jaw-thrust maneuver, and insert an oral airway.
4. Place the mask over the patient's mouth and nose, with the apex over the bridge of the nose and the base in the groove between the lip and the chin.
5. Hold the mask firmly on the face with the thumb and index finger of one hand, while placing the other three fingers under the lower edge of the jaw and behind the angle of the mandible to maintain the jaw-thrust.

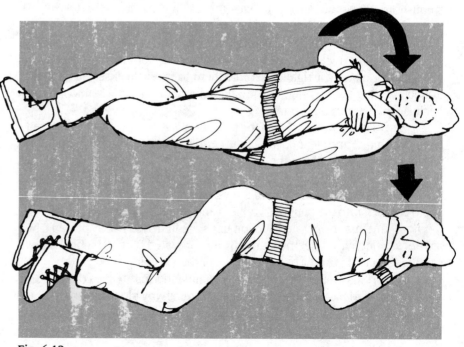

Fig. 6.12

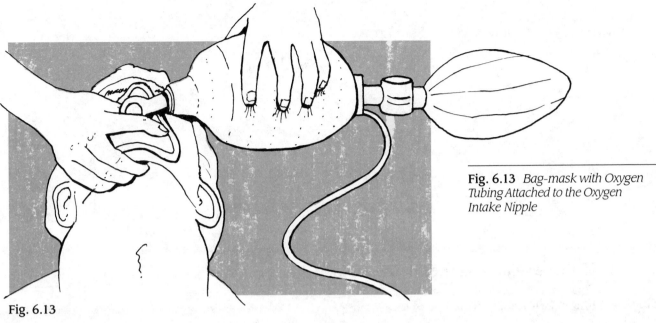

Fig. 6.13 *Bag-mask with Oxygen Tubing Attached to the Oxygen Intake Nipple*

Fig. 6.13

6. Compress the bag rhythmically every five seconds with the other hand. Observe the patient's chest to be sure it rises and falls.

A bag-mask is very difficult, if not impossible, to use during one-rescuer CPR and requires experience for use by a single rescuer during two-rescuer CPR. To maintain an effective seal over the patient's nose and mouth, one rescuer may have to hold the mask in place with both hands while a second rescuer squeezes the bag.

Indications for Oxygen Use

Administer oxygen to:
1. All patients who are in respiratory distress or are cyanotic, with the exception of those who are obviously hyperventilating (see Chapter 17). Theoretically, patients with chronic obstructive pulmonary disease (emphysema) should be given oxygen at a flow rate of no more than 2 liters per minute. Because the breathing center in the brain is driven by hypoxia, too much oxygen may curb the drive and cause the patient to stop breathing. In practice, this is more likely to occur during long-term oxygen use and probably is irrelevant in an emergency situation. Also, patients with severe emphysema are less likely to spend time in the outdoors or at alpine ski areas.
2. All patients with chest injuries other than simple rib fractures.
3. All patients who are seriously ill, i.e., those suffering from cardiac arrest, heart attack, stroke.
4. All patients who are seriously hurt, particularly with head or spinal injuries; femur, hip or pelvic fractures; multiple injuries; or severe burns, particularly of the respiratory tract.
5. All patients who are unconscious or in shock.

7

Bleeding and Shock

I'll empty all these veins, and shed my dear blood drop by drop.

—William Shakespeare
I Henry IV I.iii.

Chapter 2 covers the components of the circulatory system and the vital function of the blood in carrying oxygen from the lungs to the tissues. This function requires sufficient blood to fill the intact blood vessels. Bleeding from damaged vessels (**hemorrhage**) can reduce the blood volume significantly. **External hemorrhage** is bleeding that can be seen coming from a wound, while **internal hemorrhage** involves bleeding inside the body where it may be hard to detect.

The body of an average-sized adult contains about 6,000 milliliters (6.3 quarts) of blood. Anyone who has donated a pint of blood is aware that the loss of 500 milliliters of blood (8 percent of the blood volume) is of no consequence to a healthy adult. Loss of even 1,000 milliliters may not cause serious difficulty. However, the loss of more than 1,000 milliliters can produce the signs and symptoms of **shock**, a type of circulatory failure discussed later in this chapter.

Blood can be lost from arteries, veins, or capillaries; most bleeding is from more than one type of blood vessel. When arteries are damaged, the contractions of the heart and the high pressure within the arteries produce intermittent spurts of bright red, oxygenated blood. Venous blood, which is dark red because it is less oxygenated, flows out steadily under lower pressure. Capillary blood, also dark red, oozes out slowly because of the small size and low pressure of the capillaries. If other factors are equal, arterial bleeding is most dangerous because blood is lost faster.

EXTERNAL BLEEDING

When bleeding is external, blood is lost to the outside and can be seen on the body surface, although clothing may have to be opened to find it. Bleeding that does not involve arteries or large veins usually will stop naturally in five to 10 minutes. Even arterial bleeding may stop naturally, since a torn artery tends to respond to the injury by contracting its muscular walls and retracting back into the tissues. Nonetheless, the rescuer cannot rely on natural control of bleeding occurring before a dangerous amount of blood is lost. When a patient is bleeding heavily, every minute may count.

Most external bleeding can be controlled by **direct pressure**, which collapses and occludes (closes up) the blood vessels until normal clotting can occur. Pressure is applied locally, directly over the wound (Fig. 7.1). Other techniques which serve only as supplements to direct pressure include:

1. **Elevation and immobilization,** which promote clotting by reducing motion and lowering blood pressure at the injury site. (This technique is suitable mainly for extremity bleeding.)
2. **Pneumatic counterpressure devices** such as air splints and pneumatic antishock garments (PASGs), formerly called medical antishock trousers (MAST). (Use of PASGs requires special training and licensing.)
3. **Pressure on a major artery** proximal to the wound (pressure point). This method may decrease bleeding, but rarely stops it entirely because most wounds are supplied by more than one artery.
4. **Application of a tourniquet,** used only when all else fails and the patient's life is in danger.

Fig. 7.1 *Control external bleeding with direct pressure.*

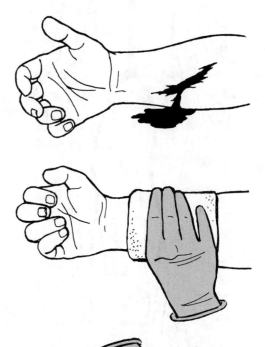

Fig. 7.1

Fig. 7.2 *Major Pressure Points*

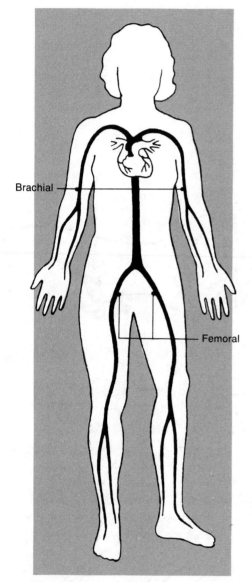

Brachial

Femoral

Fig. 7.2

Direct Pressure

To apply direct pressure, select a sterile compress large enough to cover the wound completely. Place the compress directly on the wound and apply manual pressure. If the situation is urgent and a sterile compress is not available, a clean piece of cloth or a clean sanitary napkin may be substituted. If necessary, apply pressure with a finger or hand alone. If possible, the rescuer should wear rubber gloves to prevent contact with the patient's blood or other secretions. This precaution is especially important if the skin of the rescuer's hand is broken by cuts, sores, or a rash.

After bleeding has stopped, maintain pressure by firmly applying a self-adhering roller bandage such as Kling or Kerlix over the compress.

If bleeding continues despite initial direct pressure, place additional compresses over the original ones and apply stronger pressure. Keep the wound elevated and splinted, if appropriate. If bleeding still continues, remove all compresses and inspect the wound to make sure pressure is being applied in the right place. Bleeding from a small artery at the edge of a wound may have been overlooked.

Pressure Points

If bleeding continues despite the use of these techniques, pressure point control may slow the bleeding and buy time until definitive medical care is obtained. The major pressure points are located where large arteries lie close to bone. Examples are the brachial artery in the arm and the femoral artery in the groin (Fig. 7.2). After locating the arterial pulse, use several fingers or the palm of the hand to press the artery against the underlying bone.

Tourniquet

Because a tourniquet completely occludes the blood vessels, it will cause distal tissues to die if left on too long. Even *brief* application of a tourniquet can crush the underlying tissues and permanently damage distal nerves and blood vessels. Tourniquets are not useful for trunk injuries and should not be used below the elbow or knee because nerves lying close to the surface could be easily injured. In any case, the distal extremities rarely bleed severely enough to require a tourniquet. Remember: *a decision to use a tourniquet is always a decision to risk losing a limb.* Nevertheless, a tourniquet can be lifesaving when a major extremity blood vessel is injured and bleeding cannot be controlled in any other way. Examples of such wounds include high-velocity gunshot wounds and amputations.

Tourniquet Application Technique (Fig. 7.3)

1. Fold a triangular bandage into a band to form a **cravat** 3 to 4 inches wide. Wrap the cravat twice around the extremity and tie the ends with an overhand knot. Position the cravat as far distally as possible while still keeping it above the site of bleeding.
2. Place a 6-inch stick or dowel on top of the overhand knot, and tie a square knot firmly over the stick.
3. Twist the stick until the tourniquet has tightened just enough to stop the bleeding.

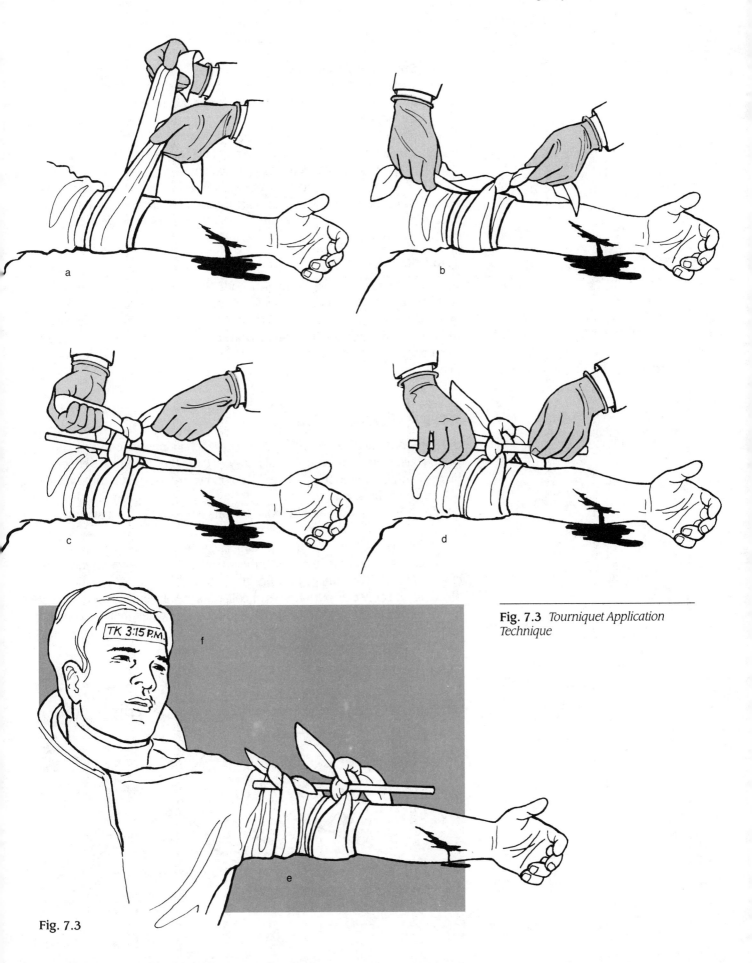

Fig. 7.3 *Tourniquet Application Technique*

Fig. 7.3

Fig. 7.4 *An air splint can be used to control external bleeding.*

4. Secure the stick in place.
5. Write the letters "TK" and the time of application on a piece of tape and fasten the tape to the patient's forehead. Be sure to inform medical personnel of the tourniquet when they take over care of the patient.
6. If bleeding is severe enough to require a tourniquet, give the patient oxygen in high concentration, if available.

Always leave a tourniquet *in plain view*. Never cover a tourniquet with a bandage or clothing. A blood pressure cuff can substitute as a tourniquet, but wire, rope or other thin materials that will cut the skin should *never* be used.

Pneumatic Counterpressure Devices

Air splints are useful for extensive skin and soft-tissue extremity injuries with widespread bleeding because they provide direct pressure to an entire extremity (Fig. 7.4). PASGs are useful mainly to control internal bleeding such as in intra-abdominal hemorrhage or fractures of the pelvis or femur. As mentioned before, special training and licensing are required to use a PASG in emergency care.

INTERNAL BLEEDING

Because internal bleeding is not directly visible, its presence must be suspected based on the mechanism of injury (see Chapter 10) and the effects of bleeding on the function of the involved body part, the circulatory system, and the body as a whole. Theoretically, internal bleeding can involve any body part; from a practical standpoint, certain types and locations of internal bleeding are more common than others.

Unless a large vessel is torn, bleeding into subcutaneous tissue and muscle usually stops promptly because these tissues contain large amounts of clot-promoting substances and because the local pressure produced by bleeding into dense tissue narrows or collapses the bleeding vessels.

However, neither of these mechanisms operates when there is bleeding into hollow organs or body cavities, or when bleeding occurs from large ves-

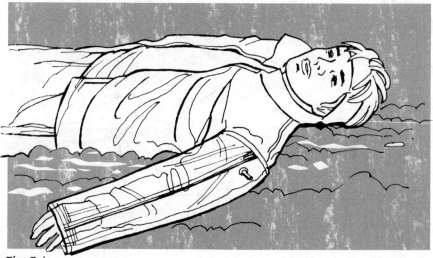

Fig. 7.4

sels, ruptured solid vascular organs, or fractured bones. In these cases, hemorrhage can be severe, prolonged, and life-threatening.

Small hemorrhages into important organs, especially those with a limited ability to swell (such as the brain), can be more devastating than larger hemorrhages into less important, more expandable organs. Internal bleeding into hollow organs may become visible at the body surface. A bleeding ulcer can produce blood in vomitus or bowel movements, and a ruptured kidney can produce bloody urine. Vaginal bleeding in pregnant women is abnormal and may mean a serious complication. Vaginal bleeding in non-pregnant women other than during the normal menstrual period may or may not be serious but should always be investigated by a physician.

Examples of Serious Internal Bleeding

1. Bleeding into the brain from a stroke or head injury.
2. Bleeding from a stomach or duodenal ulcer.
3. Bleeding from a fractured femur, fractured pelvis, or from multiple fractures.
4. Intra-abdominal bleeding caused by a trauma-induced rupture or laceration of the liver, spleen, kidney, pregnant uterus, or large vessels.
5. Intrathoracic bleeding caused by a trauma-induced rupture or laceration of the lung, heart, aorta, or large vessels.
6. Bleeding into the pelvis caused when a fetus develops in a fallopian tube instead of in the uterus (ectopic pregnancy).

Signs and Symptoms of Internal Bleeding

1. A suitable mechanism of injury (see Chapter 10) or a history of illness, such as: blunt or penetrating injury to the chest, abdomen, pelvis, or an extremity; multiple injuries; progressive indigestion; or several missed menstrual periods.
2. Progressive pain, tenderness, nausea, vomiting, rigidity, and enlargement of the abdomen following trauma.
3. Progressive respiratory distress following chest trauma.
4. Progressive enlargement, pain, tenderness, dysfunction, and possible loss of pulses in an injured limb.
5. Blood in vomitus, feces, or urine.
6. Signs and symptoms of shock following trauma when there is no external bleeding or other obvious cause of shock.
7. Bluish discoloration of the skin (ecchymosis) of the involved area (not an acute sign).

Emergency Care of Internal Bleeding

A patient with significant internal bleeding may go quickly into shock and die. Field emergency care for internal bleeding is not very effective unless intravenous therapy is available. However, proper splinting of a fractured extremity will decrease bleeding into the limb and help prevent shock. If equipment and licensed personnel are available, a PASG is useful to treat intra-abdominal hemorrhage and bleeding from pelvic and lower-extremity fractures. The most important outdoor emergency care step for internal

Fig. 7.5 *Diagram of the Three Major Types of Shock*

bleeding is to *suspect the bleeding early and rapidly evacuate the patient to a hospital*. Oxygen in high concentration should be given, if available.

SHOCK

In emergency care, the term **shock** refers to a form of rapid failure of the circulatory system and its consequent inability to deliver oxygen to the tissues. Shock frequently accompanies severe illness or injury. The signs and symptoms of shock are caused by both lack of oxygen in the tissues and the body's attempts to compensate for failing circulation.

Three components are essential for normal blood circulation: adequate blood to fill the blood vessels, a heart capable of pumping blood, and ability to control blood vessel size. When a person is in shock, functioning of one or more of these components is reduced or absent. The names of the three

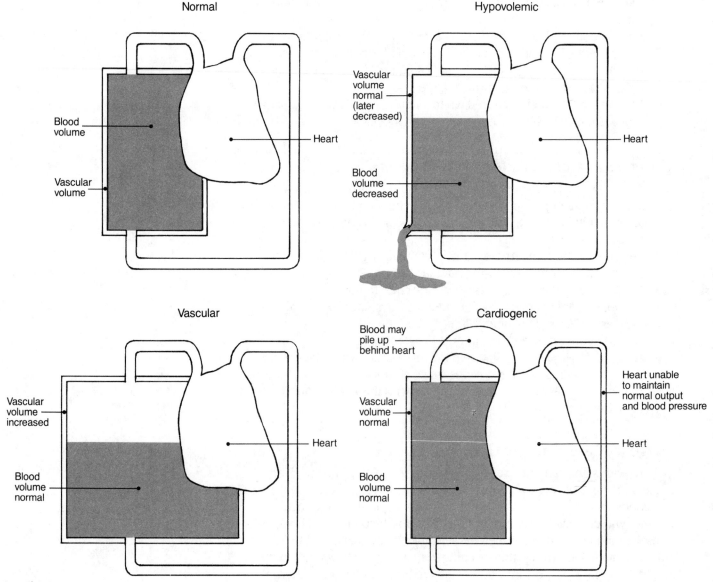

Fig. 7.5

major categories of shock—**hypovolemic**, **cardiogenic**, and **vascular** (vasogenic)—reflect the failure of each respective component (Fig. 7.5).

Hypovolemic shock is caused by a decrease in circulating blood volume. The fall in volume, which is usually rapid, may result from the loss of *whole blood* (as in external or internal hemorrhage) or the *fluid portion of the blood* (as in dehydration from vomiting, diarrhea, or severe burns). The loss of more than 1,000 milliliters (1.1 quarts) may cause moderate shock, marked by a fast pulse and low blood pressure when the patient sits up or attempts to stand. A 1,500-milliliter (1.6 quarts) blood loss causes clinical shock, marked by a fast pulse and low blood pressure even when the patient is lying down. A blood loss of more than 2,000 milliliters (2.1 quarts) causes severe shock with unconsciousness.

Cardiogenic shock occurs when the pumping function of the heart fails. It is caused by weakness of the heart muscle itself, as in a heart attack or chest injury; from ineffective contractions of a normal muscle, as in a too-rapid heartbeat; or from blockage of blood going from the heart, as in a blood clot, or to the heart, as in fluid or blood in the pericardium.

Vascular shock occurs when the mechanisms that normally control blood vessel tone fail, causing the vessels to relax and enlarge. Consequently, the normal blood volume becomes inadequate to fill the vessels. This state can be caused by conditions that directly affect the blood vessel wall, such as severe infection, metabolic illness such as diabetic ketoacidosis, and severe allergic reactions. Vascular shock also can be caused by interruption of the nerve pathways that control the blood vessels, as in patients with spinal cord injury. In cases of simple fainting, an emotional shock or other stimulus triggers nerve impulses that rapidly relax the vessels.

Shock because of failure of one component alone is rare (except in simple fainting) since the components are interrelated and failure of one eventually affects the others. For example, in a hypothermic patient, shock occurs because dehydration lowers the blood volume and cold temperature weakens heart muscle contraction, slows the heartbeat, and interferes with blood vessel control. In severe infections, the toxic products of bacterial growth injure the heart, cause the blood vessels to leak, and injure the muscles of the vessel walls, interfering with ability to maintain vascular tone. In hemorrhagic shock, lack of oxygen affects the contraction of the heart and ability of blood vessels to maintain their tone.

The severity of a case of shock depends on whether its causes are temporary or permanent and whether they can be controlled. Even treatable shock can be fatal if not attended to promptly. After a certain time, vital organs are irreversibly injured by lack of oxygen and the mechanisms that control vascular tone are paralyzed by substances produced by altered metabolism. This state is called **irreversible shock** because even the best treatment started at this point may not reestablish effective blood circulation and promote organ recovery.

The most common causes of shock in the outdoor environment are trauma with internal or external bleeding, dehydration, and heart attack.

Regardless of the underlying cause, the signs and symptoms of shock tend to be similar because they reflect the effects of hypoxia and compensatory attempts to maintain circulation to vital organs. The common denominator in all three forms of shock is a *reduction in effective circulating blood volume*, which tends to cause a *fall in blood pressure*. This stimulates corrective changes, which increase heart rate and output per beat to pump more blood; contract blood vessels in the shell (skin, muscles, and extremities) to shunt blood to the core, maintain blood pressure, and maintain circulation to vital organs; and stimulate breathing, so that more oxygen can be extracted by the lungs and each unit of blood can carry more oxygen.

These changes cause the skin to become cold, clammy, pale, or cyanotic. The patient develops shortness of breath and an increased pulse rate. The pulse becomes weak and thready if shock progresses. The kidneys reduce urine output to conserve the water and salts needed to maintain the plasma volume. Oxygen lack in the brain causes confusion, anxiety, nausea, and mental dullness; oxygen lack in the muscles causes fatigue and weakness.

If the causes of the shock can be treated or removed, the compensatory changes may be sufficient to maintain normal tissue oxygenation and the patient will recover. If the causes continue, compensation eventually fails and the patient will die.

In the early stages of shock, the compensatory changes may maintain circulation at a close-to-normal level (at least when the patient is lying flat and the heart does not have to pump against gravity), the pulse and breathing rates may increase only slightly or not at all, and blood pressure may remain normal. Later, as compensatory efforts become more stressed, the classic signs and symptoms of shock develop. Shock should be *anticipated* when a suitable mechanism of illness or injury exists.

Signs and Symptoms of Shock

1. Restlessness and anxiety.
2. Rapid pulse, which later becomes weak and thready.
3. Cold, clammy, pale skin, which later becomes cyanotic.
4. Profuse sweating.
5. Abnormal respirations. These usually are rapid and shallow at first, and later become labored and gasping.
6. Dull or lusterless eyes, dilated pupils.
7. Thirst.
8. Nausea, occasionally vomiting.
9. Weak muscles. Patient complains of feeling very tired and weak.
10. Falling blood pressure. In the early stages of shock, the patient's blood pressure and pulse may be normal while lying down but abnormal when sitting up.
11. Change in consciousness. Confusion and mental dullness may progress to stupor and coma.
12. Signs and symptoms of the underlying condition that caused the shock.

Emergency Care of Shock

1. The first priority in shock, as in any serious illness, is to secure and maintain the upper airway. Give rescue breathing if required.
2. Control obvious bleeding.
3. Administer oxygen in high concentration, if available.
4. Elevate the lower extremities about 12 inches, except in cases of cardiogenic shock or when contraindicated by the type of injury.

5. Keep the patient warm but not excessively warm, which may worsen shock.
6. As a general rule, keep the patient supine to lessen the work of the heart. In some cases, a shock patient may also have lung congestion from heart failure or lung disease and should be supine because of shock but may need to sit up because of inability to breathe when lying flat. In this situation, use the Rothberg position, in which the patient's upper body is raised at a 45-degree angle, the abdomen is flat, and the lower extremities are elevated by flexing the hips at about 15 degrees.
7. Splint any suspected fractures.
8. Do not give the patient anything to eat or drink.
9. Check and record vital signs at frequent intervals.
10. If shock is caused by a suspected fracture of the pelvis or femur or by intra-abdominal hemorrhage, rescuers who have the proper training, experience, licensing, and equipment can use a PASG.
11. If needed, give other special emergency care for specific causes of shock, e.g., care for hypothermia (Chapter 19).
12. Because there is no specific field emergency care for most causes of shock, the patient must be transported to a hospital as soon as possible. The rescuer should always *anticipate* the development of shock in injuries and illnesses known to frequently lead to shock.

Table 7.1

SUMMARY OF EMERGENCY CARE OF SHOCK
1. Give basic life support, as necessary.
2. Control bleeding, if present.
3. Give oxygen.
4. Elevate lower extremities, except in cardiogenic shock.
5. Support body temperature.
6. Keep patient lying down unless short of breath.
7. Splint fractures.
8. Give nothing to eat or drink.
9. Check and record vital signs at regular intervals.
10. Give special care for specific types of shock.
    a. Hypothermia (see Chapter 18).
    b. Use of a PASG for specific types of shock by specially trained rescuers.
11. Rapidly evacuate patient to a hospital.

SPECIAL TYPES OF SHOCK

Simple Fainting

Simple fainting, sometimes called psychogenic shock, is a common and benign form of acute vascular shock that can have either physical or emotional causes. Stimuli such as pain, the sight of blood, or a strong emotion such as fear can trigger nerve reflexes which produce sudden enlargement (dilation) of blood vessels. Sitting or standing for a long time without moving,

Fig. 7.6 *Example of a Kit Carried by People Subject to Anaphylactic Shock*

especially if it is hot, can cause blood to pool in dilated blood vessels, resulting in a loss of effective circulating blood volume, which causes the blood pressure to drop. As cerebral blood flow decreases, the person loses consciousness and collapses to the floor or slumps over his or her chair.

The causes of this type of shock are transient, and the patient will regain consciousness as soon as the supine position allows cerebral blood flow to increase. Be sure the patient is lying flat and, if the fall was hard, assess the person for injuries. Move the patient to a cool place if the environment is hot. Advise the patient to rest before normal activity is resumed.

Anaphylactic Shock

Anaphylactic shock is an emergency condition that may cause rapid death unless treated promptly. It is an immediate and overwhelming allergic reaction, usually to an insect sting, drug, or food. Common offenders are bee and wasp stings, penicillin, aspirin, seafood, nuts, and berries. Contact with the offending substance (known as the **allergen**) causes the release of histamine and other substances from the injured tissues. In turn, blood vessels leak and smooth muscle in the bronchi and other organs go into spasm. The patient develops hives; massive swelling of the face, tongue, and upper respiratory tract; wheezing; nausea; vomiting; cramps; and diarrhea. The condition may progress rapidly to convulsions, coma, and death.

The emergency antidote for anaphylactic shock is **epinephrine** (adrenalin) by injection. Rescuers who are not properly trained and licensed cannot legally give injections. However, many people in danger of anaphylactic shock from bee stings or other sources carry kits containing pre-loaded syringes of epinephrine with directions for use (Fig. 7.6). The rescuer may assist the patient in injecting the drug. Every minute counts. The patient will need a second injection of epinephrine five to 10 minutes later if he or she does not improve promptly. The patient then should be taken to a hospital as soon as possible and may require oxygen, rescue breathing, or CPR on the way.

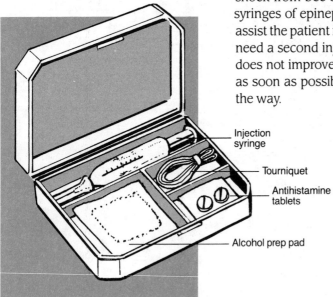

Injection syringe

Tourniquet

Antihistamine tablets

Alcohol prep pad

Fig. 7.6

8

Skin and Soft-Tissue Injuries, Burns, and Bandaging

But a certain Samaritan went to him, and bound up his wounds, pouring in oil and wine.

—Luke 10:33

This chapter presents the general principles of injuries to the soft tissues, which include the skin, subcutaneous tissues, muscles, and tendons. The hard tissues – the bones, joints, and their component ligaments – are discussed in Chapter 9. Before starting this chapter, review the sections on the skin and muscles in Chapter 2.

One of the major functions of the skin is to *protect the body from infection* by forming a barrier between the underlying tissues and infectious organisms. Bacteria, viruses, and fungi are everywhere in the environment and are normally found on the skin's surface. Any illness or injury that breaks the skin may lead to **infection** as well as bleeding.

Soft-tissue injuries are divided into two types: open and closed. A **closed injury** may damage the skin and deeper tissues but does not involve a break in the skin; an **open injury** involves a break in the skin as well as damage to the tissues beneath it.

Closed injuries include **contusions**, **hematomas**, and **muscle strains**. Open injuries include **abrasions**, **lacerations**, **incisions**, **avulsions**, and **punctures**.

CLOSED SOFT-TISSUE INJURIES

Contusions, also known as bruises, are caused by blunt trauma. The underlying tissues are crushed and small blood vessels are torn, causing local bleeding. Blood accumulates under the skin, producing a characteristic bluish discoloration known as **ecchymosis**. Capillary damage allows the fluid part of the blood to leak into the surrounding tissues, leading to a type of swelling called **edema**. The body's response to tissue damage is **inflammation**, a condition marked by swelling, pain, heat, redness, and loss of function. A severe contusion may damage larger blood vessels and cause a tumor-like collection of blood in the tissues called a **hematoma**. Hematomas also are found at the site of fractures, strains, and other injuries involving large blood vessels.

Strains, or muscle pulls, occur when a muscle is severely stretched or torn. Strains usually are not caused by blunt trauma but by a violent movement of an extremity, which creates a pull strong enough to damage a muscle. Injury to small vessels and capillaries causes swelling and ecchymosis.

Emergency Care of Closed Soft-tissue Injuries

Cold causes blood vessels to contract, which retards further bleeding and swelling. Elevation and splinting or use of a sling may be indicated, especially for injuries where underlying fractures or sprains are suspected.

Control bleeding and swelling of closed soft-tissue injuries by applying cold packs and pressure and by elevating the injured part. Place ice, snow, or a cloth soaked in cold water in a plastic bag. Wrap the bag in a towel and apply it to the injury for about 20 minutes per waking hour for the first 24 hours. Apply pressure by wrapping the site of injury firmly with a self-adhering roller bandage or rubberized bandage. Do not apply ice or snow directly to the skin or wrap the injured site so tightly that circulation is restricted. Cold compresses should not be applied to a patient who is hypothermic or in a cold environment.

Fig. 8.1 *Types of Open Injuries*

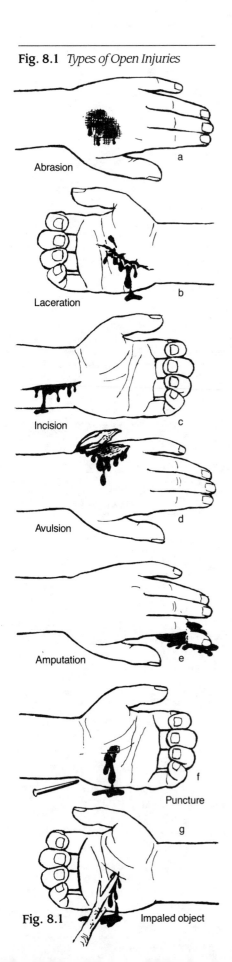

Abrasion   a

Laceration   b

Incision   c

Avulsion   d

Amputation   e

Puncture   f

g

Fig. 8.1   Impaled object

Patients with severe closed soft-tissue injuries of a lower extremity usually are unable to walk and will need to be evacuated by litter or toboggan. Patients with lesser injuries may be able to walk if the damaged extremity is supported by being wrapped in a rubberized bandage.

Table 8.1

SUMMARY OF EMERGENCY CARE OF CLOSED SOFT-TISSUE INJURIES

1. Apply a pressure bandage.
2. Apply a cold compress.
3. Elevate the injury.
4. Splint the injury, if appropriate.
5. Assist with evacuation as necessary.

OPEN SOFT-TISSUE INJURIES (Fig. 8.1)

Abrasions (Fig. 8.1a) are superficial injuries caused by moving contact between the skin and a parallel rough surface. This mechanical process, also called planing, scrapes off the epidermis but usually not the dermis. Abrasions ooze blood and plasma from injured vessels. Large abrasions are very painful because many pain nerves are irritated. Common examples of abrasions are "road burn" in cyclists and "floor burn" in gymnasts.

Lacerations (Fig. 8.1b) are tears in the skin that may also involve deeper tissues. Bleeding may be profuse or mild, depending on the size and number of blood vessels injured.

Incisions (Fig. 8.1c) are "clean" lacerations caused by a knife, ski edge, or other sharp object. They are more regular and linear than lacerations and usually bleed more because the cleanly cut blood vessels constrict and retract less effectively.

Avulsions (Fig. 8.1d) are pieces of skin torn loose from underlying tissues and left hanging by a flap. If the skin is torn completely loose, an avulsion is called a **soft-tissue amputation**. If a part containing a bone is severed, it is called an **amputation** (Fig. 8.1e).

Punctures (Fig. 8.1f) are wounds caused by a sharp, narrow object such as a knife, ski pole tip, or ice pick. Punctures also can be caused by high-velocity blunt objects such as bullets. The apparent damage caused by a puncture is often deceptive; the entrance wound may be small with little bleeding, giving no clue to the extent of damage to organs and blood vessels beneath. Bullets and long, sharp objects may penetrate completely through a body part; thus the rescuer also should search for exit wounds. An **impaled object** (Fig. 8.1g) is one that protrudes from a wound.

Tetanus can be a serious complication of open soft-tissue wounds. This disease is caused by a soil bacterium introduced into open wounds. As the bacteria grow, they produce a toxin that provokes serious muscle spasms and interferes with breathing. Puncture wounds are fertile ground for the tetanus organism, which flourishes in an oxygen-poor environment. Wounds that are deep and small in diameter are more likely to be oxygen-free. All open wounds are susceptible, however, especially those contaminated by soil. To prevent tetanus, people should be fully immunized in infancy and have a booster immunization of toxoid every 10 years. A booster should be given following an open wound if the patient has not received a booster within five years. Unimmunized patients or those whose immunization has lapsed should receive human tetanus immune globulin.

Emergency Care of Open Wounds

1. To protect against accidental exposure to the AIDS or hepatitis viruses, rescuers should wear rubber gloves when caring for patients with open wounds.
2. Inspect the wound. If necessary, remove overlying clothing, preferably by cutting or ripping along a seam.
3. Control bleeding by direct pressure. Elevation, splinting, or pressure point control may occasionally be required as well, although a tourniquet is rarely needed.
4. Guard against further contamination of the wound.
5. All open wounds are considered contaminated, even though no obvious contamination can be seen. The wounds of skiers and other oversnow travelers usually are quite clean. If the patient will receive definitive medical care within a few hours, the wound need not be washed, although any loose pieces of dirt, bark, and other foreign matter should be removed with sterile forceps. Forceps can be sterilized by heating them over a lit match or cleaning them with rubbing alcohol or an antiseptic such as povidone-iodine solution (Betadine). Next, cover the wound with a sterile dressing held in place by a bandage.

   If it will be more than a few hours before the patient will receive definitive medical care, the wound should be cleaned more thoroughly. Be certain all bleeding is controlled. Cover the wound with a sterile compress and wash the surrounding skin with Betadine or another antiseptic solution (first question the patient about allergies to iodine and other chemicals).

   Next, generously irrigate the wound with clean, warm water or, preferably, with sterile physiological saline solution. Dry the wound with a sterile compress and, if it is small, close the wound with butterfly bandages or Steristrips. If the wound is large, leave it open. Next, apply a sterile compress large enough that its edges extend at least 1 inch past the margins of the wound. Hold this dressing in place with a bandage or tape. If the wound is large and painful, splint and elevate it as well. Small lower-extremity wounds can be supported with an elastic roller bandage if the patient must walk. In general, all open wounds except the most trivial should be seen by a physician; this is especially true of wounds on the face.

   Physiological saline solution, also called normal saline solution, is a 0.9-percent solution of ordinary table salt in water. This concentration of salt water has the same osmotic pressure as normal human tissue and does not cause pain or injury when used to irrigate an open wound or keep tissue moist. Sterile physiological saline solution can be purchased in bottles or bags and stored in the first aid room or rescue cache.

6. Puncture wounds cannot be adequately cleaned and should always be seen by a physician. If underlying organs have been injured, the patient must be rapidly transported to a hospital.

7. All abrasions should be gently washed with soap and clean water before bandaging. Sterile compresses that have nonadhesive material on one side (such as Telfa) are less painful to remove than ordinary compresses.

8. For avulsions, replace the flap in the wound in its normal position before applying direct pressure to control bleeding. If time permits (i.e., bleeding is minimal), first clean the flap and the wound (see 5. above). During bandaging, place the sterile compress over the repositioned flap rather than directly on the raw wound.

9. With modern surgical techniques, it frequently is possible to reattach amputated parts. Always preserve such parts and send them along with the patient to the hospital. Wrap the part in a sterile dressing moistened with sterile physiological saline solution and place it in a plastic bag. Put this bag in a second plastic bag containing ice and water. Keep the part cool but do *not allow it to freeze.*

10. Do not remove impaled objects unless they obstruct the airway. Any motion may damage important underlying structures and removal may cause uncontrollable bleeding. Do not exert pressure directly on an object at the entrance wound, nor on tissues close to its sharp edges. Large objects that interfere with patient handling may be carefully cut off with a pipe cutter or similar device. Bandage the wound with a bulky dressing so that the impaled object is immobilized. Because surgery will be required to remove the object, give the patient nothing by mouth and arrange prompt transportation to a hospital.

Table 8.2

SUMMARY OF EMERGENCY CARE OF OPEN SOFT-TISSUE INJURIES
1. Don rubber gloves.
2. Inspect the wound. If necessary, remove overlying clothing.
3. Control bleeding by direct pressure.

Additional measures as necessary:
4. Prevent further contamination.
5. Cleanse the wound.
6. Apply a sterile compress and bandage.
7. Elevate and splint the injured part.
8. Arrange for tetanus prophylaxis (measures to guard against tetanus).
9. Treat the patient for shock.
10. Special types of wounds:
    a. Wash abrasions.
    b. Replace avulsions.
    c. Preserve amputated parts.
    d. Bandage impaled objects in place.

Fig. 8.2 *Three Types of Burns*

BURNS

A burn is a wound of the skin or mucous membranes caused by excessive thermal, electrical or radiant energy. Certain chemicals cause similar injuries, which also are called burns. Burns are divided into three types: thermal, chemical, and electrical. Eye burns are discussed in Chapter 13.

Thermal Burns

There are many dangerous sources of heat that can cause burns. In the outdoors, burns can be caused by forest fires, campfires, tent fires, stove explosions, and excessive exposure to the ultraviolet rays of the sun. The amount of damage from heat and ultraviolet light depends on the temperature or intensity, length of exposure, and the size and location of the contact area. To date, nothing better than the human eye has been devised for estimating the seriousness of a burn based on its physical characteristics and the amount of body surface involved.

Burns are divided into first, second, and third degree according to the depth of the damage (Fig. 8.2).

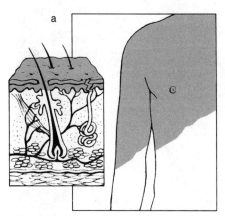 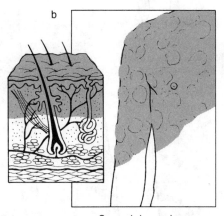 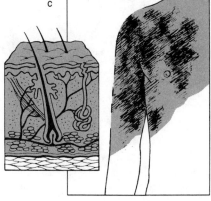

Fig. 8.2   First-degree burn   Second-degree burn   Third-degree burn

First-degree burns involve the superficial layers of the epidermis. The skin is red, tender and painful, and may be swollen. No blisters form (Fig. 8.2a).

Second-degree burns involve the epidermis and part, but not all, of the dermis. Swelling and blister formation occur (Fig. 8.2b).

Third-degree burns penetrate the epidermis and dermis into the subcutaneous tissue. The involved skin is "cooked" and appears to be dead; it is dry, thickened, leathery, and charred or otherwise discolored. Because nerves and blood vessels in the skin are destroyed, no blisters form and the area is numb (Fig. 8.2c).

A burned area may contain all three degrees of injury, usually with third-degree burns in the center, surrounded by second-degree burns and an outer rim of first-degree burns. The *size* of the burned area is very important; size can be roughly estimated by applying the **Rule of Nines** (Fig. 8.3). In adults, the head and neck represent 9 percent of the body surface area; the front and back of the trunk, 18 percent each; each arm, 9 percent; each leg, 18 percent;

Fig. 8.3 *Rule of Nines*

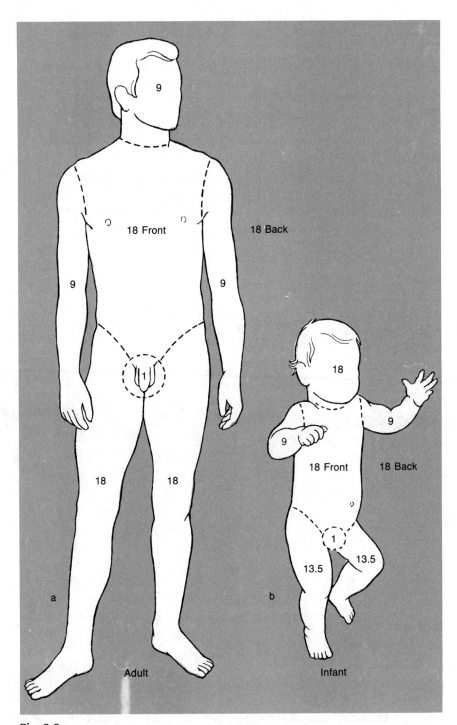

Fig. 8.3

and the genital area, 1 percent (Fig. 8.3a). In infants and small children, the head is relatively larger and the legs relatively smaller; the head makes up 18 percent, and each leg, 13.5 percent (Fig. 8.3b).

The severity of thermal burns is classified as **critical**, **moderate**, or **minor** depending on the extent and depth of the burn, the age and general health of the patient, and involvement of critical areas, such as the respiratory tract, hands, feet, or genitals.

Classification of Burns

1. Critical
   a. Burns of any degree complicated by injury to the respiratory tract, fractures, or other major injuries.
   b. Third-degree burns of the face, hands, feet, or genital area.
   c. Third-degree burns of more than 10 percent of the body surface.
   d. Second-degree burns of more than 25 percent of the body surface (20 percent in children and the elderly).
2. Moderate
   a. Third-degree burns of 2 to 10 percent of the body that do not involve the face, hands, feet, genitals or respiratory tract and are not accompanied by fractures or other serious injuries.
   b. Second-degree burns of 15 to 25 percent of the body in adults (10 to 20 percent in children and elderly).
   c. First-degree burns of 50 to 75 percent of the body surface.
3. Minor
   a. Third-degree burns of less than 2 percent of the body surface, if no critical areas are involved.
   b. Second-degree burns of less than 15 percent of the body surface in adults (less than 10 percent in children and the elderly).

Emergency Care of Thermal Burns

1. Immediately put out the fire. If a person's clothing catches on fire, tell him or her to drop to the ground and roll.
2. Move the patient away from the burning or smoke-filled area; cut away smoldering clothing or soak it with cold water.
3. Immerse hot skin in clean, cold water or cover it with a cold, wet, clean cloth for about 10 minutes. This will halt any residual burning of the skin and underlying tissues and relieve pain. However, burns of greater than 20 percent of the body surface area should *not* be cooled.
4. Burned skin is sterile. Avoid contamination and protect blisters to prevent them from rupturing.
5. Estimate the extent and depth of the burn and note any involvement of critical areas.
6. Cover the burn with a dry, sterile dressing or, if it is extensive, with a clean sheet or pillowcase. Do *not* put any type of grease, lotion, or antiseptic on burned skin.
7. Splint a burned extremity.
8. Transport the patient promptly to a hospital.
9. Watch for respiratory distress in patients who have suffered smoke exposure, those with facial burns, and those with burns classified as moderate or critical. Give oxygen in high concentration, if available, to such patients. Anticipate and treat shock when burns are extensive. Look for fractures and other significant injuries, especially if the patient jumped from a building or was injured by explosions or falling debris.
10. Anyone trapped in a burning building may have suffered carbon monoxide poisoning (discussed in Chapter 18).

Table 8.3

SUMMARY OF EMERGENCY CARE OF BURNS

1. Put out the fire and/or remove the patient from the heat source.
2. Apply cold water if the burn covers less than 20 percent of the body surface area.
3. Avoid rupturing blisters.
4. Estimate the extent and seriousness of the burn.
5. Cover the burn with sterile or clean material.
6. Watch for respiratory distress and give oxygen as necessary.
7. Immobilize the burned extremity.
8. Treat the patient for shock.
9. Check for additional injuries and treat them.
10. Transport the patient to medical care.

Chemical Burns

Chemical burns are most often caused by contact with strong acids or alkalis. It is essential to immediately remove the chemical. Emergency care of most chemical burns consists of prolonged rinsing of the involved area with *copious* amounts of water. Exceptions include contact with organic acids such as phenol, and with dry lime, which is more dangerous when wet and should be brushed off before the site is rinsed. Because organic acids are only partly water-soluble, use alcohol or cooking oil to cleanse such burns after rinsing with water. After rinsing the injured area, remove any of the patient's clothing that might harbor chemical residue. Then, cover the burned area with a sterile dressing and take the patient to a physician or hospital.

Electrical Burns

Electrical injury is discussed in Chapter 19. The local treatment of electrical burns is the same as for thermal burns. Electricity usually produces an entrance and exit burn. The damage caused by electricity usually appears small on the surface, but there may be extensive internal damage because electric current tends to penetrate along the paths of blood vessels. Respiratory and/or cardiac arrest may occur, necessitating rescue breathing or CPR.

DRESSINGS AND BANDAGES

The term **dressing** or **compress** refers to sterile material placed directly on a wound. The term **bandage** refers to the material that holds a dressing in place. In popular usage, bandage frequently refers to the dressing and bandage together, and bandaging designates the process of applying both the dressing and the bandage to a wound.

All open wounds require dressing and bandaging to prevent further contamination, to absorb blood and wound secretions, and to control bleeding. A dressing should extend at least 1 inch beyond the edges of the wound. In the past, a large amount of class time in first aid courses was devoted to the art of bandaging. Bandaging is easier using modern supplies such as the self-adhering roller bandage and, in modern emergency care, any combination that does the job is acceptable. However, there are a few tricks that help when bandaging geometrically difficult body areas (see page 154).

Apply bandages snugly to keep the dressing on the wound. Most bandaging requires that bandages be wrapped entirely around a body part, which introduces the danger of restricting circulation if the bandage is too tight. Leave the fingers or toes exposed distal to an extremity wound so that signs of poor circulation can be watched for.

Fig. 8.4 *Occlusive Dressing for a Sucking Chest Wound*

Special Types of Dressings and Bandages

1. Occlusive dressings
   a. For sucking chest wounds, place a universal dressing or several layers of sterile compresses directly on the wound and cover with a sterile, airtight layer of plastic, foil, or Vaseline gauze. Seal

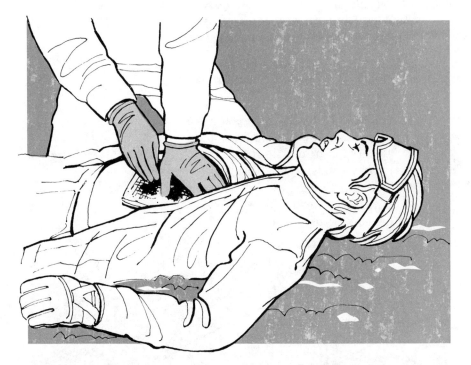

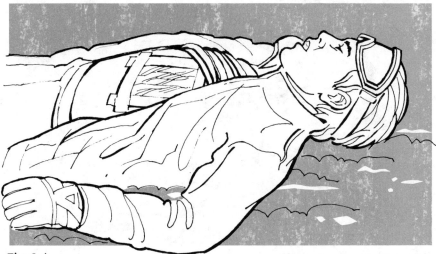

Fig. 8.4

Fig. 8.5 *Pressure Dressing*

Fig. 8.6 *Stabilizing Dressing for an Impaled Object*

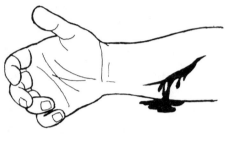
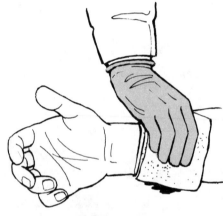
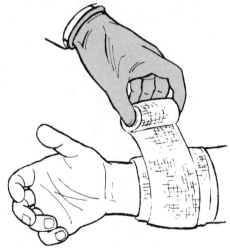

Fig. 8.5

the edges tightly to the skin with adhesive tape, preferably while the patient holds his or her breath after a maximum exhalation (Fig. 8.4).

b. Cover open abdominal wounds that expose organs with a universal dressing or several layers of sterile compresses moistened with sterile physiological saline solution or, in a pinch, with clean water. This will keep the organs from drying out. Cover the moist dressing with a piece of sterile, airtight material taped to the abdomen.

2. Pressure dressings (Fig. 8.5), used to maintain direct pressure on a bleeding wound, consist of one or more sterile compresses held in place by a firmly applied self-adhering roller bandage. A rubberized bandage such as the Ace bandage can be used instead, but the danger of accidentally interfering with circulation is greater.

3. Stabilizing dressings (Fig. 8.6), used to stabilize an impaled object, consist of a thick layer of sterile compresses held firmly in place by tape or self-adhering roller bandages.

Commonly Used Dressings and Bandages

1. Dressings (Fig. 8.7a)

   a. Sterile, nonadhesive pads come in several sizes and are covered on one side by a semipermeable plastic material (Telfa, etc.). These pads are used to cover small wounds or as the first layer for larger wounds.

   b. Sterile gauze pads, available in many sizes ranging from 1-inch by 1-inch to 4-inches by 8-inches, are used to cover small- and medium-sized wounds.

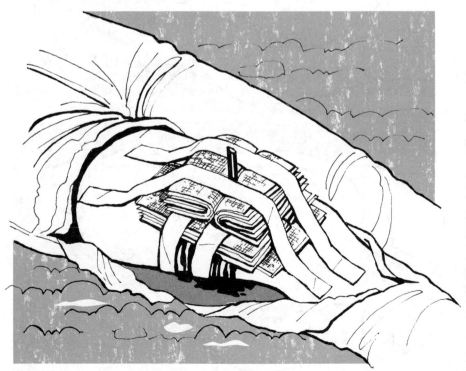

Fig. 8.6

c. Universal dressings, 9-inch by 36-inch pads made of thick absorbent material, are used to cover large open wounds.

d. Vaseline gauze (gauze impregnated with petrolatum) is available in long narrow strips used to pack bleeding noses, and in standard-sized dressings. It is airtight and nonadhesive.

e. Handy, small, prepackaged bandage strips (Bandaids, etc.) are ideal for minor cuts and blisters. These strips combine a compress with a bandage.

f. Prepackaged materials such as butterfly bandages and special paper tape (Steristrips) are used for wound closure. Butterflies can be improvised in the field from adhesive tape; the part to be laid on the wound should be sterilized by heating it over a lit match. The application technique is illustrated in Figure 8.7b.

2. Bandages (Fig 8.7c)

a. Triangular bandages are large, triangular pieces of cloth that measure about 55 inches at the base and 36 inches to 40 inches along each side. They can be used as-is to form slings or can be folded lengthwise to form long, narrow cravats several inches wide. Cravats can be used as bandages, swathes, splints for fractured ribs, and supports for sprained ankles and knees. They also are used for tourniquets.

b. Self-adhering roller bandages are a useful modern version of the venerable gauze roller bandages. They come in several widths and, because the material sticks to itself, extensive taping is not necessary to secure the ends. Self-adhering roller bandages also are slightly elastic and, when used as pressure bandages, cause less danger to the circulation than rubberized bandages.

c. Elastic (rubberized) bandages in different widths are used to support a sprained wrist, ankle, or knee. Use them with caution on a patient who is not alert enough to complain if the bandage is too tight, causing pain or numbness. Self-adhering roller bandages have mostly replaced rubberized bandages for bandaging wounds.

d. Adhesive tape comes in several widths; the most useful for field use is the 2-inch width, which can be torn lengthwise if 1-inch widths are needed. Use cloth tape rather than plastic or paper tape. Some people are allergic to tape; ask the patient before applying tape. Adhesive tape is most useful in taping blisters, splinting sprained ankles and fractured ribs, and securing dressings to flat or slightly curved surfaces (such as the chest, back or abdomen) where a roller bandage or cravat is unsuitable. Adhesive tape does not stick well when cold or when the skin is wet. In cold weather, the adherence of the tape can be improved by warming it against the rescuer's body or heating it briefly over a lit match. It is best to shave hairy skin before taping it. Never wrap tape completely around an injured extremity, because the tape can act as a tourniquet if swelling occurs.

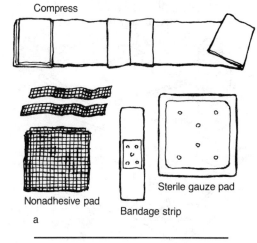

Fig. 8.7 *Various Types of Dressings and Bandages*

Compress

Nonadhesive pad

Sterile gauze pad

Bandage strip

a

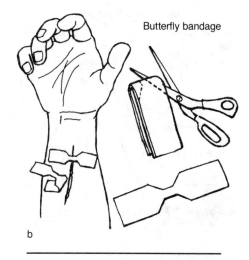

Butterfly bandage

b

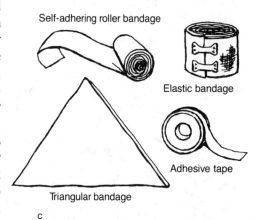

Self-adhering roller bandage

Elastic bandage

Adhesive tape

Triangular bandage

c

Fig. 8.7

Fig. 8.8 *Improvised Bandages and Dressings*

Fig. 8.9 *Application of a Figure-of-eight Bandage to the Knee*

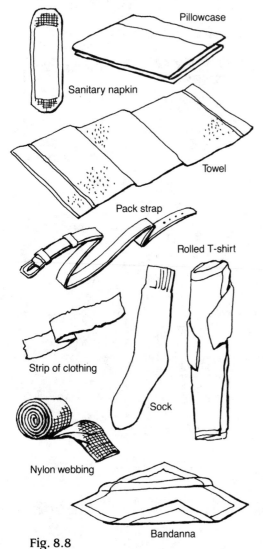

Fig. 8.8

Improvisation of Bandages and Dressings

In an emergency, dressings can be improvised from any clean cloth, such as pillowcases, sheets, towels, and sanitary napkins (Fig. 8.8). Never place loose cotton directly on an open wound because the fibers are difficult to remove. Pack straps, belts, strips torn from clothing, cord, or nylon webbing can be used to improvise bandages. Kerchiefs and bandannas can be used as cravats and triangular bandages. Rolled T-shirts also can be used as cravats, and clean socks can be used as hand or foot bandages. Plastic sandwich or garbage bags can be placed over sterile compresses to make an occlusive dressing.

Special Techniques for Problem Surfaces

Moving joints (Fig. 8.9) require a special technique because joint motion, even if only occasional, tends to shift the bandage to a position above or below the joint and loosen adhesive tape. The preferred bandage material is self-adhering roller bandage, which is elastic enough to stretch with joint motion rather than move. Apply this material in a figure eight. Make several circular turns around the limb above the joint, overlapping the upper end of the dressing. Bring the bandage diagonally across the dressing and make several similar turns around the limb below the joint. Next, bring the bandage diagonally back up over the dressing and make several turns around the limb above the joint. Repeat this process until the dressing is snug. Use tape or a safety pin to anchor the loose end above or below the joint, not over or behind it.

Joints should be bandaged in the most comfortable position. Usually, the knee is bandaged while slightly flexed and the ankle and elbow while flexed to just under 90 degrees.

Tapering cones such as the upper arm, forearm, thigh, or leg are best wrapped with a self-adhering roller bandage (Fig. 8.10). Make several turns around the limb below the dressing and then continue up, over and above the dressing, with each turn overlapping the one below by half an inch to three-fourths of an inch. Complete the bandage by making several overlapping turns above the dressing and anchoring the loose end. If the patient must walk on a bandaged lower extremity, anchor the bandage to the skin above the dressing with several vertical strips of tape.

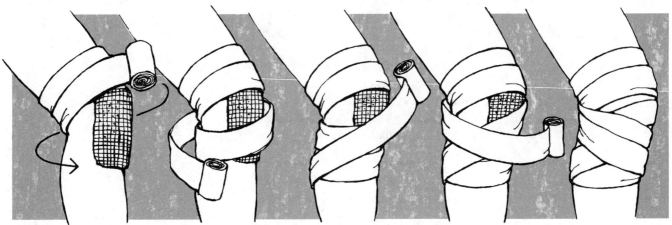

Fig. 8.9

Bandages tend to slip off the **head** because it is spherical. Compresses can be anchored with a bandanna-style triangular bandage or with the patient's hat. Fold a triangular bandage (Fig. 8.11) twice along the long side to make a 2-inch hem. Place the bandage on top of the patient's head with the triangular tail below the occiput (back of the skull) and with the hem across the forehead just above the eyebrows. Wrap the two ends of the hem around the sides of the head above the ears, cross at the occiput, and bring them around the opposite sides of the head to the forehead. Then tie the ends snugly with a square knot. Tuck the tip of the tail into the hem at the occiput. The bandage should be snug and wrinkle-free over the top of the head. Anchor the outer surface of the compress beneath the bandage with a safety pin sterilized over a lit match. Anchoring with the patient's hat works better if the sweatband is directly over the wound, or, if available, use a snug-fitting ski or stocking hat (Fig. 8.12).

Because the **hands** are seldom still, even when injured, bandages tend to work loose easily. An effective technique is to immobilize the hand com-

Fig. 8.10 *Application of a Self-adhering Roller Bandage to the Forearm*

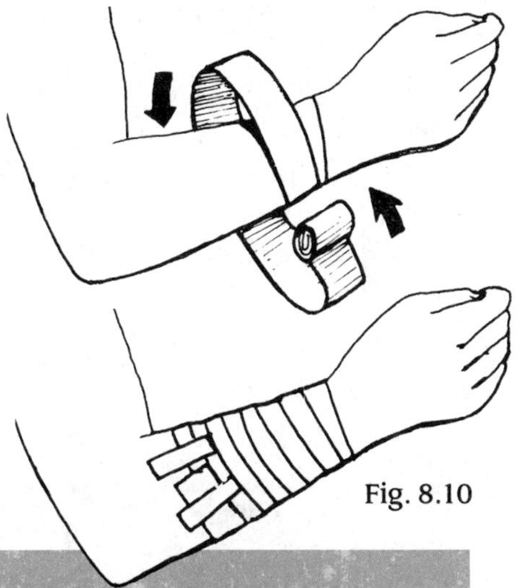

Fig. 8.10

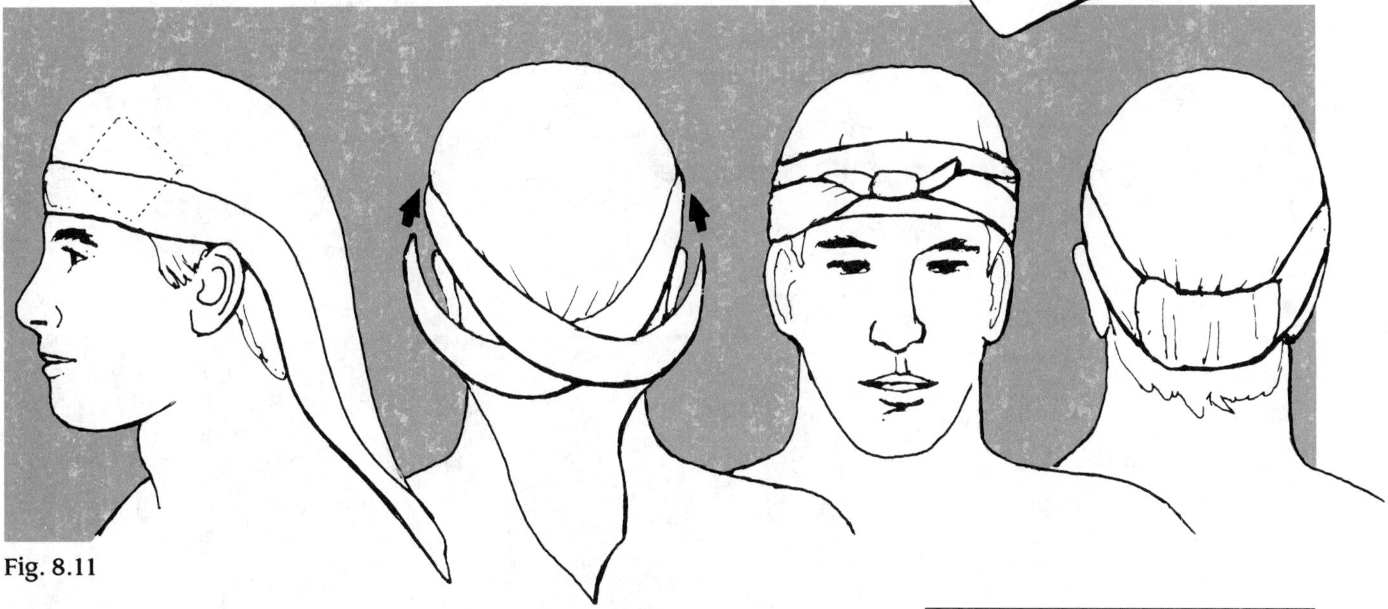

Fig. 8.11

Fig. 8.12

Fig. 8.11 *Application of a Triangular Bandage to the Head*

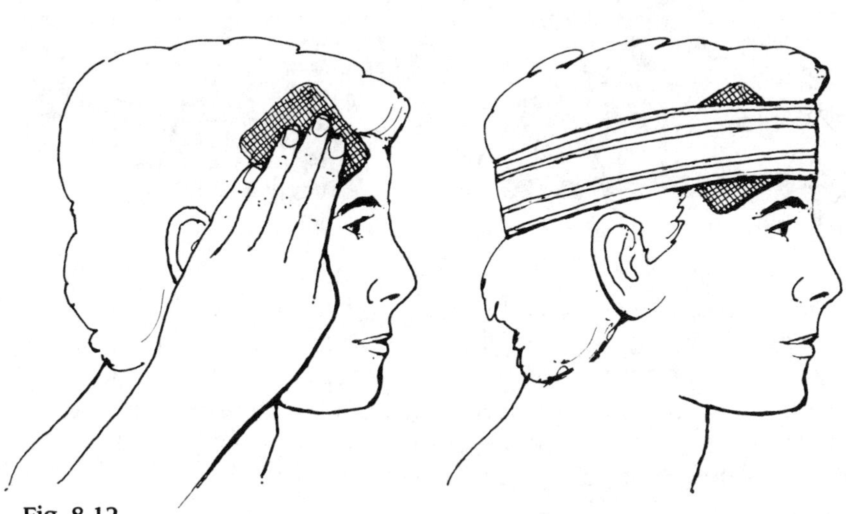

Fig. 8.12 *Use of a Headband to Secure a Dressing*

Fig. 8.13 *Bulky Hand Dressing*

Fig. 8.14 *Figure-of-eight Bandage Modified for the Hand*

pletely by cupping the fingers over a wad of gauze held in the palm, then wrap the entire hand with a roller bandage or a cravat to form a "bulky hand dressing" (Fig. 8.13).

When the fingers must be free, an alternate technique suitable for wounds of the palm or back of the hand is to make a modified figure-of-eight bandage out of a self-adhering roller bandage (Fig. 8.14). Anchor the bandage with several turns around the palm of the hand. Then, run the bandage diagonally across the back of the hand and secure it at the wrist with several circular turns. Repeat this sequence several times until the compress is firmly anchored.

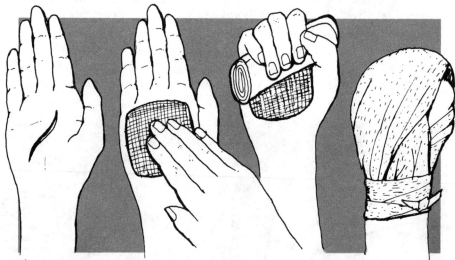

Fig. 8.13

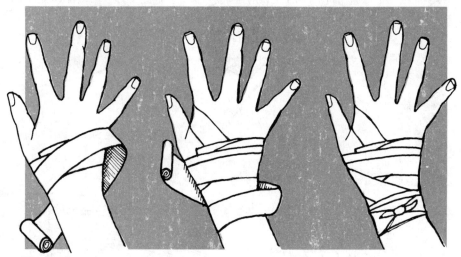

Fig. 8.14

Because **fingers** are hard to bandage, bandage strips (Bandaids, etc.) should be used whenever possible. Large finger wounds can be bandaged with a bulky hand dressing. An alternative is to modify the figure-of-eight bandage used for the hand (Fig. 8.15). Anchor the compress on the finger with multiple turns of a narrow, self-adhering roller bandage, which can be improvised if necessary by cutting a wider bandage lengthwise. Bring the bandage diagonally across the back of the hand, anchor it with several turns around the wrist, then bring it across the back of the hand again from the opposite side of the wrist to loop the finger. Repeat until the bandage is snug. Secure the loose end at the wrist.

In general, it is best to use a bandage whose width approximates the diameter of the part being bandaged:

a. Finger: 1 inch wide
b. Hand, wrist, small foot: 2 inches wide
c. Forearm, lower leg, foot: 3 inches wide
d. Upper arm, small thigh: 4 inches wide
e. Thigh, chest: 6 inches wide

Fig. 8.15 *Figure-of-eight Bandage Modified for the Finger*

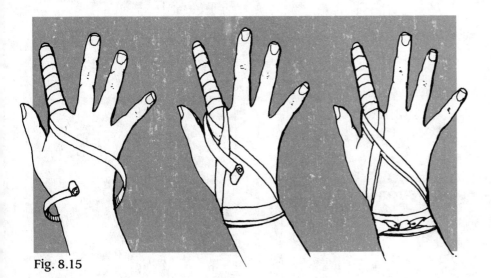

Fig. 8.15

9

Emergency Care of Bone and Joint Injuries: General Principles

The broken bone, once set together, is stronger than ever.

–John Lyly
Euphues

This chapter presents the general principles of emergency care of bone and joint injuries. The care of specific fractures, dislocations, and sprains of the upper and lower extremities and pelvis will be discussed in Chapters 11 and 12. The care of injuries of the neck and back will be covered in Chapter 14.

Before reading this chapter, review the anatomy and physiology of the musculoskeletal system in Chapter 2.

The three major types of bone and joint injuries are fractures, dislocations, and sprains.

FRACTURES

The term **fracture** is used for any break in the continuity of a bone. A fracture can range in severity from a hairline crack difficult to see on X-ray films to severe disruption with marked displacement and multiple fragments. The number of separate fragments, or **amount of comminution,** is roughly proportional to the magnitude, type, and direction of the forces involved in the injury.

Fractures can be classified in several ways:

Closed or Open Fractures

A **closed fracture** is one in which the overlying skin is intact (Fig. 9.1a). Most fractures are closed.

An **open fracture** involves a wound of the overlying skin (Fig. 9.1b), which can occur when the sharp ends of the fractured bone break the skin from within or when an object such as a bullet penetrates from the outside. A blunt force that fractures a bone also can produce a wound of the over-

Fig. 9.1 *Types of Fractures*

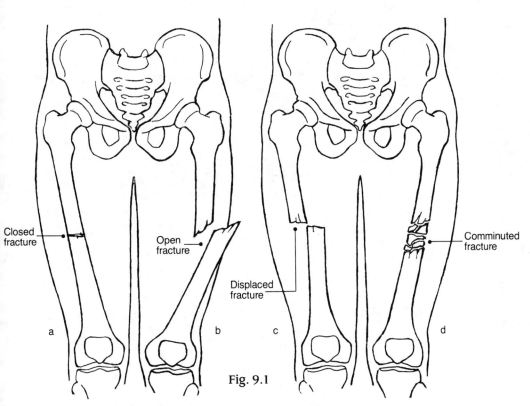

Closed fracture

Open fracture

Displaced fracture

Comminuted fracture

a   b   c   d

Fig. 9.1

Fig. 9.1 *Types of Fractures*

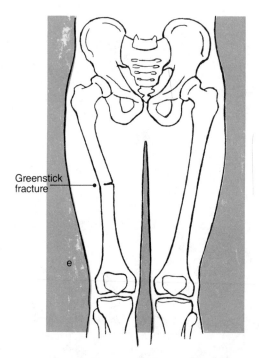

Greenstick
fracture

e

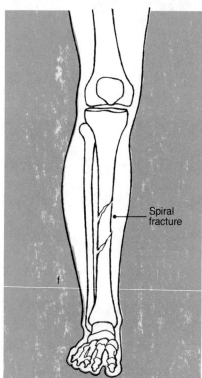

Spiral
fracture

f

Fig. 9.1

lying skin that does not necessarily connect anatomically with the fracture. Nevertheless, any fracture with an overlying skin wound is regarded as open. The skin wound may be tiny or large, and the bone can be visible or not visible in the wound.

Open fractures are very serious injuries. Bleeding tends to be more severe than in closed fractures and, because the fracture site is exposed to outside contamination, there is considerable danger of infection. Infections associated with open fractures may be difficult to treat and can cause life-long disability.

Displaced or Non-displaced Fractures

In a **displaced fracture,** the bone ends are moved out of their normal in-line position (Fig. 9.1c). Displacement, which is suspected based on the amount of **deformity** at the fracture site, can be minimal or marked. The distal part of the limb may be angulated or rotated, and the entire limb may be shortened because muscle spasm has caused the bone fragments to override.

A **non-displaced fracture** may or may not be deformed, although there usually is swelling and tenderness at the fracture site. X-ray examination may be required for diagnosis (Fig. 9.1a).

Fractures also can be classified as **simple, comminuted, greenstick, spiral, transverse,** and **stress.**

1. A **simple fracture** has only one fracture line (Fig. 9.1a, 9.1c).
2. A **comminuted fracture** has two or more fracture lines with three or more fragments (Fig. 9.1d).
3. A **greenstick fracture** is an angulated fracture through part of the bone shaft that occurs most commonly in the distal forearm and ankle. Because a greenstick fracture can occur only in elastic bones, it is seen only in children (Fig. 9.1e).
4. In a **spiral fracture,** the fracture line spirals around the shaft of the bone. These fractures are caused by rotational (twisting) forces; a common example is a spiral fracture of the lower leg bones, which can occur during a rotational fall when the skier's foot is fixed and the rest of the body can rotate (Fig. 9.1f).
5. In a **transverse fracture** (Fig. 9.1a), the fracture line is at or close to a right angle to the long axis of the bone. A common example is a transverse fracture of the lower leg bones, which can occur when a skier's bindings do not release during a forward fall over the ski tips.
6. A **stress fracture** is a hairline fracture caused by repeated small traumas to a bone. Stress fractures of the feet and legs are common in long-distance runners and should be suspected in patients who experience chronic localized pain made worse by running or walking.

When the topic of fractures is first studied, it is easy to focus on the dramatic aspects of the bone injury. For example, X-rays may reveal interesting and sometimes startling abnormalities. However, do not forget that significant soft-tissue damage can occur, particularly to nerves and blood vessels. Nerves and vessels can be injured by both the initial trauma and by the sharp ends of the fractured bone. Such damage contributes greatly to the resulting pain and disability.

Signs and Symptoms of Fractures

Any person who complains of pain after an injury is suspected to have a fracture. A child with a fracture may have *no* signs or symptoms other than pain.

Indications of a Fracture

1. **A suitable mechanism of injury** (see Chapter 10). A fracture should be suspected whenever there is trauma of suitable type and magnitude.
2. **Pain.** Pain may be mild but more typically is severe. The patient usually will be able to point to the site of pain with one finger. Pain almost always increases if the injured part is moved.
3. **Tenderness.** Tenderness usually is confined to the injury site and can be found by gentle palpation.
4. **Deformity.** Deformity is not always obvious. The injured extremity should be compared with the opposite, uninjured one.
5. **Sound.** The patient may have heard the bone snap.
6. **Function.** Usually, the patient loses partial or complete use of the limb. Occasionally, however, the patient is able to move the limb with little or no pain.
7. **Swelling and ecchymosis.** Bleeding into the tissues from the disrupted blood vessels causes swelling. As the blood works its way to the skin surface, ecchymosis develops. These signs take time to develop and may not be present initially.
8. **Crepitus and false motion. Crepitus** is a grating sensation caused by the broken bone ends grinding against each other. Limb motion where there is no joint is called **false motion**. These signs should *not* be deliberately elicited.
9. **Wounds.** Open fractures involve an open wound; sometimes exposed bone ends can be seen in the wound.

Within a few hours after a bone is fractured, a swelling composed of blood and inflammatory cells forms around and between the bone ends. The blood clots and, within a few days, other cells, including fibroblasts, begin to grow out into the clot, eventually uniting the broken bone ends with fibrous tissue. At first, this union is weak, but soon it begins to calcify and gradually become stronger. This calcified tissue, called a **callus,** eventually becomes as strong or stronger than the original bone.

Before a strong callus has been formed, motion at the fracture site can rebreak the bone and delay or prevent healing. Thus, a splint or cast must be used to prevent motion, allow proper healing, and control pain.

DISLOCATIONS

A **dislocation** is a disruption of a joint that occurs when the joint is forced to move beyond its normal range. Dislocations may be either complete or incomplete and may be associated with a fracture. During a dislocation, the joint capsule and ligaments are stretched or torn, and the bones of the joint may be completely displaced from their normal positions. A dislocated joint

Fig. 9.2 *Dislocations and Appear-ances of Shoulder and Hip Joints*

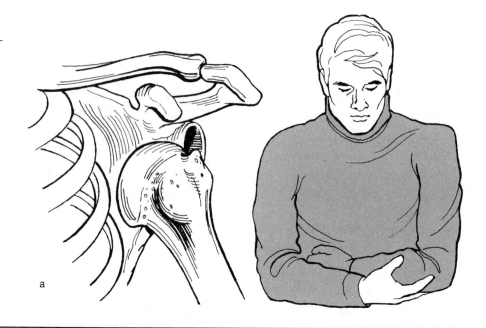

a

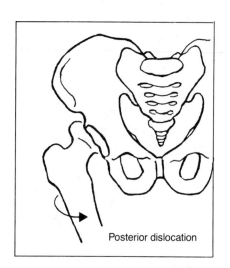

Posterior dislocation

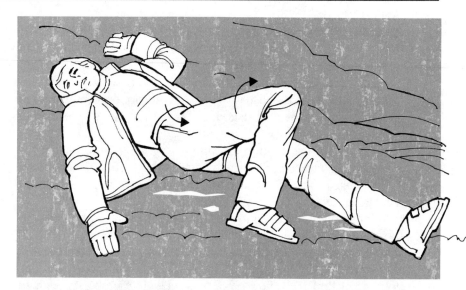

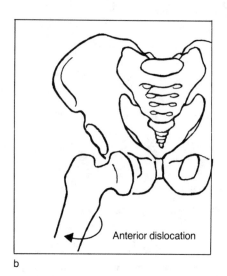

Anterior dislocation

b

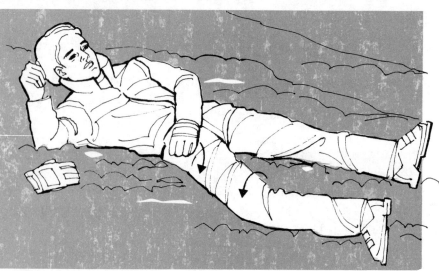

Fig. 9.2

frequently is locked in the displaced position, making an attempt to move it very painful.

The most commonly dislocated joints are those with less stability and a wide range of motion (e.g., the shoulder, Fig. 9.2a) and those whose location and type of use make them more susceptible to forces that can cause dislocation (e.g., the elbow, small joints of the fingers, the patella, and the ankle). Dislocations of the hip (Fig. 9.2b) also are common and usually are accompanied by a fracture of the deep joint cup (acetabulum). Dislocations of the knee and elbow are serious injuries because they frequently involve damage to nerves and blood vessels that can lead to loss of the limb.

Signs and Symptoms of Dislocations

It may be difficult to distinguish dislocations from fractures. However, a bone can be **dislocated** only where it forms a joint with another bone, but it can be **fractured** at any point. Fractures and dislocations can occur together.

Indications of a Dislocation

1. The **mechanism of injury** is one that can cause a dislocation (see Chapter 10).
2. **Pain** usually is more severe than would be expected for a fracture in the same area. Pain increases with any attempt to move the joint.
3. The joint has slight to marked **deformity** (comparison with the opposite side may be necessary).
4. Normal joint **motion** is lost.
5. There is **swelling** and **tenderness** over the joint.

SPRAINS

Sprains are produced in the same manner as dislocations, but by weaker forces. Stretching and tearing of the joint capsule and ligaments are less severe. The bones of the joint are not displaced and any deformity is minimal.

Sprains have three degrees of severity, depending on the extent of damage to the soft tissues supporting the joint. In **first-degree sprains,** the capsule and ligaments are stretched but not torn; in **second-degree sprains,** they are badly stretched or partly torn; in **third-degree sprains,** they are completely torn.

The most commonly sprained joints are the knee, ankle, and shoulder.

Signs and Symptoms of Sprains

1. **Tenderness,** which frequently can be located with a fingertip.
2. **Swelling and ecchymosis,** caused by edema and bleeding from injured small blood vessels.
3. **Pain** at the site of injury, which usually increases with joint motion.
4. **Loss of joint motion** because of pain.

Because the signs and symptoms are similar, it can be difficult to tell a severe sprain from a fracture. Because the goal of emergency care is the same for both–to reduce motion at the injury site–sprains should be splinted the same as fractures.

ASSESSMENT OF MUSCULOSKELETAL INJURIES

Try to determine the mechanism of the injury (see Chapter 10). Decide if the type, direction, and magnitude were sufficient to produce a fracture or dislocation or only a sprain or minor soft-tissue injury. After the primary survey has been completed and any life-threatening conditions have been treated, examine the patient's injury site or sites. Open all overlying clothing, preferably by cutting or ripping open a seam, and examine the site for wounds, swelling, tenderness, ecchymosis, and deformity. In cold weather, clothing removal may have to be minimized or postponed until the patient has been stabilized, splinted, and evacuated to a warm site such as a ski patrol first aid room.

Next, evaluate the state of the circulation and nerve supply below the injury. This is especially important with fractures and dislocations since many important nerves and blood vessels lie close to the bones and joints. Test motor function by asking the patient to squeeze your hand or wiggle his or her toes; test sensory function by determining whether the patient can feel a gentle pinch or a fingernail scrape. Check capillary refill time in a fingertip or toe tip. Check either the radial pulse at the wrist or the dorsalis pedis and posterior tibial pulses in the foot. It is difficult to examine the feet without removing shoes or boots; this may be a problem in cold weather, especially with ski injuries. If the patient can feel his or her toes wiggle, the remainder of the examination may be postponed until the first aid room is reached.

Unconscious patients present a special problem because they cannot be questioned about sensation nor asked to move. However, the patient's body can be examined for signs of injury, and the pulses and capillary refill time can be checked. The patient can be watched for spontaneous movement and for withdrawal of an extremity in response to a gentle pinch. (Injured extremities should not be tested this way.) Every unconscious, injured patient must be assumed to have an injured spine.

General Principles of Emergency Care for Musculoskeletal Injuries

The basic emergency care for all musculoskeletal injuries is **splinting.** Fractures, dislocations, and sprains may be difficult to tell apart in the field, so *if in doubt, splint.*

Purposes of Splinting

1. To prevent the jagged fragments of broken bones in fractures from grinding against each other or causing further damage to nerves, blood vessels, and other tissues.
2. To prevent accidental conversion of a closed fracture to an open fracture.
3. To reduce pain, swelling, and bleeding.
4. To prevent shock.
5. To allow greater ease in transport.
6. To prevent long-term disability and decrease rehabilitation time.

Proper splinting means immobilizing the joints *above* and *below* the injury to prevent motion from being transmitted to the injury site.

A fractured limb that is markedly deformed cannot be splinted unless the deformity is corrected. This process is called **alignment.** Careful alignment is unlikely to further damage the injured area. It is performed by gentle *manual axial* traction, meaning traction applied to the *long axis* of the extremity with the rescuer's hands and body and without mechanical devices. The fracture site should be exposed before this is done. Grasp the limb below the fracture site with both hands while an assistant supports the limb with one hand below and one hand above the break. Maintain gentle traction on the limb while straightening and, if necessary, rotating the limb into the most ana-tomically normal position possible.

Meanwhile, observe the fracture site to make sure the bone ends are not accidentally forced through the skin. Continue manual traction until the extremity has been splinted. If resistance or severe pain occurs, stop attempts to align the limb and splint it in the deformed position. The process of alignment is painful, but pain can be minimized by working smoothly and gently and by encouraging the patient to relax the muscles of the injured extremity.

Fractures of the ankle, lower leg, thigh, mid-forearm, mid-upper arm, and finger usually can be aligned safely when necessary. Attempts are not usually made to align spinal fractures or fractures near or associated with the knee, wrist, elbow, and shoulder joints, all of which should be splinted in the position in which they were found.

Because dislocations are frequently locked in the displaced condition, the type of alignment done with fractures is not possible with dislocations, and they should be splinted in the position in which they were found.

Circulation and nerve supply to the limb below the site of injury *must* be *checked* and *documented* before and after any attempt at alignment or splinting.

An injury that interrupts circulation to a limb may cause loss of the limb. An injury that damages a limb's nerve supply may cause permanent paralysis of the limb.

Signs of Loss of Circulation

1. Pulses distal to the injury are lost.
2. The part distal to the injury turns blue or white.
3. The part distal to the injury feels cold.
4. Pain worsens in the part distal to the fracture rather than at the fracture site.
5. Ability to move the part is lost or impaired.

Signs of Loss of Nerve Supply

1. Reaction to touch or pain is lost or impaired.
2. Numbness or complete loss of sensation develops distal to the injury.
3. Ability to move the limb distal to the injury is lost or impaired.

Because of the danger of tissue death or permanent disability, loss of circulation and/or nerve supply is an emergency, and the patient must be taken to a hospital as soon as possible. In the case of a fracture, if immediate medical help is not available, attempt to improve the circulation and/or nerve supply by correcting the fracture angle. Use the alignment process described earlier in this chapter. When alignment is successful, the pulses return and limb color and temperature eventually improve. Improvement in sensation and motion may take longer.

Even though dislocations in general should not be aligned, if a dislocation interrupts the circulation or nerve supply to an injured limb, the rescuer should gently attempt to change the angle of deformity. If the attempt is successful, splint the dislocation in the new position.

Dislocations of the knee and ankle present a special problem because they frequently are accompanied by severe disruption of the joint and by damage to nerves and blood vessels. A dislocated ankle often is fractured as well. In these cases, attempts at realignment and rapid transportation to a hospital are important because, if the blood supply is not reestablished within six hours, an amputation is likely.

Check and *document* the circulation and nerve supply to the limb below an injury *during the first assessment, before* and *after* alignment and splinting, and at *15-minute intervals* until the patient is transferred to the EMS system. In serious injuries with actual or potential damage to the circulation and nerve supply, the rescuer should feel the pulse and ask the patient to move parts distal to the injury (such as the fingers or toes). In less serious injuries, such as knee sprains, simply ask if the part distal to the injury is still comfortable and whether there has been any change in the way it feels. *Increasing pain* in an injured extremity may be an early indication of impaired circulation; this is an important sign that should be investigated and monitored closely.

These precautions reflect the dynamic nature of musculoskeletal injuries, which, even if properly splinted, may continue to swell, placing pressure on nerves and blood vessels.

Open fractures require special care because the overlying skin wound allows contamination of the fracture site. Before bandaging an open fracture, control bleeding by direct pressure and use sterile forceps to remove obvious foreign matter. However, the wound should not be probed. Wear sterile rubber gloves when caring for a patient with an open fracture.

It takes several hours for infection to develop in a contaminated wound. If the patient will not receive definitive medical care within this time it is preferable to clean the wound before bandaging and splinting the extremity. Cleaning is especially indicated for wounds that are very dirty. Wash the skin around the wound with povidone-iodine solution (Betadine), unless the patient is allergic to iodides, and flush the wound with sterile physiological saline. Pouring Betadine directly on the ends of a broken bone or into an open wound is controversial in emergency situations. To keep exposed bone ends moist, cover them with a sterile dressing saturated with sterile physiological saline.

On rare occasions, exposed bone ends may retract into the wound during alignment and splinting. Do not attempt to re-expose retracted bone ends or deliberately push bone ends into the wound. Remember that the purpose of traction splinting of an open fracture of the femur is to stabilize the fracture, *not* to pull the exposed bone ends back into the wound.

Shortly after the patient reaches the hospital, he or she will be taken to surgery and the injury will be opened and cleaned. Therefore, do not give the patient anything by mouth. Tell the hospital personnel *exactly* what type of emergency care was given in the field and whether the bone ends were initially exposed and retracted into the wound during splinting.

The emergency care of sprains involves providing support with a cravat or elastic bandage (see Fig. 9.11d), applying cold packs (as described for closed soft-tissue injuries in Chapter 8), and advising the patient to avoid putting weight on the injured extremity and to see a physician if symptoms do not subside within 24 hours.

Table 9.1

SUMMARY OF EMERGENCY CARE OF MUSCULOSKELETAL INJURIES

1. Expose and inspect the injury site.
2. Care for an open wound, if present.
3. If necessary, align a deformed fracture.
4. Splint the injured part.
5. Check and document circulation and nerve supply before and after alignment and splinting.
6. If circulation and/or nerve supply are impaired, attempt cautious alignment.
7. Treat sprains with support, cold packs, and by having the patient keep weight off the injured extremity.
8. Treat shock, if necessary.

GENERAL PRINCIPLES OF SPLINTING

This section presents in detail a few commonly used examples of each type of splint. Splints used by nordic ski patrols and other rescue groups that have to carry equipment on their backs tend to be lighter and simpler than splints used by alpine ski patrols and vehicle-based groups. Suggestions are included for improvising splints from natural materials and familiar equipment. However, no attempt is made to describe every variety of splint ever invented.

Splints are of three general types: **fixation, traction,** and **spine immobilization devices.** All are designed to prevent motion at the injury site, and most prevent motion at the joints above and below the site.

Either the splint or the patient should be well padded with foam or thick cloth to prevent pressure damage to superficial nerves and thin skin over bony projections. When metal splints are used, padding also prevents frostbite in cold weather and burns in hot weather. Splints should be made of a material that transmits X-rays so that complete films can be taken without removing the splint.

If possible, extremities should be splinted in the **position of function**. In the upper extremity, the shoulder is splinted next to the body, the elbow is bent to slightly less than a right angle, the wrist is bent slightly so that the hand is cocked upward, and the fingers are bent as if holding a ball. In the lower extremity, the hip should be splinted straight, the knee slightly flexed, and the ankle flexed to a right angle.

Fig. 9.3 *Types of Fixation Splints*

FIXATION SPLINTS

Fixation splints are simple devices that can be constructed from any rigid object of the proper size and shape. There are two types of fixation splints: **rigid** and **soft** (Fig. 9.3).

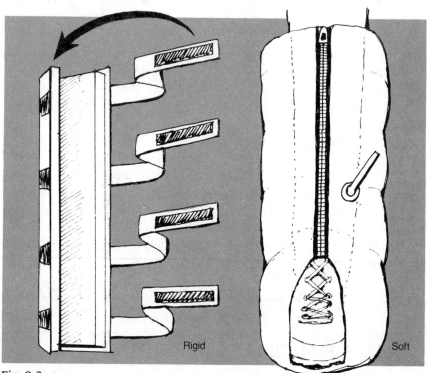

Fig. 9.3

Rigid Fixation Splints

Common examples of rigid fixation splints are plywood **"quick splints"** and **cardboard splints** for injuries to the lower extremity, and **wire, ladder,** and **malleable metal splints** for the upper extremity.

Quick splints are made of plywood padded with foam and are designed for rapid application on a ski hill so that the chilled patient can be quickly evacuated to a warm first aid room. Open the splint flat next to the injured extremity (Fig. 9.4a), loosen the patient's boot, and grasp the booted foot using slight axial traction, while an assistant provides support with one hand above and one below the injury site. The "pant leg pinch lift" (Fig. 9.4b) can be used to lift and support the extremity. Slide the splint underneath and gently lower the extremity onto the splint with the knee slightly flexed. Fold up the sides of the splint like a clamshell and secure them firmly against the extremity with laces or Velcro straps (Fig. 9.4c).

Cardboard splints are a favorite of ski patrols because they are effective, disposable, easy to apply, and inexpensive. A quick splint applied on the ski hill frequently will be replaced with a cardboard splint before the patient leaves the first aid room (Fig. 9.5). However, use judgment in deciding whether to subject a patient to a splint change. In general, do not change the splint if the patient has a very painful fracture, a bandaged open fracture, multiple injuries, or a fracture accompanied by shock.

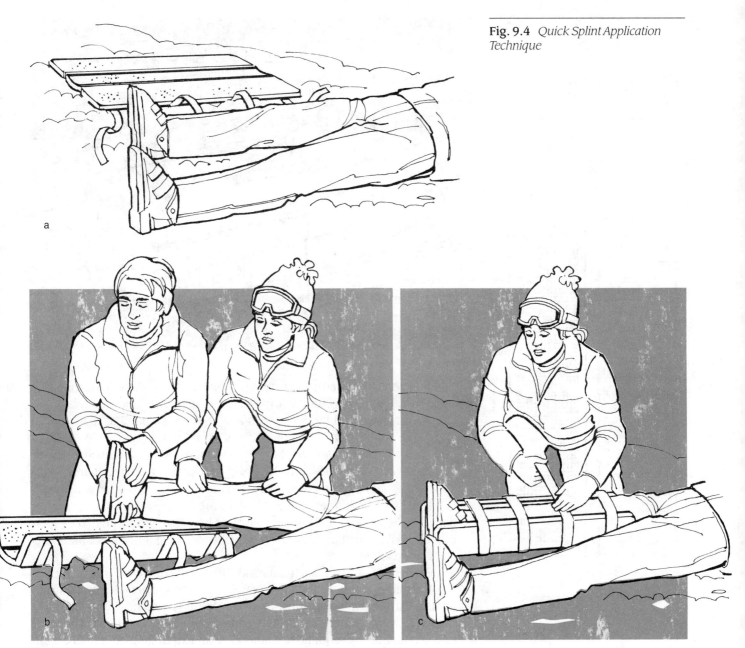

Fig. 9.4 *Quick Splint Application Technique*

Fig. 9.4

Cardboard splints can be purchased or made from sturdy single-corrugation packing box cardboard. A convenient size is 15 inches by 42 inches. Cut the splint so that the corrugations run lengthwise. Cardboard splints are tailor-made for each patient using the uninjured extremity as a guide. The splint should extend three-quarters of the way or more from knee to groin and be deep enough to contain the leg. Mark the bottom of the heel and cut the edges of the splint so that the end can be bent up at a right angle under the sole of the foot.

After removing the patient's boot, lift the injured extremity and slide the splint into position under it in the same manner as for the quick splint (Fig. 9.4b). Bend the end of the splint into position and anchor it with staples or tape. Protect the sides of the knee and ankle with padding, and place

Fig. 9.5 *A cardboard splint often replaces a quick splint in the first aid room.*

Fig. 9.6 *Wire and Ladder Fixation Splints*

Fig. 9.7 *Malleable Metal Splint*

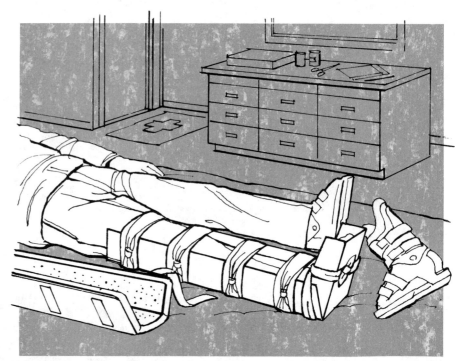

Fig. 9.5

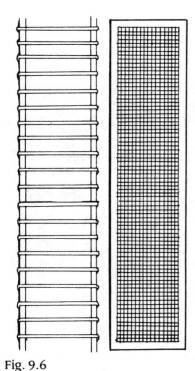

Fig. 9.6

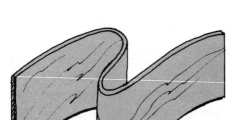

Fig. 9.7

padding under the knee to keep it slightly flexed. Fold up the sides of the splint and secure them in position with gauze roller bandage, tape, or cravats.

Wire splints and ladder splints (Fig. 9.6) can be purchased in several sizes. The smaller sizes are compact enough to fit into a ski patrol first aid belt. Commercial ladder splints (3 inches by 31 inches) are available with widely spaced rungs that allow X-rays to be taken with the splint on.

Wire splints also can be constructed from ⅛-inch or ¼-inch wire mesh. Practical sizes for homemade wire splints are 7 inches by 36 inches and 18 inches by 36 inches. The smaller splint can be rolled into a 2-inch by 7-inch cylinder. Fold 1-inch tape over all raw edges to avoid injury from the sharp ends of the wire.

Pad all wire and ladder splints and cut or bend them to fit the extremity. Lay the splints along the long axis of the extremity and bend them so that all joints are in the position of function. Then, secure the splints with self-adhering roller bandages or cravats. Depending on their strength, either one or two splints may be required to immobilize an extremity. The splints can be used doubled on one side of an extremity, placed on opposite sides of the extremity singly, or applied in a "sugar tong" shape.

Two small wire splints can be doubled over to increase their strength and used to splint upper arm or forearm fractures; position one splint on the front of the arm, the other on the back. Two large wire splints can be used to immobilize a leg or an ankle.

Malleable metal splints (Fig. 9.7) are made of soft sheet metal prepadded with thin sheets of foam glued to one or both sides. The SAM splint is one popular model. It measures 4¼ inches by 35½ inches and rolls into a 3-inch by 4¼-inch cylinder. It can be used singly or doubled, can be rounded sideways into a trough-like shape to better fit an extremity or bent into a sugar tong shape. Malleable metal splints can substitute for a wire or ladder splint or for an extrication collar. The material is soft enough to be cut, if necessary.

Soft Fixation Splints

Examples of soft fixation splints include **air splints, vacuum splints,** the **sling and swathe,** and **improvised splints** made from folded parkas, blankets, or pillows.

Air splints (see Fig. 9.3) are compact and light. While air splints are probably the best fixation splint for most wilderness rescue groups and nordic ski patrols, their relatively high cost and poor durability make them less practical for alpine ski patrols that handle large numbers of injured patients.

Air splints are double-walled bags of plastic or coated nylon. They usually have a zipper running the length of the splint. Air splints are available in sizes to fit the forearm, upper extremity, leg, or lower extremity.

To apply, unzip the air splint, lay it flat, and slide it under the extremity in a manner similar to positioning a quick splint. Fold the splint around the extremity and close the zipper. Inflate the splint by mouth, never with a pump (Fig. 9.8).

Fig. 9.8 *Air Splint*

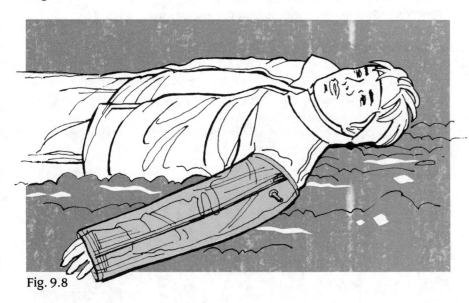

Fig. 9.8

Air splints are comfortable, need no padding, and can apply firm pressure to a bleeding wound, an advantage when a wound is so large that direct pressure by hand is difficult.

However, air splints do have a few problems. An air splint may cause the limb to perspire, which in cold weather may increase heat loss and lead to frostbite. It is essential to frequently monitor the splint and the circulation of the splinted extremity because the pressure inside an air splint may vary with changes in temperature and elevation. When an air splint is brought into a warm room from the cold, the air in the splint expands, tightening the splint. A similar complication can occur during altitude changes when an air splint is used on a patient being transported in an unpressurized aircraft. The splint will tighten on altitude gain and loosen on altitude loss. Once an air splint has been used, it should be partially inflated when stored in the cold. Otherwise, the walls of the splint may be bound together when the moisture that condenses from the breath freezes.

Vacuum splints also are double-walled airtight bags. A vacuum splint is filled with many tiny plastic pellets. After the vacuum splint is put in place, the

Fig. 9.9 *Sling and Swathe*
Fig. 9.10 *Improvised Fixation Splints*

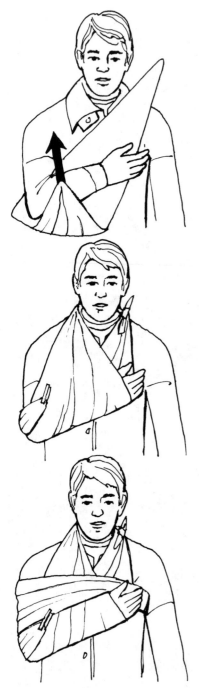

Fig. 9.9

residual air is evacuated with a suction pump, which draws the plastic pellets close together to form a rigid encasement around the injured part. Vacuum splints are expensive and somewhat bulkier and heavier than air splints.

A **sling and swathe** (Fig. 9.9) immobilizes upper-extremity injuries by using the chest wall as a splint. Bend the patient's elbow to just under a 90-degree angle and lay a triangular bandage on the chest wall under the arm. The bandage's long edge should run along the opposite mid-clavicular line just medial to the fingertips, and the upper corner should pass over the opposite shoulder. The apex should be just beyond the elbow. Bring the lower corner of the bandage anteriorly around the forearm, up over the injured shoulder, and tie the two ends together at the side of the neck. Bring the apex forward and pin it to the front of the sling. The tips of the fingers should be visible, and the forearm should be cradled in the sling with the weight of the forearm evenly distributed.

Fold a second triangular bandage to make a cravat about 3 inches wide. Wrap the cravat around the chest and arm of the patient and tie snugly under the opposite armpit. The sling and swathe is used for fractures of the clavicle and upper arm.

Improvised fixation splints (Fig. 9.10) can be made out of boards and other rigid or semirigid materials of the proper size and shape. A splint can be fashioned by rolling an inflatable mattress such as the Thermarest or a piece of Ensolite, or by folding a blanket, parka or pillow. Semirigid and soft improvised splints can be reinforced with branches or ice axes, if necessary. Padded pack straps and rolled newspapers and magazines make good splints for upper-extremity fractures.

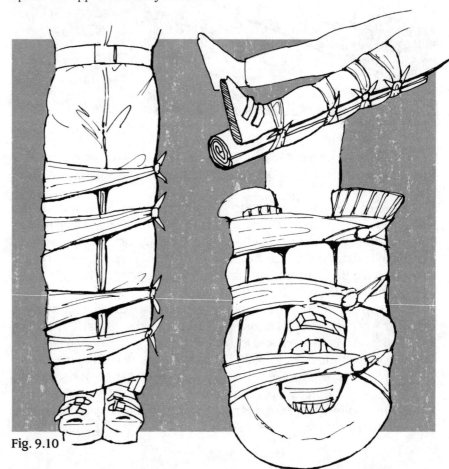

Fig. 9.10

Opposite, uninjured parts of the body can be used as splints. A fractured hip can be splinted by tying the injured lower extremity to the opposite extremity, and the chest wall can be used to splint upper-extremity fractures. A substitute for a sling can be made from a long-sleeved shirt or jacket by fastening the sleeve to the side of the garment with safety pins.

TRACTION SPLINTS

Traction splints are designed to counteract muscle spasm of the injured limb, which causes overriding of the broken bone ends, shortening of the limb, and laceration of the soft tissues with bleeding, increased pain, and the danger of shock. **Traction** consists of a pull parallel to the long axis of the broken bone and opposite to the pull of the major muscles.

In emergency care, the classic indication for a traction splint is a fracture of the midshaft of the femur. A traction splint also may be useful in oblique lower leg fractures that cause shortening and overriding of the fragments. Traction should *not* be used for fractures of the femur other than midshaft fractures or for upper-extremity injuries.

The prototype of the traction splint is the **Thomas splint** (Fig. 9.11), developed during World War I by Sir Hugh Owen Thomas. The original Thomas splint was a revolutionary device that dramatically reduced mortality from fractured femurs during that war. It consists of a rigid, longitudinal metal frame about 4 feet long, notched at the narrow end and attached at the wide end to a padded half-ring to which is fastened a strap with a buckle. The half-ring is angled to fit comfortably behind the upper thigh against the ischial tuberosity, and the strap is located so that it can be buckled in front of the thigh to keep the half-ring in place. Two people are needed to apply a Thomas-type traction splint. If the splint is adjustable, it should be measured against the uninjured side and adjusted so that the end of the splint extends 12 inches beyond the foot. To expose the injury site, remove overlying clothing (Fig. 9.12a) by cutting or ripping along a seam. Place the splint beside the injured extremity so that the long side will be on the outside of the extremity.

Prepare four cravats (or Velcro support straps) and lay them on the splint, spaced so that two will lie above the knee and two below the knee (Fig. 9.12b). Tie a 50-inch piece of ⅛-inch or ¼-inch nylon line to the end of the

Fig. 9.11 *Thomas Splint*

Fig. 9.12 *Application Technique for a Thomas Splint*
  a. *While maintaining manual stabilization, use a seam ripper to expose the injury site.*
  b. *Prepare the cravats and position the splint.*
  c. *Nylon line and a cravat are examples of two variations of a girth hitch.*
  d. *Apply a sprained ankle bandage as shown.*
  e. *Maintain manual stabilization while sliding the splint under the extremity.*
  f. *The pulley system for applying traction.*
  g. *Position cradle hitches over and around the extremity.*
  h. *The Spanish windlass is an alternative to the pulley system.*

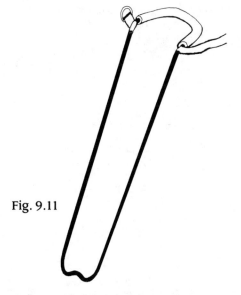

Fig. 9.11

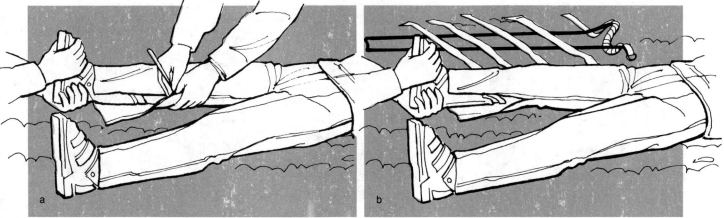

Fig. 9.12

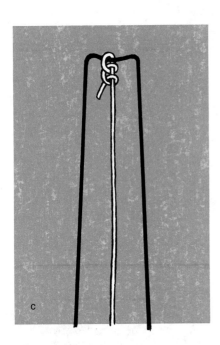

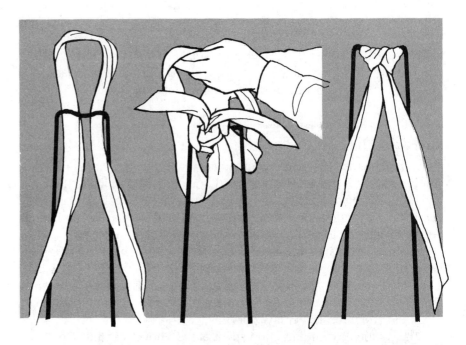

Fig. 9.12 *Application Technique for a Thomas Splint*

splint, or use a cravat (Fig. 9.12c). Next, one rescuer stabilizes the injured limb to prevent motion at the fracture site while the second rescuer puts an ankle hitch in place. This can be a sprained-ankle bandage made from a cravat or a commercial hitch made of nylon webbing (Fig. 9.13b).

To tie a sprained-ankle bandage (Fig. 9.12d), place the middle part of a 2-inch cravat in the instep of the boot of the injured extremity, forming a stirrup. The ends are crossed behind the ankle, brought around in front of the ankle and crossed again. Each end is run under the first part of the cravat on that side of the top of the foot, then pulled medially around it. The two ends are tied together in front of the ankle with a square knot. The cravat should be free of wrinkles and snug but not tight.

After the ankle hitch is in place, the second rescuer applies gentle axial traction to the foot, and the first rescuer supports the injury site while the extremity is raised several inches off the ground. A minimal amount of alignment may be necessary so that the extremity will fit into the splint. While supporting the injury site with one hand, the first rescuer slides the traction splint under the extremity until the half-ring is snugly in place against the ischial tuberosity (Fig. 9.12e).

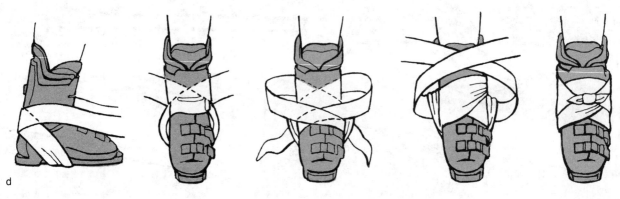

Fig. 9.12

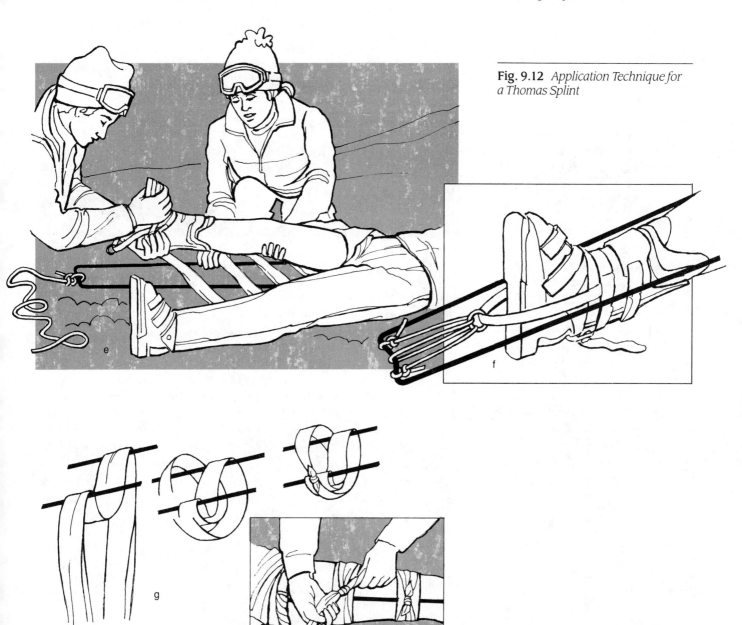

Fig. 9.12 *Application Technique for a Thomas Splint*

Fig. 9.12

Lay the end of the splint on a rock or block of wood so that it is a few inches off the ground and will not allow the patient's heel to touch the ground when the splint is in place. Maintain axial traction while the extremity is lowered onto the splint. The first rescuer buckles the strap in front of the upper thigh to hold the half-ring in place and threads the 50-inch nylon line through the stirrup of the ankle hitch, back over the end of the splint, and back through the stirrup again, forming a pulley system (Fig. 9.12f).

The first rescuer pulls the line tight and, as the second rescuer gradually releases traction, the first rescuer ties off the end of the line. The loose ends of each of the four cravats lying across the splint are reversed, brought under and around the opposite sides of the splint, over and around the extremity, and tied together at the side of the splint, forming a series of cradle hitches (Fig. 9.12g).

Fig. 9.12 *Application Technique for a Thomas Splint*

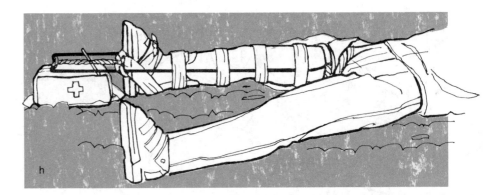

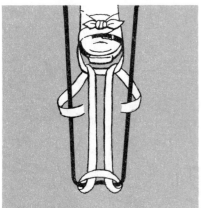

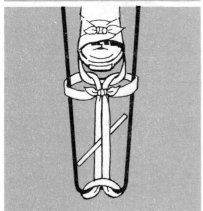

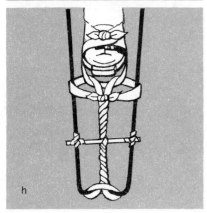

Fig. 9.12

A less-effective alternative to the pulley system described above is the venerable "Spanish windlass." In this method, a cravat or nylon cord is attached to the end of the splint at its midpoint with a girth hitch. The two loose ends are passed downward through the stirrup of the ankle bandage, run laterally around the bars of the splint, and tied together with a square knot. A short stick or dowel inserted between the two ends midway between the foot and the end of the splint is twisted to produce the desired amount of traction. The stick then is taped to the sides of the splint (Fig. 9.12h).

Commercially available modifications of the Thomas splint, such as the Hare splint (Fig. 9.13a), use Velcro straps instead of cradle hitches and a ratchet at the end of the splint to provide traction. Commercially available ankle hitches (Fig. 9.13b) are more comfortable and simpler to apply, but some are too small to fit over ski boots or heavy mountaineering boots. There are special conversion kits that give an ordinary Thomas splint some of the features of a Hare splint. Rescuers should not choose a splint that uses mechanical traction unless they know how to use it properly. If applied too tightly, such devices are uncomfortable and can cause pressure damage to the buttock or even loss of pulses in the foot from pressure around the ankle.

Several recently developed devices for traction are portable, lightweight, readily adjustable, and compact enough so that a splinted patient will easily fit into a helicopter. The Sager splint (Fig. 9.14) weighs less than 4½ pounds and breaks down to fit into a tapering package that measures 32 inches by 6 inches by 4 inches. It has a single longitudinal support that can be positioned to either the inside or the outside of the lower extremity. The Kendrick traction device is a similar splint that weighs about 20 ounces. Because of their small size and weight, these two splints are probably the best choices for wilderness rescue groups. Oversnow rescue groups may prefer to improvise traction splints from ski poles as described below.

The following is a summary of how to apply the Sager splint to the inside of the lower extremity. Also consult the manufacturer's directions.

1. Expose the fracture site and remove the splint from its case. Attach the foam-covered, T-shaped groin piece to the top of the splint. Adjust the plastic buckle so that, when closed, it will be on the front of the thigh. Estimate the necessary splint length by holding the splint next to the lower extremity so that the wheel is at the heel.

2. Slide the thigh strap under the extremity so that the groin piece is snug against the crotch and the ischial tuberosity. Patients wearing tight jeans or underclothing, especially men, may find this position uncomfortable unless the tight clothing is removed or cut open.

3. Close the buckle and tighten the thigh strap so that the groin piece is drawn sideways into the crotch.
4. Estimate the size of the ankle, and fold the number of pads (included) needed to provide padding around the ankle. Remove the patient's boot and sock, and apply the ankle harness tightly around the ankle above the malleoli. Check foot pulses before and afterward.
5. Shorten the loop of the harness connected to the cable ring by pulling on the strap threaded through the square D-buckle.
6. Extend the splint by pressing down on the red thumb piece and sliding the inner part out until the desired amount of traction is noted on the calibrated wheel. A rough guide is 10 percent of body weight up to a maximum of 22 to 25 pounds, with 10 to 15 pounds being average traction.
7. Strap the splint to the extremity by applying the three 6-inch-wide straps. Place the longest as high on the thigh as possible. Pad the area between the metal bar and the extremity. Apply the second longest strap around the knee and the shortest over the ankle harness and lower leg. Apply the figure-of-eight strap over and around the ankles to hold the extremities together.

Fig. 9.13 *Commercial Modifications of the Thomas Splint*

Fig. 9.14 *Sager Splint*

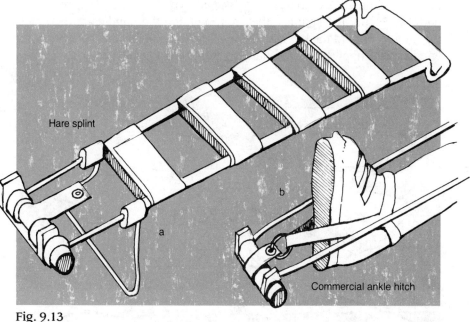

Hare splint

b

a

Commercial ankle hitch

Fig. 9.13

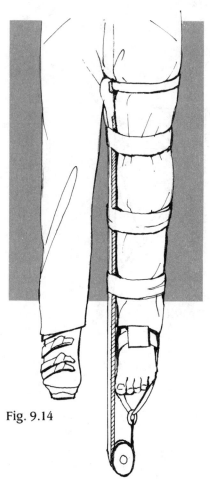

Fig. 9.14

Improvised Traction Splints

If standard traction equipment is not available, a Thomas-type of traction splint can be improvised from a single ski or from two ski poles.

For the **single-ski technique** (Fig. 9.15), purchase or prepare in advance two canvas pockets to slip over each end of the ski. Each pocket should have a grommet on one side of the base. Cravats can substitute for the pockets. To construct the splint, slip the pockets in place, with the tail of the ski toward the patient's armpit, the tip turned out, and the grommets facing the patient.

One rescuer applies steady manual traction to the foot until splinting is completed. Run a cravat around the patient's upper thigh and snug it up into the patient's groin. Tie the tails of the cravat through the grommet of the tail

Fig. 9.15 *Improvised Traction Splint Using a Single Ski*

Fig. 9.16 *Improvised Traction Splint Using Two Ski Poles*

pocket. Apply an ankle bandage or hitch to the boot. Apply traction to the boot in the manner described above for the Thomas splint, using either a nylon cord run in pulley-fashion through the grommet of the tip pocket and the stirrup of the ankle hitch, or a Spanish windlass with a cravat or cord.

Pad any areas where the lower extremity touches the ski. Wrap several wide cravats around the limb and ski from ankle to lower thigh. Support the tip of the ski to keep the patient's heel off the ground. After securing traction, stabilize the splint by wrapping cravats around the upper end of the ski and the chest, and by tying the uninjured leg to the splint.

An acceptable type of Thomas splint can be made from two ski poles, provided they are long enough. **The two-ski-pole technique** (Fig. 9.16) is the emergency traction splint of choice for ski tourers and oversnow wilderness rescue groups. Interlace or tie the pole straps together to form a half-ring no greater than one-half the thigh circumference. Join the baskets with a spreader such as an 8-inch length of ski pole that has two holes drilled in it the proper distance apart. Lay four cravats to use as cradle hitches across the two poles, apply an ankle bandage, and attach a cravat or nylon cord to the spreader.

Use manual traction in the same manner as for the Thomas splint. Slip the splint under the extremity so that the padded pole straps ride up under the buttock. Secure the splint at the groin by tying the handles of the poles together in front of the hip with a cravat. Set up a pulley device or Spanish windlass and apply traction. Finally, tighten the cradle hitches in place.

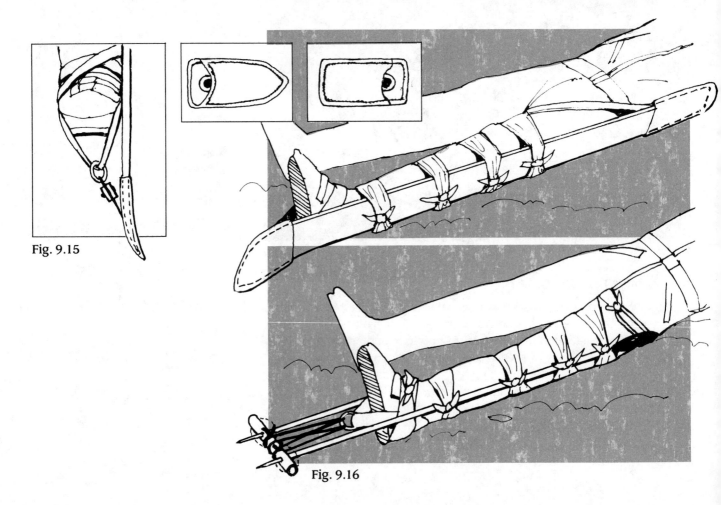

Fig. 9.15

Fig. 9.16

Traction can be applied to the lower extremity of a patient on a scoop stretcher (see **Spine Boards,** below) by using the metal bar that forms the end of the stretcher as an anchor for a nylon cord pulley or Spanish windlass. However, the patient's torso must be immobilized on the stretcher to keep the traction from pulling the patient toward the end of the stretcher. Use two cravats to immobilize the torso. Loop one around each thigh at the groin and tie them off to the side bar through a handhold.

SPINE IMMOBILIZATION DEVICES

Spine immobilization devices for neck and spine injuries include the various types of spine boards and extrication collars.

Spine Boards

In emergency care for back and neck injuries, the patient must be strapped to a spine board to prevent bending or rotating the neck or back. Spine boards also are useful for fractures of the hip and pelvis, dislocations of the hip, and in multiple fractures where individual splinting of each fracture may be impractical. Spine boards must be small enough to fit inside ski patrol toboggans and helicopters.

The board is made from ¾-inch high-density marine plyboard 72 inches by 17 inches. It is finished on both sides, sanded, and then shellacked. The handholds, which can double as strap holes, have rounded edges that measure 5 inches by 1¼ inches and are 1¼ inches from the edge of the board. Strap holes are ½ inch by 3 inches and are ¾ inch from the edge of the board. The runners are 1-inch half-rounds with tapered ends to elevate the board so that the bearers can insert their hands under the board into the handholds. The ends of the runners and the board are taped to allow the board to slide easily. The patient is secured to the board with either four adjustable straps of wide nylon webbing or a continuous lacing of 1-inch tubular nylon webbing. Rolled towels or a blanket (used to immobilize the head and neck) and extra cravats are kept in a stuff-sack stored with the board.

The aluminum scoop stretcher (Fig. 9.17) is a recent variation of the spine board. The scoop stretcher is adjustable in length and breaks apart longitudinally into two halves that are slid under the patient from either side until they meet in the middle, eliminating the need to lift or logroll the patient onto a spine board. However, the patient must be accessible on both sides for this method to work. One version of the stretcher folds in thirds so that it can be carried on a pack frame. Because the scoop stretcher is not as rigid as a spine board, it is not recommended for immobilizing patients with neck and back injuries. Special care must be taken to securely strap the patient to the stretcher so it can safely be tipped to the side if the patient vomits.

Vacuum spine boards based on the same principles as the vacuum splint also are available.

Long Spine Board Application Technique (Fig. 9.18)

The patient usually should be strapped to a backboard in the supine position. If the patient is not found in the supine position, he or she must be turned without bending or rotating the neck or back. If possible, at least four rescuers should be used for this maneuver.

Fig. 9.17 *Scoop Stretcher*

Lay the long spine board on the ground next to the patient. Using the **four-person logroll** (Chapter 14), the **straddle slide** (Chapter 14), or the **four-person direct ground lift** (Chapter 20), transfer the patient to the board. If the patient has a neck injury, apply an extrication collar (technique is described below) beforehand and continue manual stabilization of the head and neck during transfer. Check and record sensation and motion below the injury site before and after transfer.

Secure the patient's trunk and lower extremities to the board. This is somewhat difficult and requires at least four nylon straps: one around the chest just below the armpits, one around the hips, one around the thighs, and one around the ankles. Cravats also may be required.

Cross the patient's hands and tie the wrists together loosely with a cravat to keep the upper extremities from flopping to the side. Use cravats to tie the arms (which should be outside the chest strap) to the board. Put padding beneath the small of the back and the knees.

An alternative to using straps and cravats is to substitute 1-inch tubular webbing laced from one side of the board to the other back and forth across the patient's body. Double a piece about 40 feet long and attach its midpoint to the middle of the spine board at one side, using a girth hitch through a straphole. Use one end to secure the chest and shoulders and the other to secure the abdomen, hips, and lower extremities.

Secure the head by placing a head support on either side of the head and running a cravat, Velcro strap, roller bandage, or adhesive tape firmly across the forehead. Do *not* use a chin strap. A chin strap cannot adequately secure the head because of the mobility of the jaw. Also, a patient who vomits with a chin strap in place may choke. Head supports should be firm, lightweight, and noncompressible. Firmly rolled towels are ideal. Large bath towels can be folded to one-quarter width lengthwise and rolled to form cylinders 5 to 6 inches in diameter, or two smaller towels can be folded in half lengthwise and rolled.

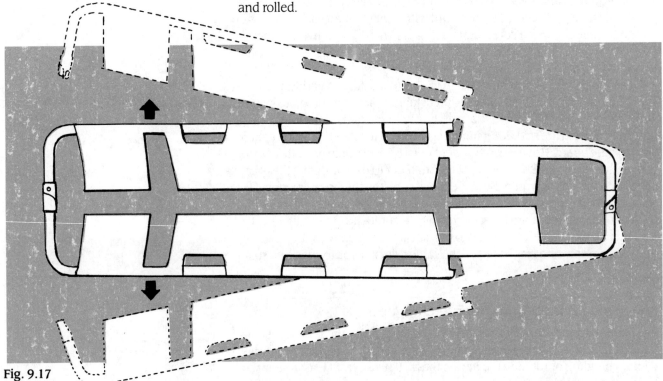

Fig. 9.17

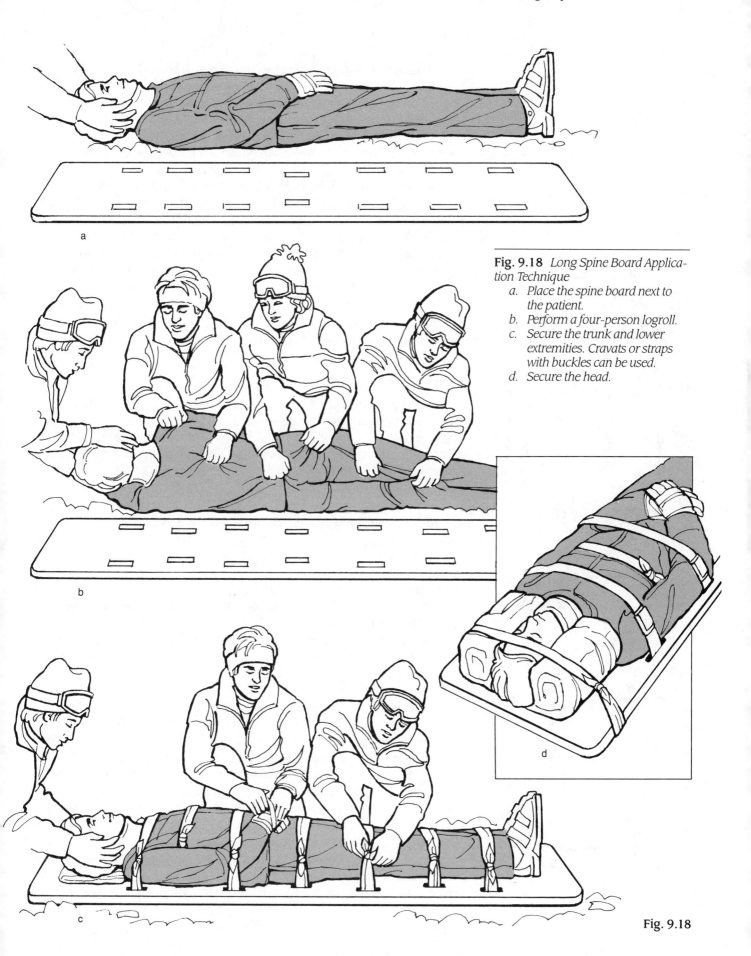

Fig. 9.18 *Long Spine Board Application Technique*
a. *Place the spine board next to the patient.*
b. *Perform a four-person logroll.*
c. *Secure the trunk and lower extremities. Cravats or straps with buckles can be used.*
d. *Secure the head.*

Fig. 9.18

Fig. 9.19 *Short Spine Board*

Fig. 9.20 *Kendrick Extrication Device (KED)*

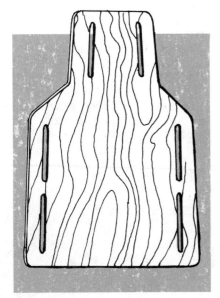

Fig. 9.19

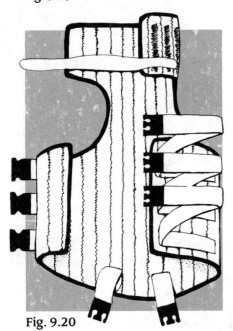

Fig. 9.20

Another good technique is to make a "horse collar" out of a rolled blanket folded into a U-shape. Do not use sandbags because, if the board is tipped on its side, their weight may make them sag and cause the neck to bend. Head immobilizers also are commercially available.

Because of individual variations in neck length and amount of back curve, it may be necessary to insert padding under the patient's head to prevent the neck from overextending. Estimate the amount of padding needed by slipping a finger behind the head to gauge the distance between the occiput and the board. While this check is being done, a second rescuer must stabilize the patient's head in the proper position. The patient should be strapped to the board with enough properly tightened straps so that the board can be tipped to the side without shifting the patient. Tipping may be necessary to aid in airway management and to avoid aspiration if the patient vomits.

If the board will be inclined from the horizontal position, cravats or straps should be fastened around both thighs at the groin and around the chest under the armpits to keep the patient from sliding.

Short Spine Boards

Short spine boards were developed to evacuate patients with spine injuries found sitting in wrecked automobiles. They are equally valuable for immobilizing the necks and spines of patients who must be extricated from awkward positions, such as extricating climbers from narrow ledges or crevasses, skiers from thick timber or tree wells, and cavers from narrow cave passages.

A short spine board (Fig. 9.19), which can be made from a piece of marine plyboard, should measure about half the length (36 inches) of a long spine board.

To position the short spine board, one rescuer stabilizes the patient's head and neck, while a second rescuer puts an extrication collar in place. Continue manual stabilization until the patient is immobilized on the short board. Slide the short board behind the patient so that its bottom is level with the patient's hips.

Secure the board to the patient's torso with cravats or straps. One strap goes around the chest under the armpits and a second strap goes around the abdomen below the costal arches. The patient's arms are placed at his or her sides and secured with a third cravat around the chest and upper arms.

Place a rolled towel on each side of the patient's head, and secure the head to the board with a cravat or adhesive tape across the forehead.

Next, carry the patient to a site where he or she can be fastened to a long spine board. The two-person seated carry (Chapter 20) is a suitable method to use. *Do not* use the board as a handle for moving or lifting the patient. A more practical device for wilderness rescue groups is a portable short spine board made of nylon strengthened with vertical slats. The board has longitudinal rigidity but can be rolled into a small cylinder for backpacking. Two examples are the Kendrick extrication device (KED) and the Oregon spine splint.

The Kendrick extrication device (Fig. 9.20) was the first to be developed. It weighs about 6½ pounds and rolls up into a package about 32½ inches by 9 inches by 5 inches. A patient extricated with a short spine board in place should be fastened to a long spine board or placed into a litter such as the Thompson or SKED before being transported.

The following is a summary of how to apply the KED. Also consult the manufacturer's directions.

1. Continue to stabilize the head and neck until the KED and an extrication collar have been applied.
2. Open the KED flat on the ground next to the patient. With a rescuer on either side of the patient, slide the device into place behind the patient's back. Place the smooth side (without the Velcro) next to the back, and center the KED along the spine. Loosen the chest restraints. Pull the leg restraints from behind the patient and lay them out of the way.
3. Wrap the chest flaps around the patient and loosely buckle the middle and lowest chest restraints. Use the lift handles to raise the KED until the tops of the chest flaps press firmly under the patient's armpits. Now, tighten the two lower restraints.
4. Apply the leg restraints by passing them under each thigh, pulling the ends up between the legs, coupling the buckle to the same side, and tightening both restraints. Do not use leg restraints if a femur fracture is suspected.
5. Fill any gap between the KED and the patient's neck with the supplied pad or other padding. Wrap the head flaps around the patient's head and hold them in place by fastening the Velcro straps over the forehead. Couple and tighten the upper chest restraint. Check all other restraints and tighten if necessary.

A spine board can be improvised from a long sturdy board, a door, or two skis fastened rigidly side by side with crosspieces such as thick tree branches.

Extrication Collars

An extrication collar (Fig. 9.21), formerly called a cervical collar, provides firm, rigid support around the neck to prevent the head from turning and the neck from bending. This support protects the spinal cord from damage by sharp fragments of a fractured vertebra. Unfortunately, all currently available collars allow excessive movement in flexion, extension, rotation, and lateral bending. Therefore, *do not rely upon the collar alone to stabilize a neck injury*. An extrication collar must always be accompanied by manual stabilization or fixation to a spine board. The most important function of an extrication collar is probably to *call attention to the presence of a neck injury*.

Use only *rigid* extrication collars. An easily portable collar is the Stifneck, which can be folded flat. The SAM splint, mentioned above, can be molded into a suitable extrication collar. Collars also can be improvised from a rolled blanket or parka reinforced with a wire splint.

Fig. 9.21 *Stifneck Extrication Collar*

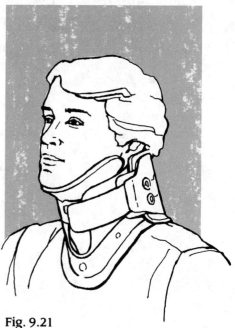

Fig. 9.21

10

Mechanisms and Patterns of Injury

Accident, n. An inevitable occurrence due to the action of immutable natural laws.

−Ambrose Bierce
The Devil's Dictionary

Injuries in the outdoors are not random examples of the workings of capricious Fate, nor are they the deliberate actions of malevolent gods. The production of injuries is governed by certain laws of physics, anatomy, and physiology. Knowledge of these laws enables one to *understand* how injuries occur and why some injuries are more common than others; *predict* the types and severity of injuries likely to have resulted from an accident based on observation of the accident scene; and *anticipate* the development of life-threatening complications.

The ease with which body parts are injured depends on their tissue characteristics, the mechanics of their construction, their location, and the manner and frequency of their use.

An elastic tissue such as the skin will deform when a force is applied to it. As the force increases, the threshold of injury eventually will be exceeded, and the skin will be torn or contused. Because skin is soft and elastic it can be easily deformed without injury, but it also is more susceptible than harder tissues to cuts and punctures. On the other hand, the hardness and inelasticity of bone make it more resistant to cuts and punctures but less resistant to fracture from deforming forces. Solid organs, such as the spleen and liver, are more susceptible to rupture from deforming forces than are hollow organs, such as the stomach or bladder. However, hollow organs may be more easily injured when they are distended with fluid. Flexible organs that are rigidly anchored, such as the aorta, are more susceptible to injury from shearing forces than are organs that can move within body cavities, such as the intestines.

Organs that are protected by parts of the skeletal system, such as the brain, spinal cord, and the organs of the chest and pelvic cavities, are less prone to injury than less-protected organs, such as those of the abdominal cavity. The usual activities of daily life injure the extremities more often than the trunk. The extremities are susceptible to injury because they are frequently in motion, are located more peripherally, have less protection, and often are used to protect the trunk from injury, e.g., extending the arms to break a fall. The shoulder joint, which has a shallow cup and a wide range of motion, is more often injured than the hip joint, which has a deep cup and a narrower range of motion. If the mechanics of a fall allow the development of a fulcrum point, a long, narrow extremity can function as a lever, focusing and multiplying the forces many times.

Most injuries are associated with motion–either motion of the body itself or motion of another object that impacts the body. Therefore, the student should be familiar with the physical laws of motion and with the laws of kinetic energy in particular.

The term **force** is used for any action that changes the state of rest or motion of a body to which it is applied. A **body** is any mass of matter that is distinct from other masses of matter. **Energy** is the capacity for doing work. It can be either **potential energy**, which is derived from the position of a body in a gravity field with respect to its own parts or to another body, or **kinetic energy**, which is energy created by motion.

The terms **trauma** (the plural is traumata) and **injury** frequently are used interchangeably. Both refer to damage to the body by an external force. However, in this chapter, trauma refers to the end effect of a force applied to the body, and injury will refer to the actual body damage produced.

Newton's First Law of Motion states that a body at rest will tend to remain at rest and a body in motion will tend to remain in motion unless acted upon by an outside force. For example, a moving skier will continue to move in a straight line unless he or she applies energy through the leg muscles to produce a turning motion (Fig. 10.1a) or collides with an obstacle such as a tree (Fig. 10.1b).

The Law of Conservation of Energy states that energy can neither be created nor destroyed but may be changed from any form to any other form. For example, the energy of a moving object that strikes the body does not just disappear; it **dissipates** as it deforms and injures the body tissues. The amount of injury is roughly proportional to the amount of energy that has to be dissipated.

The amount of kinetic energy of a body in motion is equal to one-half the product of the mass of the body times the square of the velocity. Thus, when E_k = kinetic energy, M = mass, and V = velocity, $E_k = M/2 \times V^2$.

The important thing to remember about kinetic energy is that it increases in *direct* proportion to the increase in mass but is compounded as the *square* of the velocity as velocity increases. For example, a 150 pound (68 kilogram) skier traveling at 15 miles per hour (24 kilometers per hour) has a kinetic energy of 16,875 units. A skier who weighs one-third more (200 pounds or 91 kilograms) and is traveling at the same speed has a kinetic energy that is one-third greater (22,500 units). A 150-pound skier traveling at 30 miles per hour (48 kilometers per hour) has *four times* (not twice) the kinetic energy (67,500 units). If a skier hits a tree, the kinetic energy is dissipated by crushing or tearing the skier's body. Thus, hitting a tree at 30 miles per hour can theoretically cause *four times* as much damage as hitting a tree at 15 miles per hour. (However, remember that the skier can be just as dead after a 15-mile-per-hour collision as after a 30-mile-per-hour collision.)

Another important type of kinetic energy is the energy of a falling body. Because of the force of gravity, a falling body increases its speed by 32 feet per second every second, regardless of its mass.

Kinetic energy causes injury because it is applied to the body in the form of a force. Forces have both strength (magnitude) and direction. They act on the body to speed up (accelerate), slow down (decelerate), and/or change the direction of its motion.

TYPES OF TRAUMA

Changes in speed or direction can lead to the following types of **trauma**: **penetration, compression** (blunt trauma), **bending, rotational,** and **stretching**. Bending trauma is further divided into **hyperflexion** and **hyperextension**. Pure examples of injuries caused by one force and one type of trauma are unusual; most serious injuries involve more than one force and type of trauma.

The specific injury depends on the magnitude and direction of the force or forces, the type of trauma, and the body part involved. The effects of trauma can be modified by wearing protective devices such as helmets and seat belts. The type of surface that impacts the body and the rate of **deceleration** or **acceleration** also are important. Landing in deep powder snow after a fall is less dangerous than landing on ice or concrete. Because the rate of

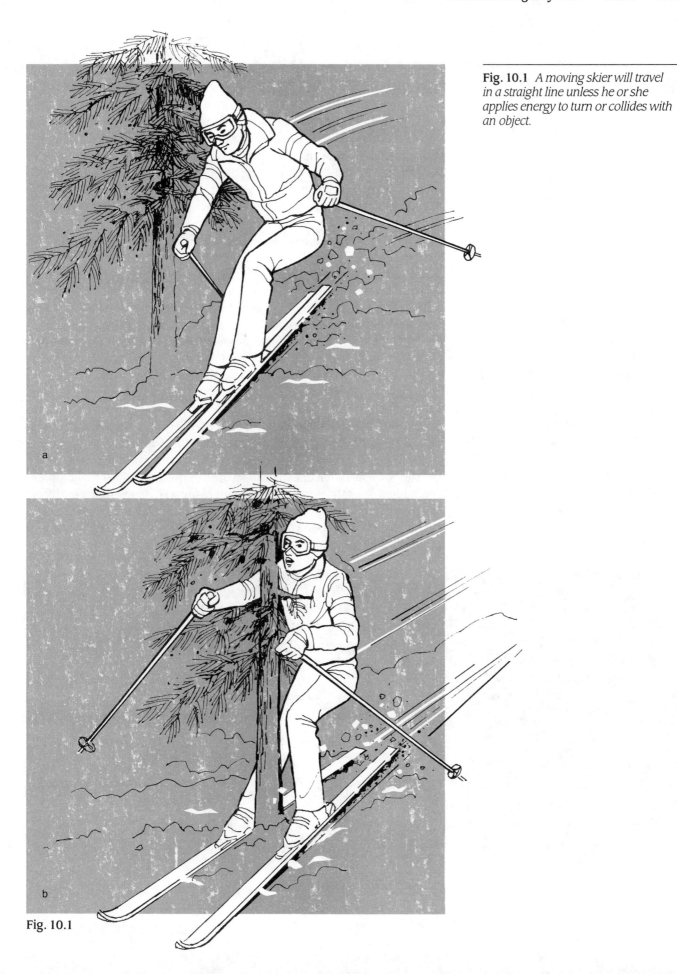

Fig. 10.1 *A moving skier will travel in a straight line unless he or she applies energy to turn or collides with an object.*

Fig. 10.1

Fig. 10.2 *Compression and penetration traumata are produced when a collision stops motion abruptly.*

deceleration is slower, it is less dangerous to be in a car that runs into a soft snowbank or a stand of thick bushes than to be in a car that hits a brick wall at the same speed.

Penetration and compression traumata are caused by similar forces. The difference is that, in penetration trauma, the wounding object is smaller in diameter and/or the force of impact is relatively greater, so that the force per unit area is great enough to drive the object through the skin. Damage to deeper tissues may be much greater than indicated by the size of the entry wound. Penetration trauma can be caused by bullets, ice axes, ski pole tips, arrows, and other sharp objects moving at moderate to high speeds, or by a moving body striking a narrow, pointed object such as a broken tree limb (see Fig. 10.1b).

In compression trauma, the wounding object is larger in diameter and/or the force is weaker, so that the skin is not broken (Fig. 10.2). However, compression trauma frequently damages tissues beneath the skin, causing a closed wound such as a contusion or hematoma.

The types of trauma and the various actions of forces can be further defined using several common accident patterns. An example of **deceleration** is a head-on collision between a skier and a tree. As the skier strikes the tree, the body comes to an abrupt halt, and its kinetic energy is dissipated through the production of various types of trauma (Fig. 10.3). The specific types of trauma depend on the skier's speed, the position of the skier's body as it strikes the tree, the angle of impact, the rate of deceleration, the skier's physical condition, and whether the skier is wearing protective clothing.

The body parts that directly impact the tree trunk are subject to compression trauma (blunt trauma), which squeezes the soft tissues, rupturing blood vessels and producing contusions and hematomas. Compression trauma can break underlying bones, such as the skull and ribs, and bruise or rupture internal organs. A glancing blow or impact with a sharp part of the tree, such

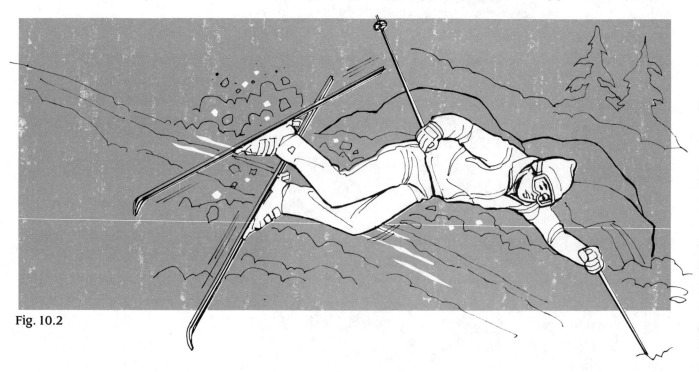

Fig. 10.2

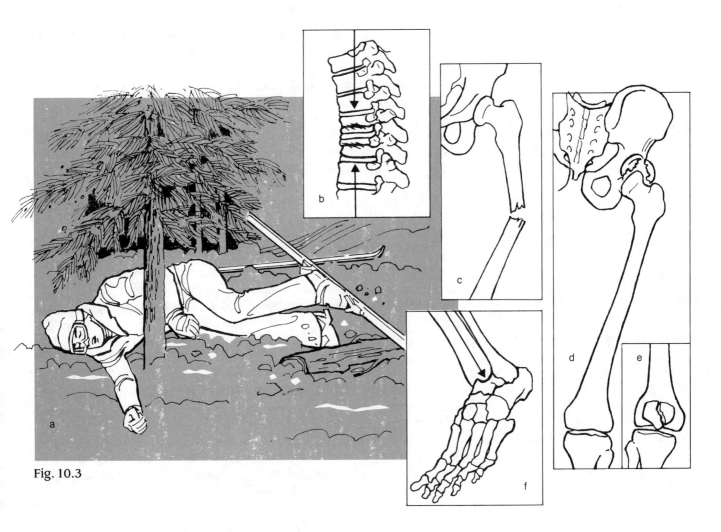

Fig. 10.3

as a broken branch, can produce a laceration, abrasion, or penetration trauma. An open chest or abdominal wound can result from penetration trauma.

If the skier strikes the tree at an angle that impacts the mid-torso and bends the upper and lower parts of the body like a horseshoe around the tree, the **hyperflexion** type of **bending trauma** can result (Fig. 10.3a). This type of trauma can cause wedge fractures or fracture-dislocations (see Fig. 10.3b) of the spine as well as the types of compression and penetrating trauma described above. If the skier strikes the tree with the midthigh, hyperflexion trauma can produce a midshaft fracture of the femur (Fig. 10.3c). Striking a tree with a bent knee can bring the femur to a sudden halt while the pelvis and the rest of the body continue to move forward. This situation, which is also common in automobile accidents when an occupant's knee strikes the dashboard, can cause a femur fracture or a fracture-dislocation of the hip joint (Fig. 10.3d) as the force is transmitted up the femur and pops the head of the femur out through the rear of the acetabulum. The patella also can be fractured as a result of compression trauma (Fig. 10.3e).

If this skier's other foot is wedged under a log for a half hour or longer before it is freed, the resulting tissue damage is a slowly developing type of compression trauma called a **crushing injury** (Fig. 10.3a, 10.3f). A crushing

Fig. 10.3 *Types of Injuries Produced by a Collision*
- *a.* *Hyperflexion Type of Bending Trauma*
- *b.* *Vertebra Compression Fracture*
- *c.* *Midshaft Femur Fracture*
- *d.* *Hip Fracture-dislocation*
- *e.* *Patella Fracture*
- *f.* *Foot Fracture (can be accompanied by a crushing injury caused by constant compression trauma)*

Fig. 10.4 *A ski pole basket that catches on a tree can cause hyperextension and stretching trauma.*

injury involves both direct tissue injury and secondary injury when pressure on the blood vessels causes circulatory disturbance.

Because many organs are somewhat free to move inside body cavities, they can be injured by **secondary collisions**. When the body suddenly stops moving, internal organs continue to move forward until they collide with the body wall or until their movement is stopped by the tightening of their attachments. Secondary collisions can injure the brain within the cranial cavity, the heart and aorta within the chest cavity, and the liver, spleen and intestines within the abdominal cavity.

An example of **acceleration** is when the speed of a vehicle suddenly increases when it is struck from the rear by a faster-moving vehicle. Unless an occupant's seat is equipped with a properly positioned headrest, the occupant's neck can be subjected to the **hyperextension** type of **bending trauma**. This type of trauma can cause stretching and compression injuries to ligaments and tendons (whiplash) and can even fracture the cervical spine. If a body part is struck violently and suddenly bent, it tends to develop compression injuries on the side that was struck and stretching injuries on the opposite side.

The dislocated shoulder suffered by a skier who catches a pole basket on a tree while skiing with the pole straps around the wrists is a mixed type of injury that includes **hyperextension and stretching trauma**. The shoulder joint is externally rotated, hyperabducted, and pulled apart by the resulting forces (Fig. 10.4).

The **hyperflexion** type of **bending trauma** can result in wedge-shaped (compression) fractures of one or more thoracic or lumbar vertebrae when the body is forced into forward flexion. This may occur when a climber falls, lands hard on the feet and pitches forward. Stronger forces of this type also can cause a fracture-dislocation of the spine.

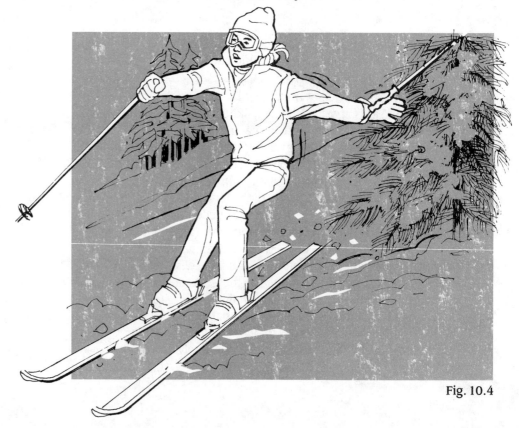

Fig. 10.4

Rotational trauma is well known to ski patrollers, who are familiar with the twisting type of fall that can cause a knee sprain or a spiral fracture of the tibia and fibula (Fig. 10.5).

An example of the injury produced by **stretching trauma** alone occurs when a person with long hair is scalped after the hair is caught in moving machinery such as a surface ski lift.

Injuries frequently are multiple, partly because of the continued dissipation of forces over time. The climber who suffers a hard fall may fracture both heel bones and the pelvis as well as the spine. Then, as energy continues to dissipate, the climber may pitch forward and land on outstretched hands, fracturing one or both wrists.

The amount of damage is proportional to the amount of energy involved. For example, if ski bindings do not release, an easy fall may produce a simple fracture of the tibia (Fig. 10.6), while a fall at high speed may cause a comminuted fracture of the tibia (Fig. 10.7). A high-velocity rifle bullet causes much more internal damage and a larger exit wound than a low-velocity pistol bullet of the same caliber.

One of the most valuable benefits derived from the skills of analyzing and understanding mechanisms of injury is the ability to predict potential internal injuries. This ability is most important in compression trauma, where visible signs of injury on the body surface may be minimal and the signs and symptoms of serious internal injury may not have had time to develop.

Compression trauma to the head frequently produces a double injury to the brain: the first injury occurs when the brain strikes the inside of the skull on impact; the second occurs when the brain bounces back and strikes the inside of the skull on the opposite side. This combination is called a contrecoup injury.

Fig. 10.5 *A twisting fall can produce rotational trauma.*

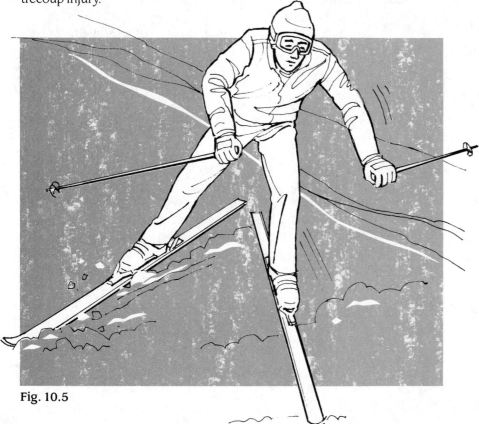

Fig. 10.5

Fig. 10.6 *Tibia Fracture*

Fig. 10.7 *Comminuted Tibia Fracture*

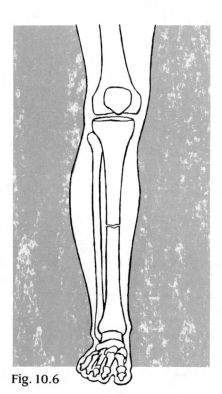

Fig. 10.6

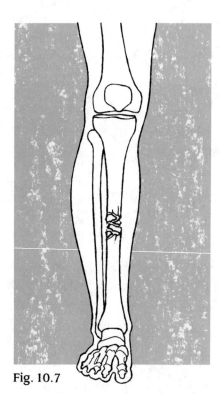

Fig. 10.7

A decelerating force may cause a compression injury of the chest wall with contusions and multiple broken ribs and also may shear off the movable aortic arch from the more fixed thoracic aorta. This type of chest injury also can contuse the heart by squeezing it between the sternum and the spine. Such a contusion can cause the pumping function of the heart to fail or can tear the heart muscle and cause bleeding into the pericardial sac around the heart (pericardial tamponade, see Chapter 15).

In the abdomen and pelvis, compression trauma can fracture the pelvic bones, and the sharp ends of the bones can lacerate the bladder (Fig. 10.8) and pelvic blood vessels. Deceleration and shearing forces also can rupture abdominal organs – particularly the pancreas, spleen, liver and kidneys – producing serious intra-abdominal bleeding.

Injuries tend to occur in predictable types and combinations. Injuries caused by automobile accidents tend to group according to the vehicle's velocity, the seat the injured person was occupying, whether the seat belt was fastened, whether the impact was direct or rotational, and whether it came from the front, rear, or side.

Most non-vehicular outdoor injuries are related to the type of terrain and the mode of transportation. Skiing is more dangerous than relatively safe outdoor activities such as walking and snowshoeing, because the increasing velocity inherent to the sport can lead to high-speed collisions and falls. Another danger is that a ski acts as a long lever attached to the foot. Hikers who slip or fall can suffer lacerations, abrasions, contusions, sprains, and fractures. Mountain hiking and technical mountaineering introduce the possibility of falls from heights with serious, multiple injuries. As a rule of thumb, a fall from three times or more a person's height will cause critical injury.

Less frequently, falling trees or tree limbs and lightning strikes cause injuries. Water sports introduce a different type of terrain and mode of transportation. Important considerations are the kinetic effect of rapidly moving water, trauma caused by collisions with rocks or other stationary objects, and injuries resulting from being struck by a boat or lacerated by a propeller.

Ski-related accidents will be covered in Chapter 21 because of the volume of data, the unusual characteristics of these injuries, and the existence of a well-organized and trained rescue system.

Careful inspection of the accident scene and mental reconstruction of the sequence of events reveals a good deal about the type, location, and severity of possible injuries. The probable speed at which the injured person was moving or the height from which he or she fell will give an indication of the amount of kinetic energy involved. This knowledge helps in predicting whether the forces were strong enough to produce fractures and serious internal injuries or whether less serious injuries should be expected.

The position of the injured person at impact and the parts of the body that were struck offer clues to the presence and location of possible internal injuries. Blood on the ground near the victim will alert the rescuer to the presence of one or more open wounds and the possibility of shock. In automobile accidents, the location and amount of damage to the vehicle gives an indication of the amount of kinetic energy involved and provides clues about the type and location of body impact. A broken windshield suggests that one or more occupants struck the windshield with the head, raising the possibility of head cuts and lacerations, brain injuries, skull fractures, and

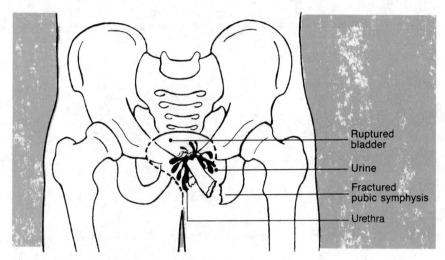

Fig. 10.8

Ruptured bladder

Urine

Fractured pubic symphysis

Urethra

Fig. 10.8 *Fractured pelvic bones can lacerate the bladder.*

neck injuries. A broken steering wheel or bent steering column indicates the possibility of a fractured sternum, crushed chest, flail chest, or injuries to the heart and lungs.

Determining the **mechanism of injury** is part of the first impression made as the rescuer arrives at the accident scene, the primary survey after dealing with emergency problems, and the secondary survey as the rescuer searches for additional injuries. By acquiring experience and a feel for the likely types of injuries, the rescuer can ensure that few injuries will be missed.

Even though understanding the significance of the mechanism of injury does not replace good assessment skills, it is an additional tool especially important in predicting the possibility of spinal cord injuries and internal injuries to the head, chest, abdomen, and pelvis that may cause internal bleeding.

Early recognition of internal bleeding may depend on the rescuer's alertness and careful monitoring of the patient based on an understanding of the mechanism of injury and its significance. When first seen, patients may be free of symptoms and have a normal or equivocal assessment despite having suffered a serious injury that is potentially fatal or permanently disabling. When the mechanism of injury suggests a possible spinal cord injury, the patient must be immobilized on a spine board even if pain is minimal and paralysis or loss of sensation is absent. Internal injuries of the head, chest, abdomen, and/or pelvis are notorious for initially appearing to be minor.

11

Specific Injuries to the Upper Extremity

Until homo sapiens becomes more sapient
I can see no prospect of his ever avoiding the foolishness
of war or of his learning that two automobiles cannot
occupy the same spot at the same time,
especially when they come from opposite directions.
Broken bones and lacerated wounds are therefore
likely to require surgical attention for as long as
this would-be clairvoyant can see into the future.

—Evarts A. Graham, M.D.
Postgraduate Medicine 7:154, 1950

The care of soft-tissue injuries in general is discussed in Chapter 8 and the principles of the care of bone and joint injuries are discussed in Chapter 9. This chapter describes the care of **specific sprains, fractures, and dislocations** of the upper extremity. Before reading this chapter, review Chapters 8 and 9 and be familiar with the appropriate sections on anatomy, physiology, and topographic anatomy in Chapters 2 and 3.

In the outdoors, upper-extremity injuries usually result from a fall on a shoulder or outstretched hand, although skiers can suffer these injuries during collisions as well. Fractures, dislocations, and soft-tissue injuries such as lacerations, contusions, and sprains can occur. The extent and type of injury depends on the age of the patient; the characteristics of equipment, if any; the type, direction, and magnitude of the forces involved; the position of the upper extremity at the time of impact; and the characteristics of the ground, snow, or other surface.

A fall on an outstretched arm can sprain the shoulder, elbow, wrist, or hand; dislocate the shoulder, elbow, wrist, or fingers; or fracture the clavicle, humerus, forearm bones, or bones of the hand.

Fig. 11.1 *A fall with the arm adducted can cause a sprain.*

Fig. 11.2 *A fall with the arm partly abducted concentrates force on the clavicle.*

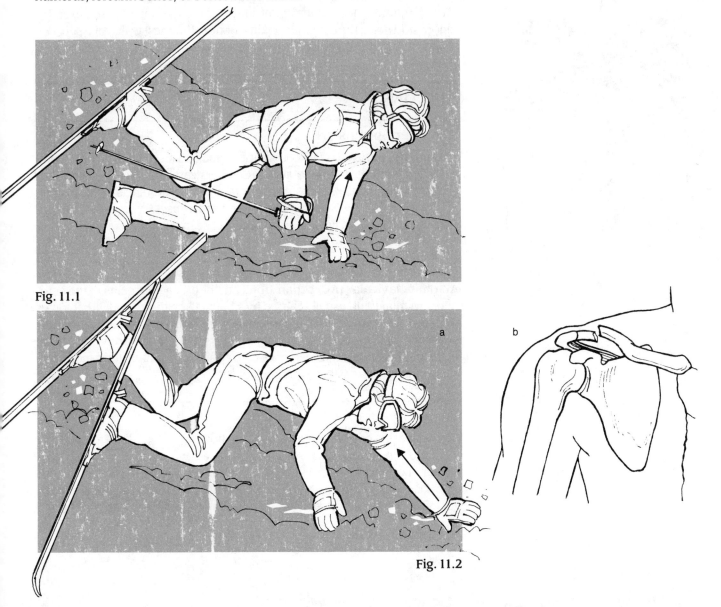

Fig. 11.1

Fig. 11.2

Fig. 11.3 *Anterior Dislocation of the Shoulder and Fracture of the Upper Humerus*

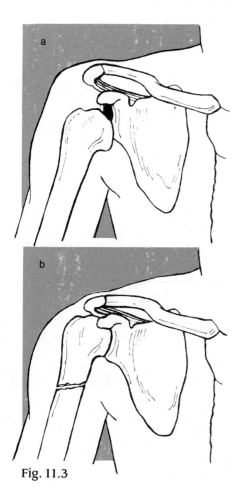

Fig. 11.3

When the arm is in the **adducted** position, the head of the humerus moves upward against the arch formed by the lateral end of the clavicle and the acromion of the scapula. A patient who falls with an arm in this position (Fig. 11.1) is more likely to sprain the shoulder joint or the acromioclavicular joint than to injure other parts of the shoulder girdle.

If the patient falls with the arm **partly abducted** (Fig. 11.2a), force is directly transmitted to the clavicle, which is likely to be fractured (Fig. 11.2b). If the arm is **fully abducted** and **externally rotated** (a common position when holding a ski pole or ice ax), the force of the fall is transmitted to the joint capsule. In young people with strong bones, this frequently produces an anterior dislocation of the shoulder (Fig. 11.3a). In elderly people, whose bones are more fragile than the tendons and ligaments of the shoulder capsule, a fracture of the upper end of the humerus is more common than a shoulder dislocation (Fig. 11.3b).

In many types of upper-extremity injury (fractures of the clavicle, humerus, and forearm; dislocations of the shoulder joint; and severe sprains of the shoulder, elbow, and acromioclavicular joints) pain increased by motion causes the patient to self-splint the injured extremity in a characteristic manner. The patient internally rotates the upper arm, flexes the elbow, and holds the extremity against or near the chest wall while supporting the forearm with the opposite hand.

SPRAINS

Shoulder Sprains

Shoulder sprains are common injuries usually caused by a fall on an outstretched hand as described above. Climbers can sprain a shoulder if they slip when their hand is anchored above their head. The joint is tender, painful and may be slightly swollen; pain is increased by use. Emergency care consists of applying cold packs and, in severe cases, a sling.

AC Separations

Acromioclavicular (AC) separations are third-degree sprains of the acromioclavicular joint, usually caused by a hard fall on the shoulder that forces the shoulder downward. Comparison with the smooth slope of the opposite, normal shoulder reveals an obvious, tender, shelf-like deformity at the point of the injured shoulder. Emergency care consists of limiting joint motion by supporting the arm with a sling and applying cold packs.

Elbow Sprains

Elbow sprains have the same causes as shoulder sprains, but are less common and *should be X-rayed* since they may be confused with non-displaced fractures or partial dislocations. They are most common in children. The elbow is slightly swollen, tender, and painful; pain is increased by use. Emergency care consists of applying cold packs and splinting with a sling and swathe.

Wrist Sprains

Wrist sprains are less common than wrist fractures. The wrist will be swollen, tender, and painful to use. Emergency care consists of applying cold packs and, for a severe sprain, splinting with a rigid splint that extends at least to the elbow and holds the hand in the **position of function** (Fig. 11.4). The arm is supported by a sling. Wrist injuries should be X-rayed because wrist sprains are difficult to tell from fractures of the small wrist bones.

Hand and Finger Sprains

Hand and finger sprains also are common. The most common upper-extremity injury in skiers is "skier's thumb," also called "gamekeeper's thumb." This is a sprain of the medial ligament at the base of the thumb (first metacarpophalangeal joint) caused when the skier tries to break a fall with an outstretched hand while holding a ski pole. Because of the position of the hand around the ski pole grip, the thumb is bent backward on impact with the snow. Twenty to 30 percent of these sprains are accompanied by a small fracture at the base of the first thumb joint, and many involve a ligament tear that is severe enough to require surgery; therefore, all patients with skier's thumb should be seen by an orthopedic surgeon. The injury can be splinted with a bulky hand dressing or taped so that it is held in adduction (Fig. 11.5).

Sprains of the hand and other fingers are less common. Mild sprains do not require treatment; severe sprains are splinted with a bulky hand dressing.

FRACTURES

Clavicle Fractures

The **clavicle** is one of the most frequently fractured bones in the body. The patient complains of pain in the shoulder area and attempts to self-splint the injury as described above. Examination reveals a dropped shoulder, swelling and tenderness over the clavicle, and often reveals a deformity when compared to the normal opposite side (Fig. 11.6a).

Emergency care consists of splinting with a sling and swathe (Fig. 11.6b) or a figure-of-eight bandage (Fig. 11.6c, 11.6d). The latter bandage is more comfortable because it holds the shoulders back and keeps the fractured ends of the clavicle in a more normal position. The figure-of-eight bandage also allows limited use of the injured extremity, a useful feature if the patient has to self-evacuate on foot. The figure-of-eight bandage is made from a 3-inch rubberized bandage or several cravats tied end to end. The bandage is passed several times across the back and over, around and under each shoulder to form a figure eight. The patient's armpits should be well padded.

Scapula Fractures

A strong force is required to fracture the **scapula**, which lies across the side of the upper back and is protected by large overlying muscles. The mechanism of injury usually is a direct blow, e.g., landing on the back after a hard fall. Anticipate and search for other injuries, particularly injuries of the adjacent

Fig. 11.4 *Splint a wrist sprain with the hand in the position of function.*

Fig. 11.5 *Sprained Thumb Taped in Adduction*

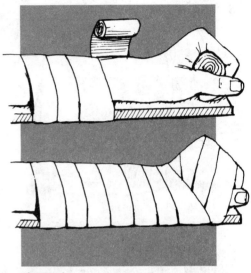

Fig. 11.4

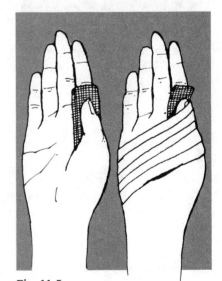

Fig. 11.5

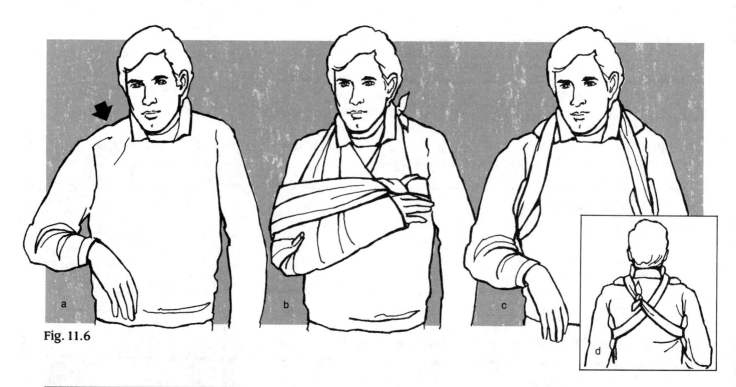

Fig. 11.6

Fig. 11.6 *Clavicle Fracture*
  a. Deformity over the Clavicle
  *b. Fractured Clavicle Splinted with
       a Sling and Swathe*
*c.,d. Fractured Clavicle Splinted with
       a Figure-of-eight Bandage*

chest wall and lungs. Examination reveals tenderness, swelling, and ecchymosis over the scapula, with pain on attempted use of the upper extremity. Emergency care consists of immobilizing the area with a sling and swathe.

Upper Arm Fractures

The humerus, or bone of the upper arm, usually is fractured in one of three places: just below its head, at its midshaft, or just above the elbow.

Fractures below the head of the humerus are more common in elderly people and may be confused with shoulder dislocations or severe sprains. Examination reveals swelling, tenderness, and ecchymosis in the deltoid muscle area.

Emergency care consists of splinting with a sling and swathe. In fractures below the head of the humerus, the bone ends are rarely displaced or angulated and, as in most other fractures near a joint, alignment should *not* be attempted.

Midshaft fractures of the humerus tend to occur in younger adults. These fractures usually involve marked swelling, angulation, and instability. The radial nerve may be injured where it winds around the back of the humerus, causing wrist drop. Examination discloses swelling, tenderness, and ecchymosis. If angulation is severe, the fracture should be aligned before splinting.

To align the fracture, support it with a hand just above the fracture site, grasp the two humeral condyles with the other hand, and exert gentle axial traction. After alignment, apply a padded rigid splint to the outside of the upper arm, and incorporate the splint into a sling and swathe. Occasionally, a second rigid splint must be placed on the inside of the upper arm to provide stability. As with any fracture, if pain or resistance occurs during alignment, stop the process and splint the injury in the angulated position using a sling and swathe plus a pillow or folded parka placed between the upper arm and the chest (Fig. 11.7).

Fractures above the elbow (Fig. 11.8) are common and may be difficult to distinguish from elbow dislocations. These fractures are important injuries because they frequently are accompanied by nerve or blood vessel injury. Examination usually reveals marked swelling and deformity of the elbow area, with tenderness, pain, and ecchymosis. Be sure to check nerve function and circulation distal to the elbow.

Emergency care consists of splinting the injury in the position found. The best method is to use two rigid splints, one on either side of the extremity, which are attached to the upper part of the upper arm above and the mid-forearm below so that they form the base of a triangle whose apex is the elbow (Fig. 11.9). Loop a cravat around the neck and tie it to the wrist to support the weight of the extremity.

If there are signs of impaired circulation such as a cold pale hand, pain in the hand and forearm, an absent or weak radial pulse, or poor capillary refill, the situation is an emergency and the patient must be transported to a hospital as soon as possible. If transportation will take more than 30 minutes, attempt to improve circulation by gently aligning the fracture. Exert axial traction by grasping the upper forearm with both hands and pulling gently downward while an assistant steadies the upper arm. Splint the extremity in the position that produces the strongest pulse. If the first attempt is unsuccessful or causes resistance or severe pain, make no further attempts at alignment and splint the arm in the most comfortable position.

Forearm and Wrist Fractures

Forearm and wrist fractures are common, especially in children and the elderly. Examination reveals swelling, tenderness, ecchymosis, pain on motion, and usually some deformity. The common **Colles' fracture** at the end of the radius produces a characteristic deformity, called a "silver fork deformity" because of its resemblance to an upside-down fork.

Fig. 11.7 *A pillow sling and swathe will support an angulated humerus fracture.*

Fig. 11.8 *Fracture above the Elbow*

Fig. 11.9 *Two padded board splints will stabilize a fracture above the elbow.*

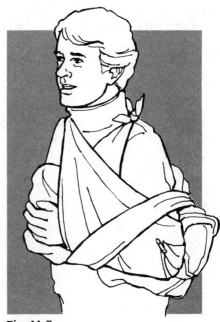

Fig. 11.7

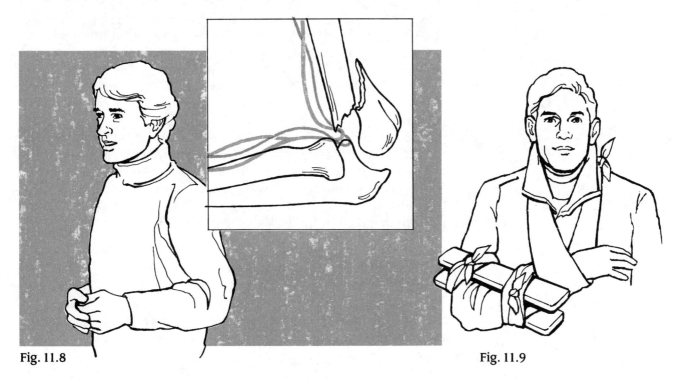

Fig. 11.8

Fig. 11.9

Emergency care consists of splinting the injury with a rigid forearm splint that also should support the hand and hold it in the position of function as described under wrist sprains (see Fig. 11.4). Use a sling to support the forearm.

Hand Fractures

Fractures of the hand are important injuries because a functional hand is so necessary for normal living. The hand contains a large number of bones, muscles, nerves and blood vessels, which are crowded together with little padding or protection. Hand and wrist injuries, other than superficial lacerations, should be seen by a physician. Fractures of the bones of the hand usually produce an obvious deformity along with swelling, tenderness, ecchymosis, and loss of function. Emergency care consists of immobilizing the entire hand with a bulky hand dressing and a rigid forearm splint, as described under forearm fractures.

DISLOCATIONS

Shoulder Dislocations

The **shoulder** is the most commonly dislocated joint in skiers and probably in outdoor enthusiasts in general. The injury usually is caused by a fall on an externally rotated outstretched hand, causing the head of the humerus to lever out of its socket using the acromion as a fulcrum. Some individuals have recurrent shoulder dislocations with each one stretching the joint capsule further, making it easier to dislocate the next time. The dislocated head of the humerus frequently can be felt in the armpit.

The most common type of shoulder dislocation is an **anterior dislocation**. In this type of dislocation, the patient attempts to splint the upper extremity by holding the upper arm slightly away from the chest, with the elbow bent and the forearm supported by the opposite hand. In the rare case of a **posterior** or **inferior dislocation**, the patient will hold the arm in front of the body away from the chest or over the head.

When the shoulder is examined, it looks and feels more square than a normal smooth, round shoulder. There is tenderness over the shoulder, and the patient resists attempts to move the shoulder because of pain. Emergency care consists of splinting the injury in position with a sling and swathe. A rolled blanket or parka may be needed as padding between the upper arm and the chest if the arm cannot be brought against the chest without pain (Fig. 11.10a). The patient usually is more comfortable when transported sitting rather than lying down. During transportation by toboggan, another person may have to sit behind and support the patient (Fig. 11.10b).

Elbow Dislocations

Elbow dislocations are serious injuries because of the possibility of nerve injury and circulatory impairment. The patient should be taken to a hospital as soon as possible. The radius and ulna usually are displaced posteriorly, producing a marked deformity with the point of the elbow more posterior than normal. The elbow joint usually is locked in slight flexion. Examination reveals marked swelling, tenderness, deformity, and pain on attempted motion. It is important to check the radial pulse and the motion and sensation of the wrist and hand.

Emergency care consists of splinting the injury in the position found, as described in the section on fractures above the elbow (see Fig. 11.9). Evidence of impaired circulation and/or nerve injury justifies an attempt to realign the elbow using gentle axial traction as described in the same section.

Wrist Dislocations

Wrist dislocations are uncommon and may be accompanied by a fracture. Examination reveals marked swelling and deformity, with pain on attempted motion of the joint. Emergency care consists of immobilizing the injury in the position found, using a rigid splint to protect the forearm and hand (see Fig. 11.4).

Finger Dislocations

Finger dislocations are common injuries. Examination shows a grossly deformed finger joint, locked in flexion, with pain on attempted motion. Swelling can be minimal or extensive. Emergency care consists of immobilizing the injury in the position found, usually with a modified bulky hand dressing and a rigid forearm splint to prevent wrist movement.

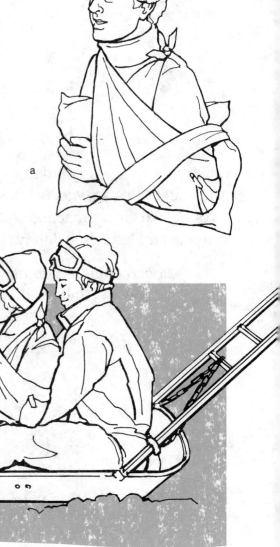

Fig. 11.10 *Care of a Dislocated Shoulder*
  a. The injury can be splinted with a pillow in the armpit.
  b. During transport by toboggan, a patroller may need to sit behind and support the patient.

a

b

Fig. 11.10

12

Specific Injuries to the Lower Extremity and Pelvis

Children, you are very little,
And your bones are very brittle;
If you would grow great and stately,
You must try to walk sedately.

—*Robert Louis Stevenson*
    "Good and Bad Children"

Injuries to the lower extremity and pelvis are not rare in outdoor enthusiasts, particularly skiers. Knee and ankle injuries are probably the most common lower-extremity injuries, with knee sprains being the most commonly reported skiing injury. Lacerations, contusions, and other soft-tissue injuries occur in the lower extremity as they do in other areas of the body. As with the upper extremity, lower extremity and pelvic injuries are mainly caused by falls, collisions, and direct blows. The extent and type of injury depend on the age of the patient; the type, direction, and magnitude of the forces involved; the position of the lower extremity at the time of injury; the condition of the snow or other ground surface; and whether skis or other equipment that increase the length of the lever arm are involved.

When the hip is abducted, a direct blow to the side of the hip or to the knee can drive the head of the femur directly into the acetabulum, fracturing it (Fig. 12.1). With the hip in other positions, forces transmitted along the femur can fracture the pelvis at other places; these fractures usually involve the weaker, thinner ischial and pubic bones (Fig. 12.2). A blow to the side of the iliac crest can fracture the crest or, depending on how the force is transmitted, fracture other parts of the pelvis. An antero-posterior blow to the pelvis also will tend to fracture the weaker parts of the ischial and pubic bones (Fig. 12.3).

Hip fractures (actually fractures of the upper end of the femur) usually are caused by falls in which compression, tension, rotational, and shearing forces are generated. Midshaft fractures of the femur usually are caused by direct

Fig. 12.1 *A blow to the lower extremity with the hip abducted may transmit force directly to the acetabulum.*

Fig. 12.2 *When the hip is adducted, force is transmitted to other parts of the pelvis.*

Fig. 12.3 *Effect of an Antero-posterior Blow to the Pelvis*

Fig. 12.4 *This type of motorcycle accident can fracture both femurs.*

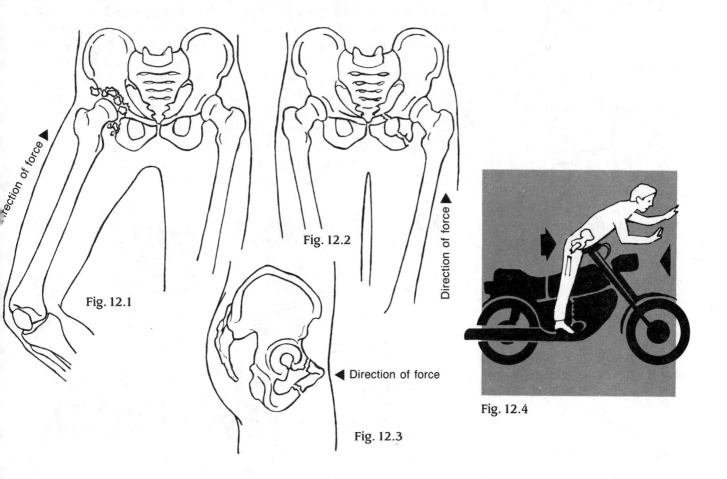

Fig. 12.2

Fig. 12.1

Direction of force

Direction of force

Fig. 12.3

Fig. 12.4

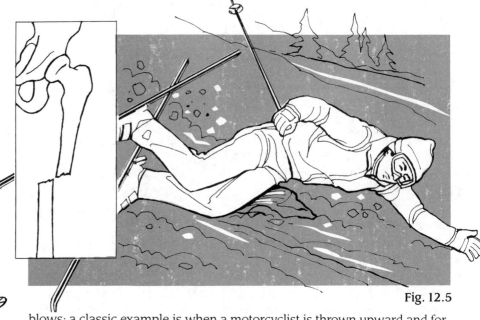

Fig. 12.5

Fig. 12.5 *This type of skiing accident can fracture the midshaft of the femur.*

Fig. 12.6 *Results of a Fall with the Foot Abducted and Externally Rotated*

Fig. 12.7 *Results of a Fall with the Foot Adducted and Internally Rotated*

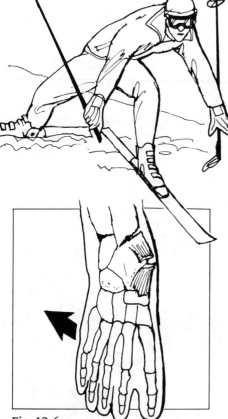

Fig. 12.6

blows; a classic example is when a motorcyclist is thrown upward and forward, striking the handlebars of the motorcycle with both thighs and fracturing both femurs (Fig. 12.4). Skiers can fracture a femur in a hard fall against a rock (Fig. 12.5), and climbers can fracture a femur in a long, hard fall.

The causes of knee-joint injuries and leg fractures are discussed in detail below and in Chapter 21.

The ankle usually is injured in one of three ways. The first method is when the foot is forced into abduction and external rotation, e.g., by falling when the foot is fixed by a ski binding or trapped between rocks. Such a fall can tear the medial ligament of the ankle, fracture the tip of the medial malleolus, or fracture the fibula just above the lateral malleolus (Fig. 12.6). The second situation occurs when the foot is forced into adduction and internal rotation, e.g., when the patient trips–the mechanism that produces the most common type of ankle sprain (Fig. 12.7). The lateral ligament may be stretched or torn, and the tip of the medial malleolus may be fractured. The third situation involves vertical compression of the type that occurs when landing on the feet after a hard fall. Vertical compression can crush the lower end of the tibia, fracture the large bones of the foot (the talus and calcaneus), and damage ligaments and soft tissues (Fig. 12.8).

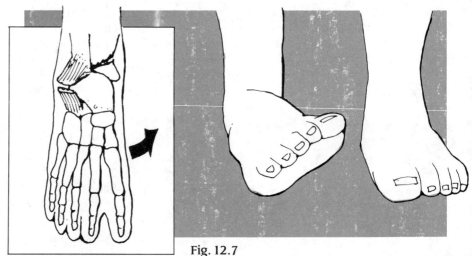

Fig. 12.7

Before continuing with the material on specific sprains, fractures, and dislocations of the lower extremities and pelvis, please review Chapters 8 and 9 and the appropriate sections on anatomy, physiology, and topographic anatomy in Chapters 2 and 3.

SPRAINS

Knee Sprains

Knee sprains are common in participants in many outdoor sports and recreational activities, particularly skiers. Because of the knee's importance, the student should be thoroughly familiar with its anatomy (Fig. 12.9) and function, discussed briefly in Chapter 2. The knee is a **modified hinge joint**. Although its motion is mainly in the single plane of flexion-extension, some degree of rotation of the tibia on the femur can occur during full flexion and full extension.

The bones of the knee joint are the **femur** proximally, the **tibia** distally, and the **patella** anteriorly (Fig. 12.9a and b). The **fibula** is only indirectly involved in the knee joint.

The riding surfaces of the knee are the convex **condyles** of the femur, which are semicircular and covered with cartilage, and the concave **tibial plateau**, also covered with cartilage, on which the femoral condyles sit. The C-shaped **medial and lateral cartilages** (menisci) sit atop the tibial plateau, deepen its concavities, and cushion the joint. The **patella** sits in front of the knee joint in the groove between the femoral condyles.

The knee joint is enclosed by a fibrous joint capsule (Fig. 12.9c) lined by a synovial membrane that secretes lubricating synovial fluid. The medial and lateral parts of the knee joint capsule are thickened and strengthened, forming the **medial and lateral ligaments** of the knee (Fig. 12.9d), also called collateral ligaments. The front and back of the capsule are loose, permitting flexion and extension of the joint.

There are two other important ligaments of the knee joint: the **anterior and the posterior cruciate ligaments** (Fig. 12.9d and e). These originate in the groove between the femoral condyles, cross each other in an X, and insert in the middle of the tibial plateau. The anterior cruciate ligament inserts in

Fig. 12.8 *Injuries Caused by Landing on the Feet After a Hard Fall*

Fig. 12.9 *Anatomy of the Knee*

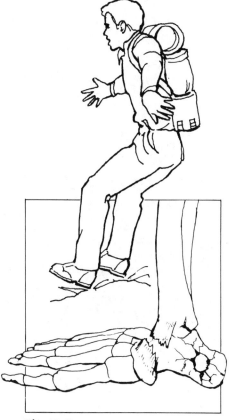

Fig. 12.8

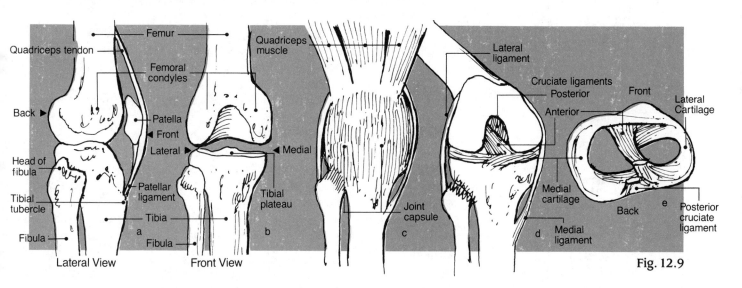

Fig. 12.9

Fig. 12.10 *Major Muscles Associated with the Knee Joint*
  a. *Quadriceps*
  b. *Hamstring*

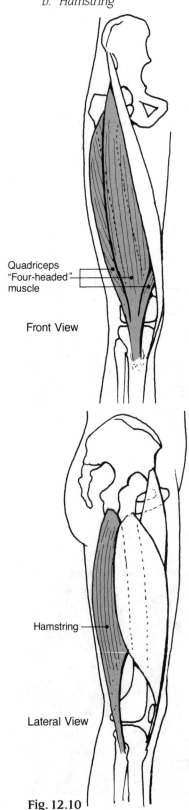

Quadriceps
"Four-headed"
muscle

Front View

Hamstring

Lateral View

Fig. 12.10

front of the posterior cruciate ligament. Because the concavities of the tibial plateau are shallow, the knee joint would be easy to dislocate if not for these four powerful ligaments and the muscles and tendons around the knee.

The major muscles associated with the knee joint are the **quadriceps femoris** ("quad") anteriorly, which attaches to the top of the patella and extends the knee, and the **medial and lateral hamstring muscles** (Fig. 12.10) posteriorly, which flex the knee. These ligaments and muscles are important in maintaining the stability of the knee joint. The lateral and medial ligaments are probably the most important in preventing medial and lateral dislocation of the knee; the anterior cruciate, in preventing forward dislocation; and the posterior cruciate, in preventing backward dislocation. Hyperextension is prevented by both cruciates, mainly the anterior cruciate, and also by the posterior part of the joint capsule.

When the knee is in *slight flexion*, most ligaments and tendons are tight and the joint is in its strongest position. When the knee joint is stabilized in this way, a rotational force of the type frequently exerted during skiing is more likely to cause a binding release than a knee injury. One of the reasons beginning skiers are told to "bend ze knees" is to maintain better control and to prevent knee injuries. The medial cartilage (meniscus), which is partly fixed by its attachment to the medial ligament, is torn more often than the lateral cartilage, which can move to some extent within the joint.

Prolonged flexion of the knee at close to a 90-degree angle, as in "sitting back" while skiing bumps, puts a severe strain on the patella. If done frequently, this eventually injures the cartilage that lines the posterior patellar surface, a condition called chondromalacia of the patella. The knee also is less stable in this position, and the relaxed anterior cruciate seems to be more prone to injury.

The patella provides an advantage in completing knee extension when the knee is partly extended (less than 30 degrees), since the patella lies on the lower end of the femur just above the condyles, holds the quadriceps tendon away from the joint, and lengthens the lever arm (Fig. 12.11a). However, in full flexion, the mechanical advantage of the patellar system is lost because the patella moves downward, sinks between the femoral condyles, and allows the quadriceps tendon to move closer to the joint (Fig. 12.11b). Modern ski boots with built-in forward lean put considerable stress on the patella. Skiers are advised to loosen their boots and stand up straight when they are not skiing.

Knee sprains continue to make up 20 to 25 percent of all reported skiing injuries in both alpine and nordic skiers. Sprains of the medial ligament are the most common, occurring with about 10 times the frequency of sprains of the lateral ligament. The anterior cruciate ligament is the next most commonly injured ligament. Minor anterior cruciate injuries are more common in women and novice skiers; severe anterior cruciate injuries are more common in advanced skiers of either sex.

Even for experienced physicians, it is often difficult to specifically diagnose knee injuries because serious ligament tears may not appear to be that severe when first seen. Successful treatment of many knee injuries depends on prompt diagnosis and surgery within a week or two; delay can cause serious problems later on. Therefore, all patients with knee injury should be seen by a physician – preferably an orthopedist – if knee symptoms do not clear up within 24 hours.

The examiner frequently can form a good idea of which ligament or ligaments have been injured by noting the circumstances of the injury and the area where the knee is tender. Severe anterior cruciate ligament injuries can occur without a fall, but frequently the patient hears or feels a pop in the knee at the time of the injury.

When examining an injured knee, look for swelling and feel for tenderness of the medial and lateral ligaments, the patellar ligament, the posterior part of the joint capsule, and the hamstring tendons.

Emergency care of a knee sprain consists of applying cold packs and immobilizing the knee with a suitable fixation splint (Fig. 12.12). Advise the patient to see a physician before putting weight on the extremity.

Fig. 12.11 *Mechanics of the Patellar System*
    a. Knee Extended
    b. Knee Flexed

Fig. 12.12 *Immobilization of a Knee Sprain with a Cravat or a Fixation Splint*

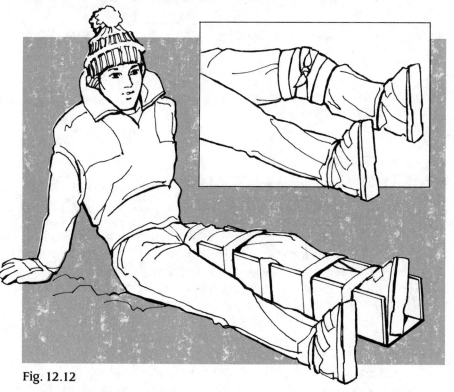

Fig. 12.12

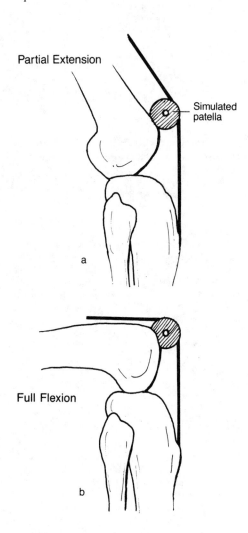

Partial Extension

Simulated patella

a

Full Flexion

b

Fig. 12.11

Ankle Sprains

Ankle sprains, another common injury, are a hazard for outdoor travelers walking on uneven ground and for alpine and nordic skiers. Although modern hiking and alpine skiing boots tend to protect the ankle, ankle sprains still are common in nordic skiers because of the low tops of nordic ski boots. As the use of higher boots and higher, stiffer telemark boots increases, the number of ankle sprains in nordic skiers probably will decrease.

Depending on the mechanism of injury and the particular ligaments injured, examination may reveal tenderness, swelling, and bruising over the top of the foot and/or around one or both malleoli. Emergency care of *mild* sprains consists of applying cold packs and supporting the ankle with a cravat ankle bandage (Fig. 12.13a) or a figure-of-eight made from an elastic bandage (Fig. 12.13b). *Severe* ankle sprains are hard to tell from fractures and should be treated with a fixation splint designed for the lower leg. All patients with severe ankle sprains or mild sprains that do not improve within a few days should see a physician.

Fig. 12.13 *Two Types of Support for
a Sprained Ankle*
  a. *Cravat Sprained Ankle Bandage*
  b. *Figure-of-eight Bandage Using
      an Elastic Bandage*

Under wilderness conditions, a patient with a mild to moderate ankle sprain may have to self-evacuate. An adhesive-tape boot may stabilize the sprain enough to allow the patient to walk or ski out (Fig. 12.14, and Appendix B).

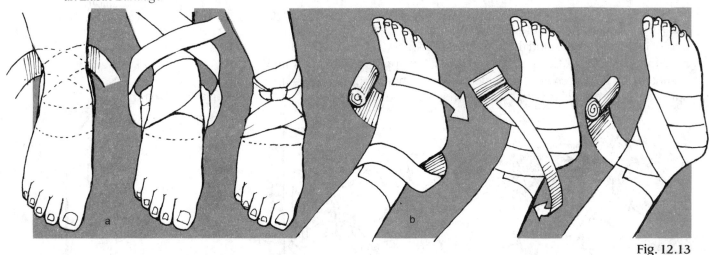

Fig. 12.13

Fig. 12.14 *Adhesive Tape Boot*

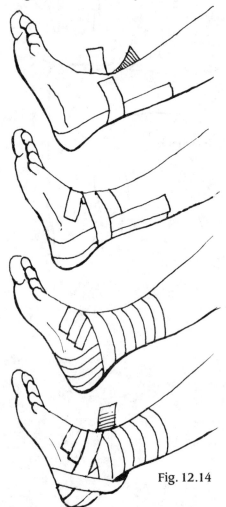

Fig. 12.14

FRACTURES

Pelvic Fractures

A pelvic fracture should be suspected when the mechanism of injury and the magnitude of the forces involved could produce such a fracture. The major hazard of pelvic fractures is damage to blood vessels and pelvic organs from sharp bone fragments. Internal bleeding from large pelvic blood vessels may be difficult to detect initially but should be anticipated in all pelvic fractures. Monitor the vital signs closely to detect early signs of continued bleeding and impending shock. Pelvic fractures also can injure the uterus of a pregnant woman, the bladder, and the urethra.

The patient with a fractured pelvis will be lying down and complaining of pain in the lower abdomen or pelvis which usually is increased by movement. Because the pelvis is a continuous ring, pressure on one part of the pelvis is transmitted to any injured area, causing pain in that area. If a pelvic injury is suspected, place one hand on each iliac crest and press gently inward with both hands, then press gently backward on the pubic bone with one hand. If the pelvis is fractured, one or both of these maneuvers should cause pain.

Emergency care of a patient with a pelvic fracture consists of immobilization on a long spine board and treatment for shock, if needed. Carefully lift the patient using a three- or four-person direct ground lift (see Chapter 20), lay the patient directly on the board, and secure him or her in place with straps, padding, and rolled parkas as necessary. The patient may prefer to lie with the knees and hips bent. A PASG is useful to control severe bleeding, if personnel trained and licensed in its use are present. Inspect any urine voided by the patient for the presence of blood. Blood in the urine (hematuria) indicates injury of the bladder or urethra and mandates transporting the patient to a hospital without delay.

Hip Fractures

A hip fracture usually refers to a fracture of the upper part of the femur. This injury, while common in elderly persons after a minor fall, is less common under outdoor conditions except with severe trauma. Skiers rarely suffer hip fractures.

A patient with a fractured hip usually complains of severe pain and is unable to move. In some cases, a patient with a hip fracture may complain of moderate pain that is increased by walking or passive manipulation of the hip joint. The involved lower extremity almost always is externally rotated and usually is shortened. The upper thigh below the groin or around the greater trochanter usually is tender when palpated.

Emergency care consists of immobilizing the patient on a long spine board as described in the section on pelvic fractures. Do not attempt to flex the hips or knees. If the hip is flexed, do not attempt to straighten it. Instead, stabilize the hip in position with folded parkas and padding as needed. If the patient must be moved before a long spine board is available, the injury can be splinted against the normal lower extremity by putting padding between the extremities and tying the legs and thighs firmly together with cravats.

Femoral Shaft Fractures

A femoral shaft fracture is best treated by traction splinting, which counteracts the spasm and pull of the large, powerful thigh muscles, prevents further damage from the sharp bone ends, and minimizes blood loss into the thigh. Examination will disclose an externally rotated and shortened limb, with a large, tender bulge in the thigh. The patient usually experiences severe pain and is unable to move. The fracture may be severely angulated.

Shock should be anticipated, since patients with femoral fractures frequently lose 500 to 1,000 milliliters or more of blood into the thigh. Nerves and blood vessels may be damaged as well. The circulation and nerve supply to the distal extremity must be monitored. If the circulation and nerve supply are impaired, there may be improvement after splinting.

Emergency care of a patient with a fractured femoral shaft usually consists of immobilizing the extremity with a traction splint (Fig. 12.15) as described in Chapter 9 and treating shock, if necessary.

A subtrochanteric fracture resembles a classic midshaft fracture of the femur but cannot be splinted with a traction splint. This type of femoral frac-

Fig. 12.15 *Alternatives for Immobilizing a Fractured Femur with a Traction Splint*
  a. Nylon Cord Pulley System
  b. Spanish Windlass

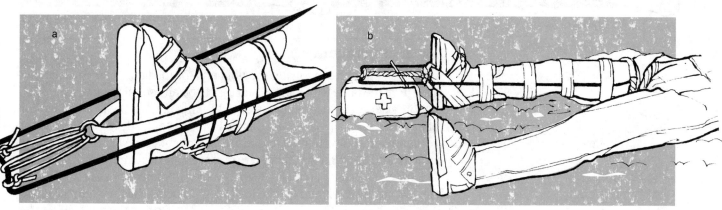

Fig. 12.15

Fig. 12.16 *Fixation Splint for a Fracture Above the Knee*

Fig. 12.17 *Technique of Gentle Alignment of a Fracture to Improve Circulation*

ture involves the upper part of the femur below the trochanters. The pull of the psoas muscle holds the proximal fragment in a flexed position; attempts to straighten the hip cause severe pain. A patient with a subtrochanteric fracture is placed on a spine board with the limb stabilized in position with rolled parkas or pillows. The patient may prefer to sit up during transportation.

Above-knee Femur Fractures

A fracture of the femur above the knee (supracondylar fracture) is a serious injury. The pull of the thigh muscles tips the lower fragment so that its jagged upper end lies against the nerves and blood vessels running down the back of the thigh, where it may injure them. Examination reveals a large, tender swelling in the lower thigh above the knee, with pain and inability to move the limb. The circulation and nerve supply below the injury should be checked and monitored. Emergency care consists of immobilizing the fracture with a lower-extremity fixation splint that extends to just below the groin (Fig. 12.16). Do *not* use a traction splint.

The patient must be taken to a hospital as soon as possible if there are signs of impaired circulation, such as a cold, pale foot, pain in the foot and leg, absence or weakness of the posterior tibial and dorsalis pedis pulses, and delayed capillary refill. If transportation will take more than 30 minutes, try to improve circulation by gentle alignment of the fracture. Do this with the patient's knee bent. Grasp the leg just below the knee and exert axial traction (Fig. 12.17). If alignment is successful, splint the extremity in the position that produces the strongest pulses. If the first attempt is unsuccessful or causes resistance or severe pain, make no further attempts and splint the injury in the most comfortable position.

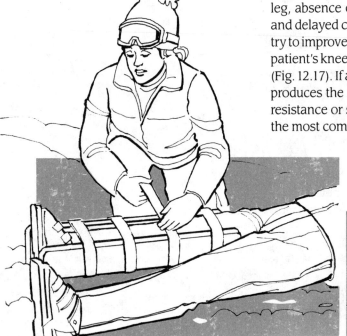

Fig. 12.16

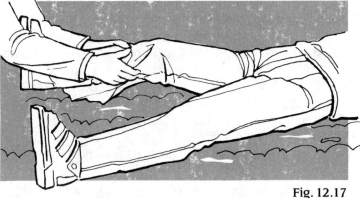

Fig. 12.17

Lower Leg Fractures

A lower leg fracture involving the tibia and/or the fibula can occur at any place from the knee to the ankle joint. Boot-top and spiral fractures are common in skiers. The extremity distal to the fracture usually is angulated or rotated. Occasionally, it may be rotated as much as 180 degrees. The patient will complain of severe pain and resist movement of the leg. Swelling, tenderness, and ecchymosis usually are present at the fracture site.

Emergency care of patients with lower leg fractures consists of applying a fixation splint designed for the lower leg. To apply the splint, the fracture must be aligned so that the foot is in its proper relationship to the leg. Grasp the foot firmly with both hands while an assistant supports the leg with one hand above and one hand below the fracture site. With the aid of gentle axial traction, the injured extremity usually can be straightened and rotated into a more normal position. The sooner alignment is done after the injury, the easier it is to perform. Check circulation and nerve function in the distal extremity before and after alignment.

Ankle Fractures

An ankle fracture actually is a fracture of the lower end of the tibia and/or fibula, although the bones of the foot occasionally may be involved. The ankle joint has two "shear pins," the lateral and medial malleoli, which usually break first when a rotational force is applied to the ankle joint, thus preventing a more extensive fracture of the shafts of the bones. Ankle fractures are caused by twisting falls and falls from heights; such fractures are now less common in skiers because of improved boot designs.

An ankle fracture may be hard to tell from a severe sprain. Examination reveals swelling, tenderness, and ecchymosis of the tissues around the ankle joint. The patient may or may not be able to move the joint. If a malleolus is fractured, gentle pressure over its tip will evoke tenderness. Emergency care consists of applying a fixation splint designed for the lower leg. A folded blanket or parka splint also is useful and comfortable.

Foot Fractures

Fatigue fractures of the metatarsals can occur in long-distance runners and in hikers who carry heavy packs for long distances. The foot also may be fractured in a fall or when struck by rocks or other falling objects. Examination reveals tenderness, swelling, ecchymosis and, occasionally, deformity at the fracture site. In the case of a fatigue fracture, the only symptom may be pain that is increased by walking. Patients with a fracture of the foot should stay off their feet. If there is little swelling, the patient's boot or shoe can be used to protect and splint the injury. Severe fractures should be splinted with a folded blanket, pillow, or folded parka.

DISLOCATIONS

Hip Dislocations

Because the hip socket is deep, the hip is rarely dislocated without fracturing the socket. The most common type of hip "dislocation" is a **posterior fracture-dislocation**. This injury can occur in auto accidents when an occupant's knee strikes the dashboard and the force is transmitted along the shaft of the femur to the posterior lip of the socket. A skier can suffer the same type of fracture-dislocation if a ski binding inadvertently releases during a rapid descent. This may allow the boot to jam deeply into the snow, bringing the lower extremity to a sudden halt while the skier's momentum carries the rest of the body forward. The posterior lip of the hip joint is torn away as the hip is dislocated posteriorly. A severe fall from a height also can dislocate a hip.

Fig. 12.18 *Dislocated Knee*

Fig. 12.19 *Axial traction improves circulation when the knee is dislocated.*

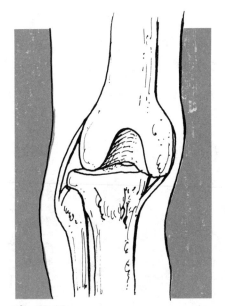

Fig. 12.18

In a posterior dislocation, the lower extremity is internally rotated and the knee is bent. In the rare anterior dislocation, the hip is slightly flexed and externally rotated and usually cannot be straightened. Attempted motion produces severe pain, and there is tenderness over the upper thigh just below the groin. The sciatic nerve, which runs behind the hip joint, may be injured when the hip is dislocated, causing paralysis of the foot, foot drop, and numbness in the lower leg and sole of the foot.

Emergency care of a patient with a dislocated hip consists of immobilization on a long spine board. The involved lower extremity is maintained in the position found with pillows, wadded jackets, straps, and cravats. Ability to preserve the head of the femur and prevent serious long-term disability diminishes each minute the head of the femur remains out of the socket. Therefore, treat this situation as an emergency and immediately transport the patient to a hospital.

Knee Dislocations

A knee dislocation is a rare but very serious injury because the blood vessels and nerves behind the knee frequently are damaged, impairing the circulation and nerve supply to the lower leg. This injury is another true emergency, and the patient must be taken to a hospital without delay.

A knee dislocation (Fig. 12.18) involves complete disruption of all or most of its ligaments. Severe trauma, usually a fall, is necessary to produce this degree of injury. The patient experiences severe pain, swelling and gross deformity of the knee, and is unable to move the knee.

Immediately check and monitor circulation and nerve supply to the extremity distal to the injury. If distal pulses are good, splint the dislocation in the position found. A clamshell type of lower-extremity fixation splint, such as the quick splint, is a good choice (see Fig. 12.16). The knee also can be splinted like a dislocated elbow, with two padded board splints, one on either side of the extremity, attached to the thigh just below the hip and to the ankle so that a triangle is formed with the knee at its apex (Fig. 11.9).

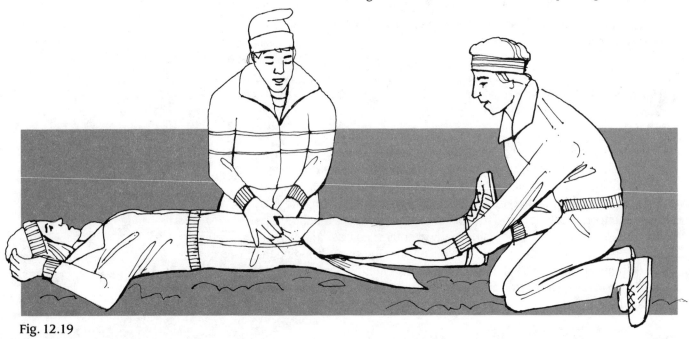

Fig. 12.19

If pulses are weak or absent and transport to a hospital will take more than 30 minutes, an attempt to restore circulation by axial manual traction is justified. Grasp the patient's ankle with one hand and the patient's calf with the other hand, while an assistant steadies the lower thigh. Then, exert gentle traction while flexing the knee slightly (Fig. 12.19). Test the pulses in the foot with the knee in the new position. If the maneuver is successful, splint the limb in the position that produces the strongest pulses. If the attempt is unsuccessful or if severe pain or resistance occur, splint the limb in the most comfortable position and take the patient to a hospital as soon as possible.

Patella Dislocations

A patella dislocation is a bizarre injury that can occur during athletic activities. The patella usually dislocates laterally and locks the knee in the flexed position, producing a marked deformity. It occasionally moves back into place when the knee is extended. Emergency care consists of splinting the injury using the same technique as for a dislocated knee.

Ankle Dislocations

An ankle dislocation is hard to distinguish from an ankle fracture and usually is associated with fractures of both malleoli. Examination reveals tenderness, swelling, and deformity of the ankle joint, with pain on motion. A severe injury can produce a flail (excessively mobile) ankle. The deformity usually will have to be aligned to allow splinting. Alignment is achieved by gentle axial traction. Splint the ankle with a lower-leg fixation splint in a manner similar to that used for a fractured ankle. If attempts at alignment are unsuccessful or produce increased pain or resistance, splint the ankle in the position found with a pillow or rolled blanket splint. Immediately take the patient to a hospital. Circulation and nerve supply to the foot frequently are impaired; in these circumstances, an attempt to realign the injury using the technique described for a knee dislocation is justified.

13

Injuries to the Head, Eye, Face, and Throat

For, as the substance of the brain, like that of
the other solids of our body, is nearly incompressible,
the quantity of blood within the head must be the same,
or very nearly the same, at all times, whether in health
or disease, in life or after death.

> –Alexander Monro
>   Observations of the Structure
>   and Functions of the Nervous System

Before reading this chapter, review the section on the anatomy and physiology of the skeletal and nervous systems in Chapter 2.

Head injuries are a major cause of death and disability. In an urban setting, head injuries are most frequently caused by motor vehicle accidents; in the outdoors, they are most often caused by falls and collisions. Such injuries can be prevented to some extent by wearing helmets when climbing, ski racing, or riding snowmobiles or mountain bikes.

The importance of a head injury depends on the amount of **brain injury**. The degree of recovery for a head-injury patient depends on the sum of the damage occurring at the time of the accident and the secondary damage caused by complications following the accident.

Head injuries can be either **open** or **closed** (Fig. 13.1). The brain can be directly injured by a penetration injury that lacerates the brain tissue or by a contusion. While rescuers have no control over this initial damage, they may have considerable control over secondary damage. The brain can be secondarily injured when blood flow is restricted as a result of increased pressure inside the rigid skull caused by swelling or bleeding. Decreases in blood flow cause hypoxia of the brain tissue. Secondary damage to the brain also can occur in patients who develop hypoxia because of airway obstruction and in patients with multiple injuries who develop shock.

A head injury by itself *does not cause shock*; if shock develops, the patient probably has additional injuries of the chest, abdomen, pelvis, or spinal cord. Any patient with a head injury should be assumed to have a **cervical spine injury.**

Field emergency care for patients with head injuries is not very effective. Transport the patient to a hospital as soon as possible. Any head injury in a patient who has lost consciousness, even momentarily, is considered significant. Most patients with serious head injuries are unconscious and remain so during emergency care. *Changes in consciousness* are important, especially if the patient is initially alert but gradually becomes more lethargic, confused, and sleepy. Consciousness should be monitored by applying the AVPU or Glasgow Coma scales (see Chapter 4). Record this information and send it with the patient to the hospital.

Review the assessment of an unconscious patient presented in Chapter 4. Information on this assessment is summarized in Table 13.1. Remember that a head injury patient may lose consciousness for a reason other than the head injury itself. For example, a patient who suffers a sudden stroke or seizure may lose consciousness, fall to the ground, and suffer a head injury from the fall.

Because an unconscious patient cannot tell the examiner how he or she feels and may be unable to perform actions such as coughing that are carried out routinely by conscious individuals, the rescuer must anticipate and prevent problems. The emergency care of a head injury patient is much the same as emergency care of a patient unconscious for any reason and is described below.

Fig. 13.1 *Head Injuries*

Penetration injury

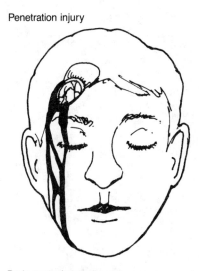

Brain contusion

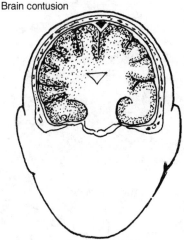

Blood clot inside the skull

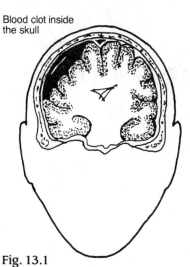

Fig. 13.1

Table 13.1

SUMMARY OF ASSESSMENT OF AN UNCONSCIOUS PATIENT

1. **First impression**. Determine the mechanism of injury.
2. **Primary survey**. "ABCD." Treat urgent problems in the following order:
   a. Airway: Open with jaw-thrust maneuver and maintain.
   b. Breathing: Give rescue breathing as needed.
   c. Circulation: Give CPR as needed.
   d. Control severe bleeding.
   e. Maintain manual stabilization of the head and neck, if appropriate.
3. **Secondary survey.** "E."
   a. Record and monitor vital signs. (Take the temperature with a low-reading thermometer if hypothermia conditions exist.)
   b. Check pupils, skin color and temperature, state of consciousness, reaction to pain and touch, ability to move.
   c. General body examination from head to toe.
      (1) Check for wounds, bleeding.
      (2) Check for other injuries.
   d. Check for medical bracelets and wallet cards.

Fig. 13.2 *Use the jaw-thrust maneuver to open and maintain the airway.*

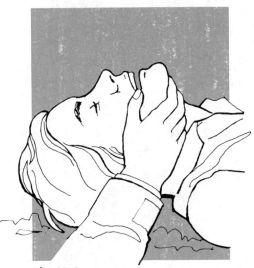

Fig. 13.2

GENERAL CARE OF UNCONSCIOUS PATIENTS

Treat problems uncovered during the primary survey. The most immediate danger to most unconscious persons is obstruction of the upper airway, most commonly caused by the tongue, although mucus, vomitus or foreign matter such as food or snow are other possible causes. Use the jaw-thrust maneuver (Fig. 13.2) to open the airway of *every* unconscious trauma patient and every patient in whom the onset of unconsciousness was unobserved. The cervical spine could have been injured by the initial trauma, or by a fall if the patient lost consciousness while sitting or standing.

Remove any foreign material using the finger-sweep method, suction or, if necessary, the Heimlich maneuver (see Chapter 5). Insert an oral airway to keep the airway open (see Chapter 6). If indicated, perform rescue breathing or, if pulses are absent, perform CPR.

Vomiting is common in unconscious patients, particularly those with head injuries, and is an important cause of airway blockage. Anticipate vomiting and watch for it constantly. If the patient is unconscious for a reason other than trauma, the semiprone (coma or NATO) position (see Chapter 6) is useful in maintaining the airway and promoting drainage of secretions from the mouth and nose; this position should be used if the patient cannot be watched constantly.

Search for external bleeding, particularly of the scalp. Control external bleeding as described in Chapter 7 and in the section on scalp lacerations below. An open skull fracture is extremely serious because of the danger of meningitis or brain infection. Protect open wounds with sterile compresses.

Give unconscious patients oxygen in high concentration to ensure that each unit of blood will carry the greatest possible amount of oxygen to the delicate brain tissues.

Assume that an unconscious trauma patient has back or neck injuries. After applying an extrication collar, immobilize the patient on a spine board. The spine board can be tipped on its side if the patient vomits. If a spine board is unavailable, the head and neck must be stabilized manually when the patient is turned on one side to vomit.

Recheck and record the patient's vital signs at regular intervals. It is particularly important to periodically observe the pupils for size and equality and to examine the ears, nose, and mouth for bleeding and drainage of clear fluid. If blood or fluid is draining, the patient should be turned so that gravity will cause this material to flow outward. Monitor the state of consciousness at regular intervals according to the AVPU or Glasgow Coma scales and document these findings in writing.

Carry out a secondary survey and treat any additional injuries.

Keep the patient lying down, and elevate the head of the spine board about 6 inches to raise the patient's head and trunk slightly higher than the rest of the body; do *not* use a pillow. This position helps to retard swelling of the brain. Keep the patient warm but not hot. Remove hard contact lenses, if present (see Chapter 4), and keep the patient's eyelids closed to prevent the corneas from drying out.

Unconscious patients may convulse. Because convulsions cannot be stopped, emergency care consists of protecting the patient from self-injury (see Chapter 18). If breathing stops temporarily during a convulsion, the only treatment required is to maintain an open airway. If the case involves a nontraumatic loss of consciousness, consider such medical illnesses as diabetes and epilepsy, and look for wallet cards and medical-alert tags and bracelets.

Table 13.2

SUMMARY OF GENERAL CARE OF UNCONSCIOUSNESS

1. Primary survey. Treat life-threatening conditions. Give CPR and rescue breathing, and control severe bleeding as necessary. It is very important to maintain the airway.
2. Insert an oral airway.
3. Give oxygen in high concentration.
4. Place the patient in the coma position in cases of nontraumatic unconsciousness or when there is no question of neck or back injury. The patient's head should be slightly higher than the feet.
5. Dress wounds.
6. Watch for vomiting. Use suction if necessary.
7. Monitor vital signs and state of consciousness.
8. Keep the patient warm but not too warm.
9. Keep eyelids closed to prevent the eyes from drying.
10. Watch for convulsions.

SPECIFIC TYPES OF HEAD INJURIES

Scalp Lacerations

Because of the generous blood supply to the scalp, a **scalp laceration** usually bleeds freely and can cause considerable blood loss. Examine the wound to see whether the skull bone or brain is exposed and whether there is an indentation that suggests a depressed skull fracture. Control bleeding by careful direct pressure. If the patient has a depressed skull fracture, exert pressure around the *edges* of the injury rather than at its center. Open skull fractures are extremely serious. Take care to avoid introducing dirt or loose hair into the wound. Do *not* irrigate scalp wounds or trim the patient's hair near the wound, since contaminants may be washed into an open fracture and hair clippings may get into the wound. However, a scalp avulsion should be cleaned, if necessary, with sterile physiological saline solution. Be careful not to wash anything into the wound. After cleaning, replace the tissue, then bandage the wound by covering it with a sterile compress held in place by a triangular bandage or stocking cap as described in Chapter 8. Infection in simple scalp wounds is unusual because of the scalp's excellent blood supply.

Concussions

A patient who has lost consciousness or has other symptoms of temporary brain dysfunction after a blow to the head is said to have a **concussion**. Symptoms can include "seeing stars," confusion, loss of memory, dizziness, severe headache, weakness, and double vision or other visual changes. Some patients are unable to remember events that occurred just before the injury. These symptoms usually are temporary and will subside without residual damage. They probably occur because the brain has been jarred, causing a temporary "short-circuit" of its electrical connections.

A concussion is significant because its symptoms are similar to early symptoms of brain hemorrhage and other serious illness or injury. The rescuer should monitor and record at regular intervals the level of consciousness, state of the pupils, and other vital signs of any patient who has symptoms of a brain concussion. In a remote setting where the patient cannot be transferred to a hospital immediately, monitoring should continue at least overnight. Any person who loses consciousness, even momentarily, should be checked by a physician.

Brain Contusions

Brain contusions involve bruising of brain tissue and swelling of the brain. Because the brain lies within a "tight, bony box," only a small amount of swelling can occur without causing an increase in pressure inside the skull. The signs and symptoms of a brain contusion are similar to but more severe than those of a concussion. Prolonged loss of consciousness, paralysis, and changes in the pupils can occur. A contusion is a serious injury, and the patient should be taken quickly to a hospital. During transport, closely monitor the patient's airway, level of consciousness, pupils, and other vital signs, and treat unconsciousness if it develops.

Bleeding Inside the Skull

Bleeding inside the skull can be caused by a head injury or by the spontaneous rupture of a blood vessel. Blood vessel ruptures can be caused by stroke, chronic high blood pressure, or the rupture of a berry-like weak spot on a vessel, called an **aneurysm**. Bleeding can occur within the brain or into the spaces between the coverings of the brain (**meninges**). The signs and symptoms are caused by both pressure on the brain and destruction of brain tissue. The neurological status of the patient may deteriorate rapidly. Monitor the patient closely and record findings at regular intervals. Quickly transport the patient to a hospital, treating unconsciousness if it develops.

Fig. 13.3 *Anatomy of the Eye*

Skull Fractures

Because a considerable force is required to fracture the skull, some degree of brain damage almost always accompanies **skull fractures**. Skull fractures can be open or closed. A frequent cause of open skull fractures is a penetrating injury from a sharp or high-velocity object such as an ice pick or a bullet. The signs and symptoms of a skull fracture are mainly those of the underlying brain damage. In addition, the patient may have a scalp wound which may expose the skull or brain tissue. Cerebrospinal fluid, which is watery and colorless or pink, may exude from the wound or drip from the nose or ear; there may be bleeding from the nose, ear, or mouth. Bleeding from a skull fracture also may be indicated by ecchymosis, usually in the skin around the eyes ("raccoon eyes") or at the tip of the mastoid process (Battle's sign). However, these signs of bleeding usually do not appear until several hours after the injury occurs.

Cerebrospinal fluid coming from the nose or ear may be overlooked if it is mixed with blood. If the discharge is allowed to drip onto a compress or other cloth, the cerebrospinal fluid will form a pink ring resembling a target around the blood.

The general emergency care of a patient with a skull fracture is similar to that of a patient with a brain contusion or hemorrhage (see above). Local wound care is discussed in the section on **Scalp Lacerations** above. Do not remove an impaled object; instead, immobilize it in place with a stabilizing dressing.

EYE INJURIES

Eye injuries have special significance because of the associated risk of blindness. An understanding of eye injuries and their emergency care requires a brief overview of the anatomy (Fig. 13.3) and physiology of the eye.

The eyeball is a hollow globe about 1 inch in diameter that lies in the eye socket of the skull. The optic nerve connects the eyeball with the brain through an opening in the back of the socket. The posterior five-sixths of the globe is formed by a dense tissue, the **sclera**, that is continuous anteriorly with the transparent **cornea**. In front, the visible part of the sclera is white and is called the white of the eye. It is covered by a transparent tissue, the **conjunctiva**, that contains small visible blood vessels. When this tissue is inflamed (**conjunctivitis**), the blood vessels enlarge, turning the conjunctiva pink or red.

The eyeball is divided into two compartments by the transparent **lens** and its supporting ligaments. The posterior compartment is filled with a jellylike fluid, the **vitreous humor**; the anterior compartment is filled with a watery fluid, the **aqueous humor**. The pressure of these two fluids maintains the globular shape of the eyeball. A laceration that allows fluid to leak out will cause the eyeball to collapse.

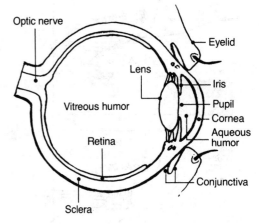

Fig. 13.3

Fig. 13.4 *Removal of a Foreign Body from the Inside Surface of the Upper Eyelid*

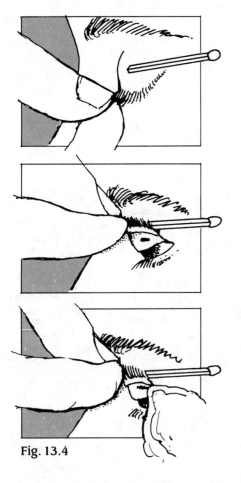

Fig. 13.4

Between the cornea and the lens lies a circular sheet of muscle, the **iris**, with a central hole, the **pupil**. The iris acts like the diaphragm of a camera, adjusting the size of the pupil to regulate the amount of light entering the eye. The outer surface of the iris is covered with pigmented cells that account for the color of the eye. The inner surface of the sclera is covered with a thin sheet of tissue, the **retina**, containing light-sensitive cells.

The eye can be compared to a simple camera. The cornea acts as a transparent lens cover, the lens of the eye corresponds to a camera lens, the iris to the camera diaphragm, and the retina to the film. The lens of the eye is elastic and can change shape to focus an image on the retina. In people over 45 years of age, this elasticity often is lost and must be compensated for by eyeglasses, usually bifocals or trifocals.

The cornea is protected by the **upper and lower eyelids** and is kept from drying out by **tears** produced by **tear glands** that lie above the outer part of each eye. The tears flow down across the cornea and drain at the inner corner of the eye through the **tear ducts** into the nasal cavity.

When evaluating an eye injury, the examiner should look for skin wounds, bleeding, swelling, ecchymosis, and abnormal prominence of one eye compared to the other. Inspect the conjunctiva for injuries or abnormal redness. Examine the pupils for size and symmetry, test with a flashlight for reaction to light, and compare the eyes to each other to detect differences in size and shape. Ask the patient to follow the movement of the examiner's finger; observe whether the patient's eyes move together and follow the finger as it is moved up, down, and from side to side.

The removal of contact lenses is discussed in Chapter 4.

Eye motion can aggravate an injured eye. Because the eyes normally move together as a unit, the only way to keep an injured eye quiet is to *cover both eyes.* Because eye injuries (except for irritation from small, easily removed foreign bodies) are a serious matter, a patient with an eye injury must be taken to a hospital emergency department or to a physician (preferably an ophthalmologist) as soon as possible. Transport the patient in the supine position.

Foreign Bodies

The conjunctiva is designed to protect the eye and is well supplied with nerves. Any object that touches the eyelashes or conjunctiva causes an instantaneous blink reflex, which is the body's attempt to keep the object out of the eye. A foreign body that penetrates these defenses and lodges on the conjunctiva causes severe pain and irritation. The eye produces tears in an attempt to flush out the object, and the eyelids go into spasm. Warn the patient never to rub or press on an eye containing a foreign body, because this can grind the object into the delicate eye tissues.

Small foreign bodies, such as cinders, frequently lodge under the upper eyelid. These can be removed using the moistened corner of a clean handkerchief after rolling the lid back (Fig. 13.4). Place a matchstick horizontally against the center of the eyelid, and lift the lid up over the stick by pulling on the eyelashes while the patient looks downward.

It is safe for a well-coordinated layperson to remove small, loose foreign bodies from the inner eyelid or conjunctiva; only a physician should remove a large or embedded foreign body, or an object lying on the cornea. Impaled foreign bodies should be stabilized in place by dry, sterile compresses. Cover the injured eye with an inverted paper cup and patch the normal eye.

Eye Lacerations

Lacerations of the eyelid require delicate suturing to preserve normal function and appearance. Bleeding from a lacerated eyelid can be controlled by gentle direct manual pressure. However, do not press on a lacerated eyeball. The emergency care of patients with eyeball lacerations and penetrating injuries consists of protecting the injured eye with a sterile dressing covered by an inverted paper cup, and patching the normal eye. Do not replace an exposed or displaced eyeball; instead, cover it with a sterile dressing moistened with sterile physiological saline solution or, if this is unavailable, with clean water. It is important to prevent the eyeball from drying out.

Eye Contusions

Blunt trauma to the eye can injure its structures and fracture the bones of the orbit. Bleeding into the eyeball may occur, and at times blood may be seen in the anterior compartment. Normal eye motion may be impaired. Emergency care consists of protecting the eye with an inverted paper cup or metal eye shield and patching the normal eye.

Eye Burns

Eye burns can be caused by heat and caustic chemicals. Sunburn of the eye (snowblindness) is discussed in Chapter 19.

Thermal burns usually involve a burn of the face that injures the eyelids, which close reflexively to protect the eyes. Eyelid burns are serious injuries that require expert care. The patient should be immediately transported to a hospital. Both eyes should be covered; the injured eye should be covered with a sterile compress moistened with sterile physiological saline solution.

Chemical burns also are serious injuries that may cause extensive destruction of delicate eye tissues. Major offenders are acids and alkalis; alkalis cause the worst injuries. Because these injuries progress rapidly, every second counts. The sole emergency care is immediate and prolonged flushing of the eye with clean water. The flushing method can consist of pouring water into the eye, holding the patient's head under a running faucet, or immersing the patient's face in a bucket while he or she blinks rapidly. The eyelids may be in spasm and may have to be forcibly held open during flushing. Flushing is continued for at least five minutes; alkali burns should be flushed for 20 minutes. While flushing, prevent the flushing solution from running into the uninjured eye. After flushing, patch both eyes, and immediately take the patient to a hospital.

Eye Changes With Head Injuries

Head injuries that damage the orbits or eyeballs or interfere with nerve or muscle function can cause **eye changes**. These changes should alert the rescuer to the possibility of a head injury and should be monitored to detect deterioration in the patient's condition. Such changes include:

Fig. 13.5 *A patient with a nosebleed should sit up and lean forward.*

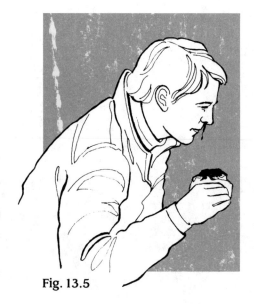

Fig. 13.5

1. Differences in the size and/or shape of the pupils (see Chapter 4, Fig. 4.10).
2. Complaints of double vision.
3. Failure of the eyes to move together or to point in the same direction.
4. Bleeding into the eyeball or orbit, which can produce visible blood in the anterior chamber of the eye or ecchymosis of the eyelids.
5. Abnormal protrusion of one or both eyes.

INJURIES TO THE FACE AND THROAT

Facial and throat injuries can be caused by the same mechanisms that injure the head and are accompanied by the same risk of cervical spine injury. Soft-tissue injuries, hemorrhage, and/or facial bone fractures may occur. The greatest danger is upper-airway blockage because of bleeding, swelling, deformities, loose teeth, dentures, or direct injury to the larynx or trachea. Vomitus, blood, mucus, and other materials obstructing the mouth and pharynx may have to be suctioned. In addition, patients with facial injuries may be unconscious and have the airway problems commonly associated with unconsciousness. Lacerations and other open injuries of the face are important from a cosmetic standpoint because they may heal with unsightly scars.

Emergency care of soft-tissue injuries of the face and neck is similar to that of any soft-tissue injury (see Chapter 8). Always examine the inside of the mouth for bleeding, broken teeth, vomitus, and foreign material.

Control bleeding by direct pressure; however, pressure should not be excessive if an underlying fracture is suspected. It may be necessary to apply pressure from both inside and outside the cheek to control bleeding from cheek lacerations. Patients who are bleeding from the mouth or nose should be positioned on one side or sitting up and leaning forward to prevent them from swallowing blood.

Bandage open wounds. Because infected wounds heal with severe scarring, dirty wounds and wounds that will not receive medical care within a few hours should be cleaned (see Chapter 8).

Cover exposed important structures such as the brain and eye with sterile compresses moistened with sterile physiological saline solution.

Control swelling with cold applications.

Preserve amputated pieces of ear or nose tissue and send them along to the hospital with the patient (see Chapter 8).

Clean an avulsed flap of skin by irrigating it with sterile saline solution; replace the flap over the wound before bandaging.

Nose Injuries

The inside of the nose is lined by a thin mucous membrane containing fragile blood vessels. The anterior part of the thin bone dividing the two halves of the nasal cavity (nasal septum) is the most common area to bleed. Bleeding can be caused by disease of or damage to the vessels, or by interference with the normal blood clotting mechanisms. Many nosebleeds occur without obvious cause; others are caused by injury to the face or head, the effects of high blood pressure or altitude, or by blowing the nose hard. People with allergies or head colds frequently have nosebleeds. Most spontaneous nosebleeds will stop of their own accord; those caused by disease or injury may be harder to stop. The patient usually is alarmed by the sight of so much blood and may become nauseated from swallowing blood. Instruct the patient to sit up and lean slightly forward so the blood will drain out of the nose rather than down the throat (Fig. 13.5).

Fig. 13.6 *Methods for Stopping a Nosebleed*

Stopping or Slowing a Nosebleed (Fig. 13.6)

1. Press the upper nostril against the septum for five minutes (Fig. 13.6a).
2. Place a pencil-sized roll of gauze between the upper lip and the teeth, and press inward on it for several minutes to shut off the artery to the septum (Fig. 13.6b).
3. Place a wad of Vaseline gauze in the bleeding nostril and press the side of the nostril against the septum (Fig. 13.6c).
4. Place an ice bag over the nose (Fig. 13.6d).

When the nose has been fractured by a blow it usually will be deformed and bleeding. For cosmetic reasons and to return the airway to normal, patients with fractured noses should see a physician. The earlier a nasal fracture is seen, the easier it is to restore the normal relationship of its parts.

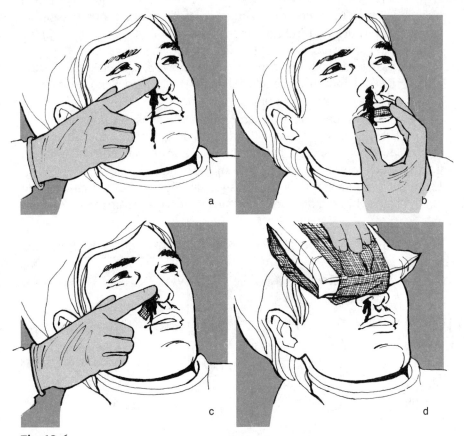

Fig. 13.6

Fig. 13.7 *Proper Method of Handling an Avulsed Tooth*

Facial Fractures

Facial fractures may be accompanied by difficulty in talking and swallowing, deformity, swelling, bite irregularity, and bleeding. The major risk is airway obstruction, which may worsen as swelling and bleeding progress.

Emergency Care of a Patient with a Facial Fracture

1. Open and maintain the upper airway, always protecting the cervical spine.
2. Use suction if necessary.
3. Insert an oral airway if the patient is unconscious. The patient may have to be turned onto one side so that copious secretions or bleeding can drain away. Remember that this maneuver, while at times necessary to prevent suffocation, may aggravate a cervical spine injury.
4. Give oxygen in high concentration.
5. Stop external bleeding with direct pressure.
6. The patient may need to be immobilized on a spine board.

Oral-dental Injuries

Lacerations inside the mouth can occur with or without injury to teeth. If bleeding occurs following the fracture or avulsion of a tooth, use sterile gauze to wipe out blood and clots, then place several gauze squares over the bleeding area. Ask the patient to bite down gently on the gauze. If this does not control the bleeding, direct finger pressure may be required. Do not let the patient rinse the mouth, since this may worsen bleeding. Send extra gauze pads along with the patient during transportation.

Facial blows may chip or fracture teeth. If a sensitive dental nerve is exposed, it should be covered with gauze to protect it from cold air. If teeth are displaced or avulsed, the patient should see an oral surgeon immediately. If an avulsed tooth can be found, it should be handled by *the crown only* (Fig. 13.7a). Do not touch, rub, or vigorously clean the tooth, although it can be gently cleaned by holding it under running water or a stream of sterile saline

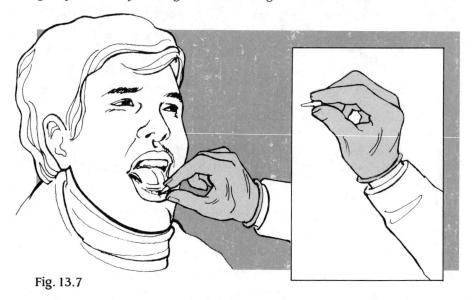

Fig. 13.7

poured from an IV bottle. Replace the tooth in the socket, if possible (Fig. 13.7b). Otherwise, send the tooth along with the patient in a container of milk, saline solution, water, or, if the patient is alert and dependable, inside the patient's cheek. If at all possible, the tooth should be reimplanted by an oral surgeon within 30 minutes; the success rate falls off rapidly if replacement takes longer.

Immobilize a fractured lower jaw by gently lifting the mandible into proper position against the upper teeth. Secure it with a cravat tied snugly under the jaw and around the head so that it can be slid off quickly if the patient retches (Fig. 13.8). A dislocated jaw usually is locked open and requires no splinting; it should be relocated only by a physician.

Fig. 13.8 *Immobilization of a Fractured Lower Jaw*

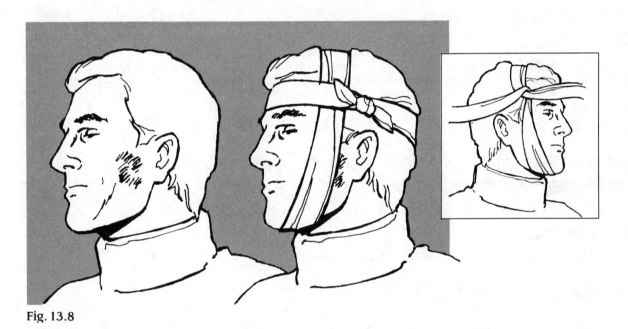

Fig. 13.8

Throat Injuries

Injuries to the soft tissues of the neck and direct injury to the larynx or trachea can cause bleeding, swelling, and upper-airway obstruction. These injuries frequently are accompanied by a cervical spine injury. Injury to the air-containing structures of the neck can cause subcutaneous emphysema, which is air in the soft tissues that imparts a characteristic crackling sensation when an examiner touches the area with a finger ("Rice Krispies" under the skin). Injuries to the larynx usually cause voice loss.

Bleeding or swelling from a throat injury may cause or worsen airway obstruction. Because this type of airway obstruction frequently cannot be managed without an endotracheal tube or a tracheotomy, quickly transport the patient to a hospital. Give oxygen in high concentration but *do not use a bag-mask* because positive pressure may force air into the damaged tissues, worsening the obstruction. For the same reason, instruct the patient to breathe slowly and quietly.

14

Injuries to the Neck and Back

And sadly reflecting,
That a lover forsaken
A new love may get,
But a neck when once broken
Can never be set.

> *–William Walsh*
> "The Despairing Lover"

Serious injuries to the neck and back are significant because they can cause major, often permanent disability if the spinal cord is involved. In urban settings, such injuries most often result from automobile or motorcycle accidents. In outdoor pursuits, these injuries can be caused by collisions while skiing, direct blows from falling rocks, dives into shallow water, falls, and cave-ins. Injuries to the soft tissues of the neck and back are discussed in previous chapters. This chapter covers injuries to the major parts of the skeletal and nervous systems found in the neck and back: the **spine** and **spinal cord**.

The spinal cord lies in a long tunnel, the spinal canal, formed by the successive arches of the vertebrae. The spinal cord is somewhat protected by the spine; however, this close association means that severe injuries to the spine are likely to involve the spinal cord as well. A spinal cord injury is a *neurosurgical emergency*.

When the patient is first seen, many times the examiner can only tell that the patient has a neck or back injury. It may be impossible to know for certain whether the spine or spinal cord is injured or, more important, *whether the spinal cord is in danger of being injured*. Nevertheless, because the consequences of missing an actual or potential spinal cord injury can be so severe, *all* neck and back injuries must be treated as spinal cord injuries. Fortunately, most spine injuries are minor, heal well, and produce no long-term disability. However, in the field, it may be impossible to distinguish minor spine injuries from unstable or displaced fractures that can cause permanent injury or death.

Before reading this chapter, please review the anatomy and physiology of the spine and spinal cord in Chapter 2.

Classification of Neck and Back Injuries

1. Injury to the skin, muscles, tendons, or ligaments *alone*, without bony spine or spinal cord injury (Fig. 14.1a).
2. Spine injury *without* spinal cord injury (Fig. 14.1b). The major purpose of emergency care is to *prevent* a cord injury.
3. Spine injury with *incomplete* cord injury (Fig. 14.1c). In this case, the patient suffers partial but not complete paralysis and loss of sensation at and below the injury site. Repeated monitoring is necessary to detect possible *progression*. The presence or absence of progression is important information for the neurosurgeon. The major purpose of emergency care is to *prevent further cord injury*.
4. Spine injury with *complete* spinal cord injury (Fig. 14.1d). The patient suffers complete paralysis and loss of sensation below the injury site. Although the outlook for recovery and improvement is much worse than for an incomplete cord injury, prompt surgery may relieve pressure on the cord permitting some recovery over time.

Signs and Symptoms of Spine Injury

1. **Pain at the injury site**. Pain may be elicited or increased by motion produced at the injured site. *Never ask a person with neck or back pain to move the body at the injured site* and never move such a patient except by techniques designed to safely place the person on a spine board.

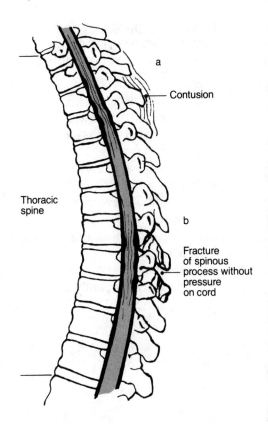

Fig. 14.1 *Types of Neck and Back Injuries (see text)*

Contusion

Thoracic spine

Fracture of spinous process without pressure on cord

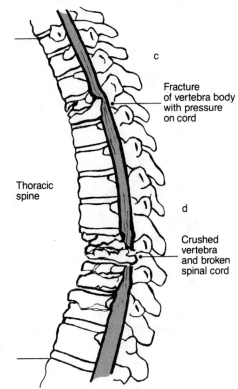

Fracture of vertebra body with pressure on cord

Thoracic spine

Crushed vertebra and broken spinal cord

Fig. 14.1

Table 14.1

SUMMARY OF SIGNS AND SYMPTOMS OF SPINE AND SPINAL CORD INJURIES

1. Spine
   a. Pain at the injury site.
   b. Localized tenderness.
   c. Associated soft-tissue injuries.
   d. Occasionally, deformity.
2. Spinal cord
   a. All of the above may be present.
   b. Loss of touch and pain perception.
   c. Abnormal sensations.
   d. Weakness or paralysis.

2. **Localized tenderness**. Gently press the spinous processes of all the vertebrae; tenderness of one or more suggests injury at that site. Unless the patient is being examined in the lateral or prone position, slide your hand under the patient's back from the side so your fingers touch the spinous processes. Do not allow the patient's trunk to turn or rotate.
3. Associated soft tissue injuries, with **tenderness, swelling, and ecchymosis**. These signs can be detected only if the patient is examined in the lateral or prone position.
4. **Deformity or unusual positions** of the spine may or may not be present.

In addition to the signs and symptoms listed for spine injuries, patients with spinal cord injury may have signs and symptoms that involve *one* or *both* sides of the body below the injury site.

Signs and Symptoms of Spinal Cord Injury

1. Varying degrees of **loss of sensation** to touch and pain.
2. **Abnormal sensations** such as numbness, tingling, or unusual types of pain.
3. **Muscle weakness or complete paralysis**.

Assessment of a Patient with a Neck or Back Injury

1. Ask the patient what happened. Consider the mechanisms of injury to determine whether the accident would be expected to produce a spine or spinal cord injury.
2. Perform the primary survey and treat urgent problems. It is particularly important to check for respiratory distress, which, if present, suggests either a concurrent chest injury or paralysis of the chest wall muscles.
3. During the secondary survey, note the strength of the pulse and the capillary refill time and, if possible, measure the patient's blood pressure since neurogenic shock can be a complication of spinal cord injury. Examine the patient in the supine position or, if the patient is found prone, carry out the initial examination with the patient in the prone position. Ask the patient to indicate the location and type of any pain and whether there is numbness, weakness, or abnormal sensations below the site of pain.
4. Next, ask the patient to wiggle his or her toes and to squeeze both your hands. Check the patient's arms and legs for perceptions of pain and touch. Look for obvious injuries of the face, head, neck and trunk, and for any obvious deformities of the spine.
5. Finally, *without moving* the patient, run your hand under the patient's back and neck, feeling for any deformity or tenderness of the spinous processes.

If abnormalities are detected during this examination, suspect a spine injury. Do not allow the patient to move; rescuers should only move the patient using proper techniques.

Many steps of the examination cannot be performed on an unconscious patient. This is irrelevant in cases of unconsciousness related to trauma, since all such patients are considered to have a spine injury.

Definitive emergency care of a patient with a neck or back injury is *immobilization on a spine board* designed to splint the body to prevent neck or back movement. When assessing the mechanism of injury, try to foresee the extrication and immobilization techniques that will be required so that hand position and rescuer location will be proper. The patient must be transferred to the spine board using proper techniques so that the neck and back are not bent or rotated. When the spine board cannot be brought in to the patient, use the extrication techniques described in Chapter 20.

The emergency care of a patient with a neck injury is identical to that of a patient with a back injury, except that with a neck injury, an extrication collar is recommended if it can be put in place without further manipulation of the patient's neck. In any case, continue manual stabilization of the head and neck until the patient is immobilized on the spine board.

Emergency Care of a Patient with a Neck or Back Injury

1. If possible, examine and immobilize the patient in the supine position to simplify maintenance of the airway, monitoring of vital signs, transfer to the spine board, and management of vomiting. In rare cases, a patient with a marked deformity of the back may be found in a position that justifies immobilization in other than the supine position. The four-person direct ground lift (see Chapter 20) is probably the best technique to use to avoid producing motion at the site of injury while transferring such a patient to a spine board.

   A patient found in the *prone* position usually is rolled as a unit into the supine position as soon as possible. This technique, called logrolling (Fig. 14.2), also can be used to roll a supine patient onto one side so that a spine board can be slid underneath. Four rescuers are required for this maneuver.

   Before logrolling the patient, control any severe bleeding. Maintain the airway (using the jaw-thrust maneuver) and make sure breathing is adequate. If the jaw-thrust maneuver fails to open the airway, the neck may have to be realigned slightly, especially if the head is turned or the neck is bent.

   To realign the neck, use gentle manual traction, turning the head toward a natural position relative to the rest of the body (eyes-front position, Fig. 14.2a). Although there is some danger of aggravating a spinal cord injury by this maneuver, the patient will die if the airway cannot be opened. Stop at several points during this procedure and repeat the jaw-thrust maneuver to see if the airway can then be opened. Realign the neck only enough to open the airway. Maintain the head and neck in the new position manually, and immobilize the head and neck in this position after the patient has been transferred to the spine board. Avoid marked flexion and extension of the neck. If the rescuer needs to reposition his or her hands, repositioning is performed with the aid of an assistant using the helmet-removal method described in step 4.

   To perform the **logroll**, first tie the patient's legs together with a cravat. The first rescuer kneels by the patient's head, facing the patient, and is responsible for stabilizing the patient's head and neck throughout the maneuver and until the patient is immobilized on the

Table 14.2

SUMMARY OF ASSESSMENT OF A PATIENT WITH A NECK OR BACK INJURY

1. First impression. Determine mechanism of injury.
2. Primary survey
   a. Significance of respiratory distress.
   b. Possibility and significance of shock.
3. Secondary survey
   a. Ask about symptoms of injury (see Table 14.1, above)
   b. Ask the patient to squeeze your hands and wiggle his or her toes.
   c. Check for sensation below the injury site.
   d. Examine the injury site without moving the patient, if possible.

Fig. 14.2 *Technique of Logrolling a Patient from the Prone to the Supine Position (see text)*

spine board. With the thumbs on the occiput behind the patient's ears, the index fingers on the jaw angles, and the remaining fingers along the jaw and cheeks, exert gentle traction to maintain the head and neck in line with the body. If the airway requires maintaining by the jaw-thrust maneuver, the jaw can be thrust forward with the index fingers. If the patient has a neck injury, an assistant puts an extrication collar in place (Fig. 14.2b).

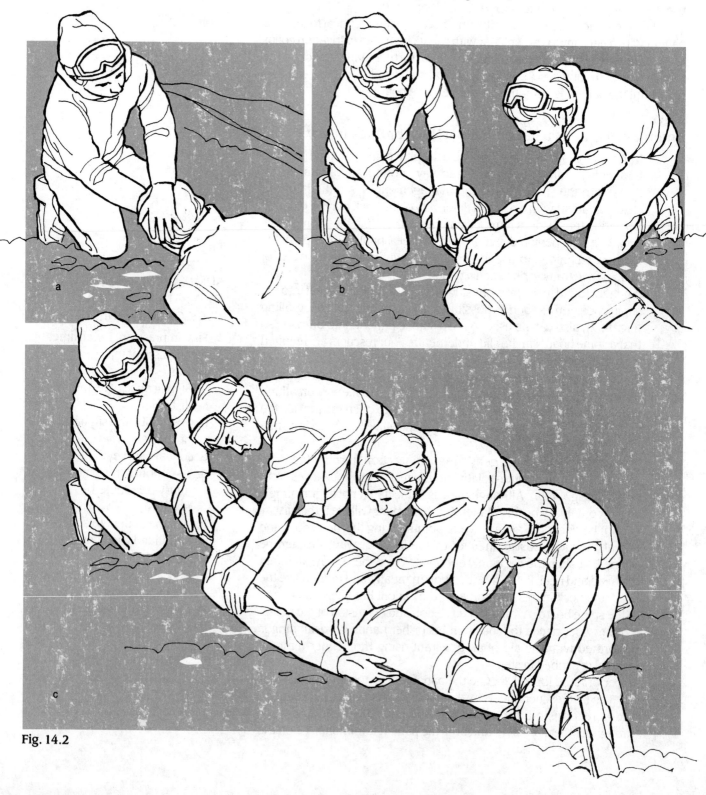

Fig. 14.2

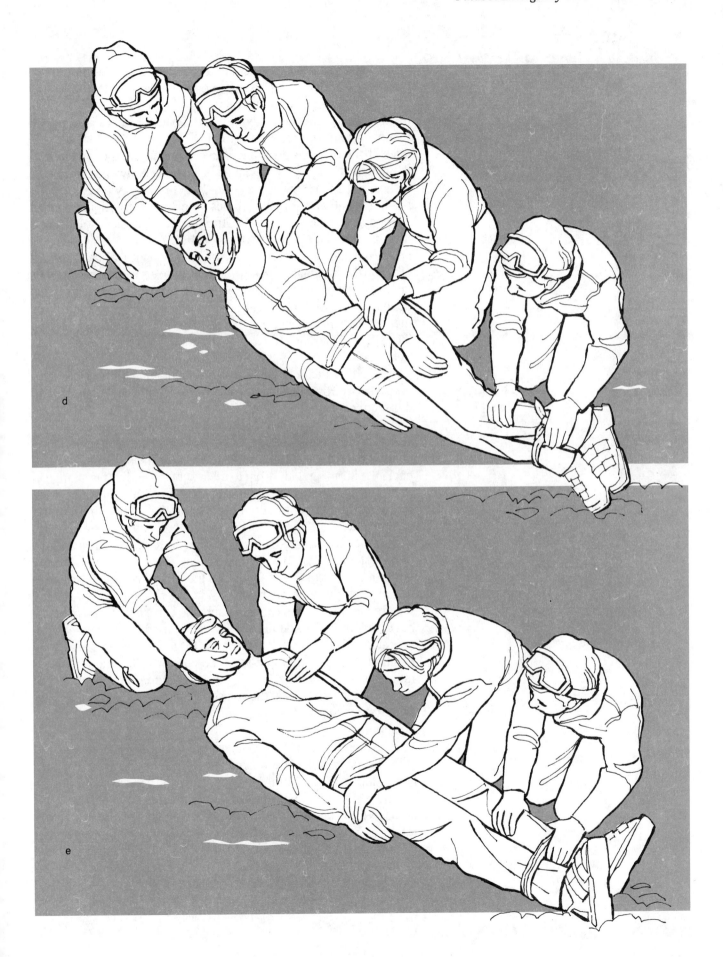

d

e

The other three rescuers kneel in a row (Fig. 14.2c) on the side to which the patient will be rolled. In older methods of logrolling, the patient's near arm would be raised over the patient's head at this point. This maneuver is no longer used because it can cause the neck to move and the thoracic spine to sag.

Instead, the patient's arms are placed along the sides of and next to the patient's body, with the palms against the body and the elbows locked, to "splint" the spine. The second rescuer, who is kneeling beside the patient's shoulders, holds the patient's arms tightly against the body by placing one hand on the patient's opposite shoulder and the other hand over the opposite forearm. The third rescuer kneels beside the patient's buttocks, with one hand on the iliac crest and the other on the midthigh. The fourth rescuer kneels beside the patient's knees, with one hand on the opposite knee and the other hand on the opposite leg just below the calf. The first rescuer is in charge and gives the signal for the other three rescuers to roll the patient slowly toward themselves, avoiding any twisting or bending of the back (Fig. 14.2d). The first rescuer turns the patient's head as the patient's body is rolled, so that the head and neck are maintained in the same relationship to the body at all times and the neck is not bent or twisted. In this manner, the patient is moved from the prone to the supine position (Fig. 14.2e).

The rescuer who is at the patient's head will need to shift the position of his or her hands by 180 degrees to maintain the patient's head and neck in a normal relationship to the rest of the body. This change in hand position requires a shift in body position, which may throw the rescuer off balance and compromise proper stabilization of the patient's head and neck. A shift can be prevented by starting the maneuver with the hands crossed so that the hand placed on the side of the patient's head to which the patient will be rolled goes around underneath the patient's face, and the other hand goes over the patient's occiput to reach the other side.

A safer method is to use an assistant who can stabilize the patient's head and neck in a manner similar to that used for helmet removal (see step 4.), allowing the first rescuer to shift to a more stable body position. The assistant kneels at the patient's side and maintains manual stabilization by cupping one hand under the patient's chin and the other hand under the back of the patient's neck and occiput. The first rescuer takes over again after regaining a comfortable position.

2. If the patient is found in the *supine* position, open the airway and stabilize the head and neck manually while kneeling at the patient's head. Place one hand firmly on each side of the head, with the fingers along the mandible and behind its angle. If necessary, the fingers can be used to thrust the jaw forward to maintain the airway. Do not rotate or bend the head excessively during this maneuver and, if increased pain or resistance occur, stabilize and immobilize the head and neck in the position found. If the patient has a neck injury, an assistant puts an extrication collar in place.

3. Give additional basic life support measures, and bandage open wounds, if necessary.
4. It may be necessary to remove helmets worn by injured climbers, ski racers, and snowmobilers. If the helmet is small and fits snugly, it need not be removed. Remove the helmet if it is large, so loose that the head cannot be immobilized, or if a face mask or visor interferes with ventilation. To avoid twisting or bending the neck, the helmet should be removed by two rescuers.

The first rescuer kneels at the patient's head, places one hand on either side of the helmet with the fingertips under the edge of the jaw, and applies gentle manual stabilization of the head and neck. The second rescuer kneels at one side, cuts or loosens the chin strap, and then cups one hand under the patient's chin with the thumb on one side of the jaw and the fingers on the other side. The other hand is cupped under the back of the neck, exerting pressure on the occiput. The second rescuer maintains stabilization while the first rescuer removes the helmet. After removing the helmet, the first rescuer resumes manual stabilization of the head as described in step 2. above; manual stabilization is maintained until the patient is secured to the spine board. If the patient is suspected of having a neck injury, an extrication collar is put on after the helmet is removed.
5. To put a long spine board in place under the patient, logroll the patient onto one side using the technique described above, or lift the patient using the **straddle-slide** (described below) or the four-rescuer direct ground lift (see Chapter 20).

When the logroll method is used, the board is placed beside the patient (Fig. 14.3), touching the patient's side, and is tipped at a 30- to 45-degree angle.

The **straddle slide** requires four rescuers. The first rescuer crouches at the patient's head and stabilizes the head and neck with gentle manual stabilization. The second rescuer straddles a long spine board.

Fig. 14.3 *Logroll Method for Placing a Spine Board Under a Patient*

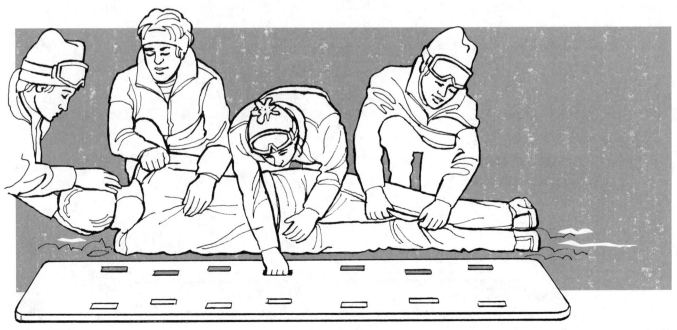

Fig. 14.3

Fig. 14.4 *A patient can be strapped to the long spine board with cravats or straps.*

placed lengthwise above the patient's head. The third and fourth rescuers straddle the patient, one behind the other, facing the patient's head. The third rescuer reaches under the patient's armpits and places a hand against each of the patient's upper scapulae. The fourth rescuer places a hand under each side of the patient's upper pelvis.

At a command from the first rescuer, the patient is lifted slightly off the ground as a unit by the first, third, and fourth rescuers, while the second rescuer slides the spine board lengthwise beneath the patient. On a second command, the patient is lowered as a unit onto the board.

The straddle slide is a difficult maneuver to perform on an incline, on uneven ground, or while wearing ski boots. Also, it requires the rescuer to bend over and lift with the legs spread far apart–a posture that can cause back injury. This method is poorly suited for short patients, because the third and fourth rescuers are stationed too close together. Use the straddle slide only in special circumstances when the logroll or direct ground lift is unsuitable because of difficulty in access or other reasons.

In some cases, the patient must be carried a short distance to the spine board using the four-rescuer direct ground lift and carry (see Chapter 20). The technique of strapping the patient to the long spine board is described in Chapter 9 (Fig. 14.4).

Once the patient has been placed on the spine board, he or she may have to be centered. Do this by pulling in the direction of the long axis of the body rather than pulling the patient sideways.

6. When a patient is found sitting or in a difficult-to- extricate position, a short spine immobilization device may be preferable. The immobilization technique is described in Chapter 9. The short spine device is designed for use *only* during extrication. The patient should be immobilized on a long spine board or strapped into a rigid litter as

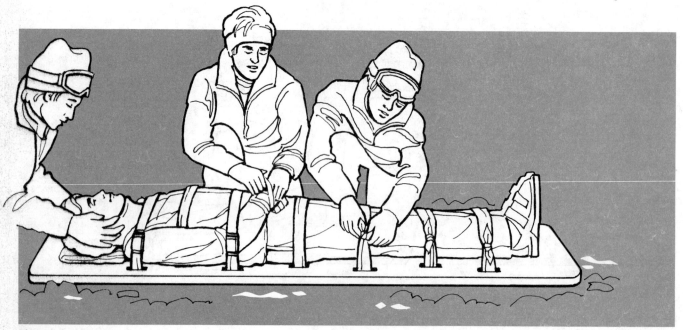

Fig. 14.4

soon as possible. Always leave the short spine board in place when the patient is transferred to the second device. Because the short spine board does not completely immobilize the spine, never lift the patient by the short board alone.

7. If available, give oxygen in high concentration to all patients with obvious or suspected spinal cord injuries.

8. If the patient is unconscious, provide the appropriate care (see Chapter 13).

9. If the patient has associated fractures, use judgment when deciding whether to splint these before or after immobilizing the patient on a spine board. In general, fractures that can be splinted without moving the patient and major ones such as open fractures and fractures of the femur should be splinted beforehand, since a patient with a spine injury is stable as long as he or she remains stationary. Splint minor fractures and fractures that are relatively painless and stable after the patient is on the spine board.

10. A patient with a cervical or high thoracic spinal cord injury may have paralysis of the chest wall and abdominal muscles and may be breathing with the diaphragm alone. The motor supply of the diaphragm comes from the **phrenic nerves**, which exit the spinal cord at the level of the third, fourth, and fifth cervical vertebrae and run down through the neck and mediastinum to the diaphragm. Their pathways can be interrupted only by injury to the chest or to the highest part of the cervical spinal cord.

When the chest wall and abdominal muscles are paralyzed, the patient's respirations will be rapid and shallow and the chest wall will not move, but the abdomen will move in and out with each breath as the diaphragm moves up and down. In this situation, monitor the patient's respiration and give the patient oxygen in high concentration. If respirations appear inadequate, the rescuer may assist breathing by using a bag-mask or pocket mask so that oxygen in high concentration can be given at the same time.

Vascular shock may occur in a patient with a spinal cord injury because of paralysis of the nerves that maintain blood pressure by controlling blood vessel tone (see Chapter 7). Hypovolemic shock also may occur because of blood loss from accompanying injuries. Emergency care consists of controlling bleeding, splinting other fractures, and elevating the foot of the long spine board about 12 inches so that the patient is in the head-down position.

When a patient has suffered multiple serious injuries, a head or chest injury may indicate elevating the patient's head and chest, but the presence of shock may indicate a head-down position. The rescuer should first treat the condition that appears to be the most life-threatening, even though some treatment requirements conflict with others.

Table 14.3

SUMMARY OF EMERGENCY CARE OF A PATIENT WITH A NECK OR BACK INJURY

1. Maintain the airway and stabilization of the head and neck.
2. In case of neck injury, apply extrication collar.
3. Logroll the patient into the supine position.
4. Give additional basic life support measures, as needed.
5. Care for any open wounds.
6. Remove the patient's helmet, if present.
7. Place the patient on a long spine board or, if appropriate, on a short spine board.
8. Give oxygen in high concentration.
9. Care for any associated fractures.
10. Monitor vital signs and state of consciousness.
11. Assist breathing, if necessary.
12. Treat shock, if present.

15

Chest Injuries

Mercutio: Go villain, fetch a surgeon.
Romeo: Courage, man; the hurt cannot be much.
Mercutio: No, 'tis not so deep as a well, nor so wide
as a church door, but 'tis enough, 'twill serve. Ask for me
tomorrow, and you shall find me a grave man.

> *—William Shakespeare*
> *Romeo and Juliet III.i.*

Chest injuries are a significant cause of death and disability. In the urban environment, these injuries most commonly result from vehicle and industrial accidents. In the outdoors they can be caused by collisions and falls while skiing, falls while climbing, direct blows from rockfall, and the like. Before reading this chapter, review the sections on anatomy and physiology of the respiratory and circulatory systems in Chapter 2.

The chest is most commonly injured by either blunt or penetrating trauma. The structures of the chest wall—skin, subcutaneous tissues, muscles, tendons, ligaments, and ribs—may be injured. Injury also may involve the chest wall plus the contents of the chest. The most important chest contents are the heart, lungs, pleura, diaphragm, and traversing structures such as the great vessels, trachea, esophagus, and important nerves.

Chest wounds can be either **open** or **closed**. **Open chest wounds** are caused by objects that penetrate the chest wall, either because they are sharp (e.g., ice axes, ski pole tips, knives) or because of their high velocity (e.g., bullets). Air enters the pleural cavity through the wound, causing normal negative pressure to be lost and the lung to collapse. Structures inside the chest can be lacerated and punctured, causing bleeding and loss of function.

Closed chest wounds are caused by blunt trauma, for example, when a skier collides with a fixed object. The skin can be either broken or unbroken. The chest wall and organs within the chest can be crushed, torn, or ripped from their attachments. Single or multiple ribs can break, and their sharp ends can lacerate blood vessels and other organs, causing bleeding and loss of organ function. Fractures of multiple ribs can loosen a section of the chest wall, causing interference with the normal ability of the chest cage to expand and contract during breathing.

Following trauma, there are certain important signs and symptoms that suggest significant chest injury has occurred.

Signs and Symptoms of Chest Injury

1. Pain at the site of injury, usually increased by breathing and coughing.
2. Respiratory distress, which can include **dyspnea** (difficult or labored breathing), **tachypnea** (increase in the breathing rate), and **hyperpnea** (increase in the breathing depth). Dyspnea also includes the patient's awareness of the need to make extra efforts to get enough oxygen.
3. Coughing.
4. Failure of one or both sides of the chest to expand normally with breathing.
5. Signs and symptoms of shock (see Chapter 7).
6. Coughing up blood (hemoptysis).
7. **Cyanosis**, a bluish discoloration of the skin, fingernails and mucous membranes that occurs because the blood is not properly oxygenated.

Table 15.1

SUMMARY OF SIGNS AND SYMPTOMS OF SIGNIFICANT CHEST INJURY

1. Pain at the injury site, usually increased by breathing and coughing.
2. Respiratory distress.
3. Cough.
4. Failure of normal chest wall motion.
5. Shock.
6. Coughing up blood.
7. Cyanosis.

Fig. 15.1 *Types of Rib Fractures*

SPECIFIC CHEST INJURIES

Rib Fractures

Rib fractures are common injuries usually caused by falls and collisions. Fractures can be single or multiple and can involve one or more ribs. The broken ends of the ribs can be displaced or non-displaced (Fig. 15.1). The fifth through tenth ribs are the most commonly fractured. The upper four ribs are protected by the shoulder girdle; the last two ribs are small, their front ends are unattached, and they are more likely to bend at their attachments to the spine than to break.

Simple forward falls usually do not cause rib fractures because people tend to break a fall with their hands; however, falling to the side and striking the ground with the arm against the body may cause lateral rib fractures. Multiple ribs can be broken during hard falls, long pendulum swings during climbs, high-speed collisions while skiing, and automobile accidents.

Several adjacent ribs fractured in more than one place can loosen a section of chest wall so that it moves in instead of out when the patient inhales, and out instead of in when the patient exhales. This condition is called paradoxical motion of the chest wall; the loose section is called a **flail chest** (Fig. 15.2).

The sharp, displaced end of a fractured rib can tear a hole in the lung (Fig. 15.3), causing air to leak into the pleural space and the lung to collapse (**pneumothorax**, Fig. 15.4). If a blood vessel is lacerated, significant bleeding can occur.

Fractured ribs are very painful, with pain typically increased by breathing and coughing. The proper treatment for a fractured bone is splinting, which reduces pain and speeds healing. Because the patient must breathe, the chest wall cannot be splinted enough to completely prevent rib motion. Fortunately, a fractured rib will heal even without complete immobilization. Advise the patient to stabilize the painful area with a hand before coughing. The pain of a broken rib usually is well-localized, and the patient often can point to the painful spot with one finger. Breathing typically is shallower and more rapid because of the pain. The patient usually prefers to sit up and tries to splint the chest by leaning to the injured side. Signs that the patient has a

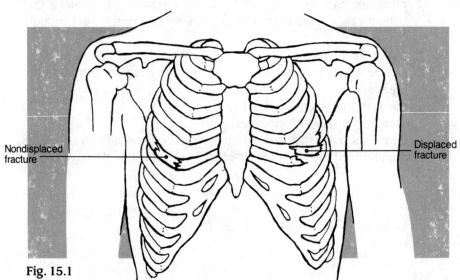

Nondisplaced
fracture

Displaced
fracture

Fig. 15.1

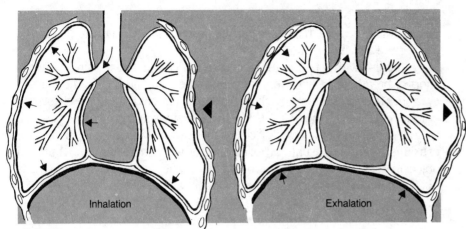

Fig. 15.2

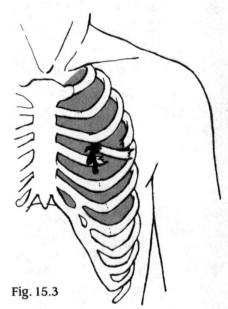

Fig. 15.3

significant lung injury rather than a simple rib fracture include shortness of breath that is severe or accompanied by cyanosis, severe cough, or coughing up blood.

A flail chest is a serious injury because it usually is accompanied by a crushing injury of the underlying lung, in addition to disruption of the normal mechanics of breathing on the injured side. The patient may develop cyanosis and severe respiratory distress. Inspection of the chest will disclose failure of the flail segment to move out on inhalation and in on exhalation.

Penetrating Injuries

Penetrating injuries occur when an object such as a knife or bullet penetrates the chest wall. The object may stop in the chest wall but usually enters the chest cavity, where it can injure any organ within the chest. The most commonly injured organs are the heart, lungs, and blood vessels. A penetrating injury can cause air and/or blood to leak into the pleural cavity. Massive bleeding with shock can occur; the bleeding may not be obvious because it is internal.

If the entrance wound is small, the wound may seal itself, but if it is larger, a **sucking chest wound** usually develops. This wound is an open hole in the chest wall that establishes a connection between the pleural space and the

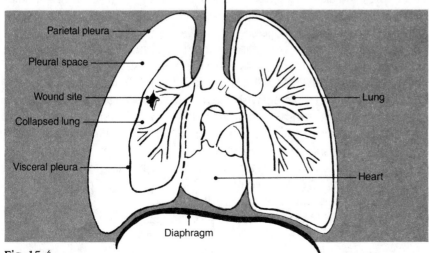

Fig. 15.4

Fig. 15.5 *Sucking Chest Wound*

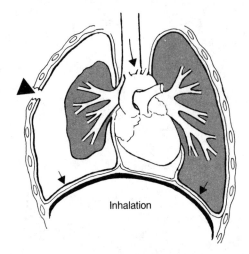

Inhalation

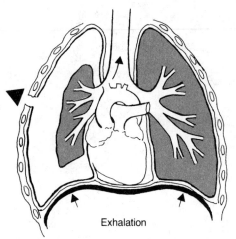

Exhalation

Fig. 15.5

outside air. The lung on that side collapses and, during breathing, air moves in and out of the hole in the chest rather than in and out of the lung through the normal airway (Fig. 15.5).

A patient with a penetrating chest injury complains of pain, is always short of breath, usually prefers to sit up rather than lie down, and may be cyanotic. The patient may cough up blood, the affected side of the chest may not move as well as the normal side, and the signs and symptoms of shock may be present. Examination discloses the entrance wound and, in the case of a gunshot wound, usually an exit wound as well. There may be an impaled object in the wound and external bleeding may be significant. If the wound is open, a peculiar sucking noise may be heard as the air moves in and out of the hole.

Compression Injuries

A sudden, massive, circumferential crushing injury to the chest causes multiple rib fractures and crushing injuries of the lungs and other intrathoracic organs. This type of trauma is seen in cave-ins and explosions. A sudden, rapid increase in intrathoracic pressure occurs that produces swelling and cyanosis of the upper body, distension of the neck veins, and bulging of the eyes. The patient may experience shock, severe respiratory distress, cyanosis, and other signs and symptoms of severe injury.

Injuries to the Back of the Chest

Trauma to the back of the chest can injure the posterior chest wall, thoracic spine, scapulae, back muscles, and underlying organs such as the lungs and kidneys. Any injured person who complains of pain in the back of the chest should be logrolled onto one side for a careful examination of this area.

Pneumothorax

The term **pneumothorax** means air in the pleural space. The normal pleural space is a closed sac with an internal partial vacuum that is essential for normal breathing. The lungs are elastic and are held in the expanded condition only because the negative pressure of the pleural space allows outside air to enter and expand them. The expanded lungs get larger during inhalation and smaller during exhalation as they follow the movements of the diaphragm and thoracic cage.

If an abnormal passage connects the pleural space with the outside air, the vacuum is lost and the pressure in the pleural space becomes equal to that of the outside air. Loss of the pressure differential causes the elastic lung to collapse and fail to expand with air when the chest cage expands. Such an abnormal passage can be either in the chest wall, where it connects the pleural space directly with the outside air, or within the lung, where it connects the pleural space with the outside air via the bronchi.

Even though a small abnormal passage usually seals itself off, the air in the pleural space takes many days to be absorbed. Larger passages do not seal by themselves, and require surgery.

Pneumothorax can be caused by spontaneous rupture of a bleb (blister-like abnormality of the lung surface) or cyst of the lung (spontaneous pneumothorax), by a penetrating wound of the chest wall, or by laceration of the lung from the sharp ends of a broken rib. The signs and symptoms are those of the condition that caused the pneumothorax and always include pain, respiratory distress, and decreased motion of the affected side of the chest during breathing.

Spontaneous pneumothorax usually occurs in young people who have congenital cysts or blebs on the lung surfaces. This condition should be suspected when a young, healthy person develops sudden chest pain and respiratory distress in the absence of a chest injury.

Tension Pneumothorax

Tension pneumothorax is a serious complication of a pneumothorax that occurs when a defect simulating a one-way valve develops at the injury site (Fig. 15.6). Each time the patient inhales, the valve opens, and air is pumped into the pleural space. When the patient exhales, the valve closes, and the air cannot escape. The pressure within the pleural space becomes higher and higher, eventually compressing the lung into a ball a few inches in diameter. The mediastinum is forced toward the other side of the chest, interfering with the function of both the heart and the opposite, normal lung. When pressure in the pleural space exceeds pressure in the venae cavae, blood can no longer flow back to the heart, and the patient rapidly goes into shock and dies.

Tension pneumothorax can occur with spontaneous pneumothorax and with both open and closed chest injuries. It occasionally occurs after a sucking chest wound is bandaged. Signs and symptoms include severe, rapidly progressive respiratory distress; a weak, rapid pulse; falling blood pressure; bulging of the chest wall tissues between the ribs and above the clavicles on the involved side; engorgement of the neck veins; deviation of the trachea to the opposite side; and cyanosis.

When the examiner thumps the affected side of the chest with the fingers, a drum-like note is heard that is higher pitched than the sound heard on the normal side. The condition progresses rapidly, and death can occur within a few minutes. To relieve a tension pneumothorax, a physician or paramedic decompresses the chest by piercing it with a large needle or a special tube.

If a patient with a sucking chest wound has been treated with an occlusive dressing and suddenly gets worse, the rescuer should suspect development of a tension pneumothorax. Pressure can be relieved by lifting a corner of the dressing.

Hemothorax

Hemothorax, or blood in the pleural space, is caused by bleeding from vessels in the lung or chest wall that have been damaged by a closed or open chest injury. Hemothorax frequently is accompanied by air in the pleural space (hemopneumothorax). The pressure of the blood partly collapses the lung. The signs and symptoms are similar to those of pneumothorax, except that significant blood loss into the pleural space may cause shock. In the field, hemothorax and pneumothorax are difficult to tell apart; a patient with a pneumothorax whose condition is worsening is probably developing either a hemothorax or a tension pneumothorax.

Fig. 15.6 *Tension Pneumothorax*

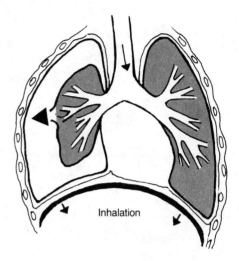

Inhalation

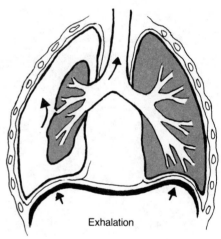

Exhalation

Fig. 15.6

Subcutaneous Emphysema

Injury to air-containing parts of the respiratory tract in the chest and neck can allow air to escape into the tissues, where it spreads as small bubbles into the subcutaneous tissues. When the involved area is examined, the examiner feels a unique crackling sensation similar to Rice Krispies under the skin. The signs and symptoms usually are those of the underlying injury, frequently a lung lacerated by a fractured rib.

Pulmonary Contusion

A **pulmonary contusion** is a lung bruise resulting from a blunt or crushing chest injury of the type experienced during hard falls, collisions, and auto accidents. A pulmonary contusion usually is accompanied by injuries to the chest wall. The injured lung develops bleeding and swelling (from edema fluid) in and between the alveoli as well as damage to the blood vessels and bronchi. The signs and symptoms are those of the causative injury and always include respiratory distress.

Myocardial Contusion

Blunt injuries to the chest may injure the heart as well as the lungs, most frequently causing a heart muscle bruise called a **myocardial contusion**. The signs and symptoms include a fast or irregular heartbeat caused by the injured muscle's tendency to produce abnormal electrical discharges. Large contusions may injure enough muscle to cause heart failure or shock.

Pericardial Tamponade

Pericardial tamponade is the accumulation of fluid in the pericardium, a fibrous sac surrounding the heart that ordinarily contains only a small amount of fluid. Penetrating injuries to the chest occasionally cause a heart laceration with bleeding into the pericardium. Pressure buildup because of increased amounts of blood or other fluid within the pericardium interferes with the heart's ability to relax between contractions and refill with blood. Less blood is ejected with each beat of the heart. As a result, blood pressure falls, and the patient may eventually go into shock.

The signs and symptoms of pericardial tamponade include a weak, fast pulse; falling blood pressure; and a progressive decrease in the difference between the systolic and diastolic pressures (drop in pulse pressure). Because of back pressure on the veins, the neck veins engorge and the face swells.

Injury to the Great Vessels

Crushing or penetrating chest injuries can damage the great vessels: the aorta, venae cavae, or their larger branches. Vessel walls may be lacerated, or entire vessels can be fractured or sheared. Such injuries usually are rapidly fatal because of massive bleeding from the large vessels.

EMERGENCY CARE OF CHEST INJURIES

Chest injuries, other than simple contusions or rib fractures, usually are serious and are emergencies. Every effort should be made to promptly transport the patient to definitive medical care. The medical facility should be notified in advance, if possible.

Fig. 15.7 *Emergency Care of an Open Chest Wound*

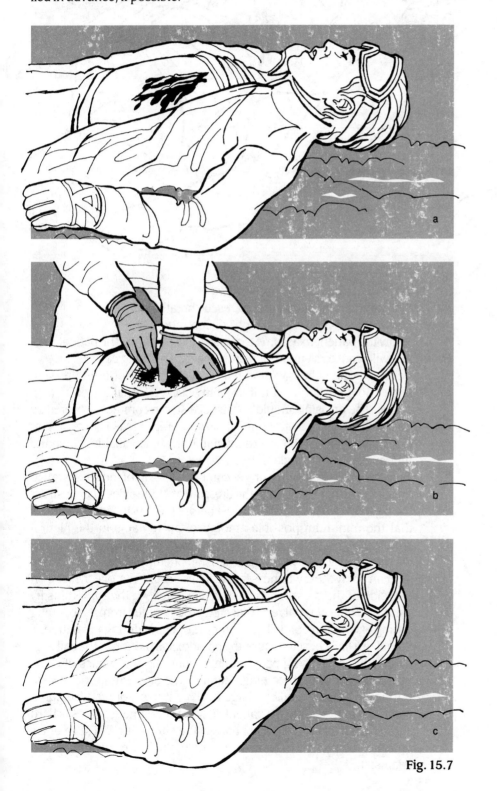

Fig. 15.7

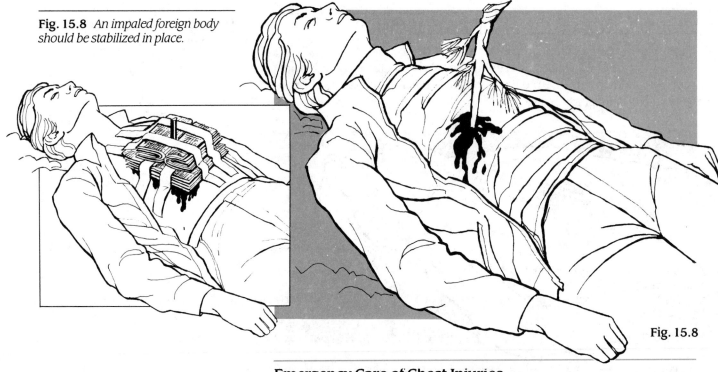

Fig. 15.8 *An impaled foreign body should be stabilized in place.*

Fig. 15.8

Emergency Care of Chest Injuries

1. Open and maintain the upper airway.
2. If breathing is inadequate, start rescue breathing.
3. If available, give oxygen in high concentration.
4. Allow the patient to assume a comfortable position. The patient usually will want to sit up, which often makes breathing easier.
5. Cover an open chest wound (Fig. 15.7a) with an airtight dressing large enough to prevent it from being sucked into the wound (Fig. 15.7b). The dressing should consist of a sterile compress covered by an airtight layer of aluminum foil, plastic wrap, a plastic bag, or Vaseline gauze (Fig. 15.7c). If airtight material is not available, substitute multiple layers of standard dressing material.

   Tape the edges of the dressing securely to the skin of the chest wall to ensure an airtight seal. Tape the dressing on three sides, then instruct the patient to exhale forcefully just before the fourth side is taped so that the minimum possible amount of air remains in the pleural space.

   On rare occasions, symptoms of tension pneumothorax will develop after an open chest wound is taped. If this occurs, remove the tape on one side of the dressing. This usually will relieve the symptoms by creating a one-way valve so that air will be expelled from the opening during exhalation but will not enter the opening during inhalation.
6. Stabilize a flail chest to reduce the paradoxical motion of the flail segment, thus decreasing pain and improving the mechanics of chest wall motion during breathing. Stabilize the segment in the inward position by taping a pillow, large thick compress, or wadded parka against it, or by having the patient lie with the segment against a hard surface such as the side rail or base of the litter. If the flail segment is anterior, the patient may be able to hold a pillow or wadded parka against it.

7. Control external bleeding by direct pressure.
8. Stabilize an impaled foreign body (Fig. 15.8) in place. A long object, such as a ski pole, can be cut off short with a pipe-cutter or similar device.
9. Observe the patient closely to detect any changes in condition. Obtain vital signs initially and at 15-minute intervals thereafter.
10. Treat the patient for shock, if necessary (see Chapter 7).
11. Simple rib fractures can be splinted for comfort and to allow a patient to self-evacuate on foot, if necessary (Fig. 15.9). Have the patient place the hand that is on the injured side on top of the head, and sit up. Place a cravat, elastic bandage, or one or two padded trouser belts around the injured area. Ask the patient to take a deep breath, exhale deeply, and hold the breath while the material is tightened around the chest and tied in place. If increased pain or respiratory distress occurs, remove the material immediately.

If evacuation will be prolonged, splint the chest with adhesive tape (Fig. 15.10). Tape the rib cage in the unexpanded position by applying tape to the injured area while the patient holds his or her breath after an exhalation as described above. If a razor is available, shave hair off the area before taping. After each exhalation, apply a long strip of 2-inch-wide adhesive tape from the midline in front to the midline in back. Six to eight strips are required; they should overlap each other like shingles on a roof. The nipple should be protected with gauze before tape is laid over it.

Fig. 15.9 *Emergency Care of a Simple Rib Fracture*

Fig. 15.10 *Adhesive Tape Splint for a Rib Fracture to Permit Self-evacuation*

Table 15.2

SUMMARY OF EMERGENCY CARE OF CHEST INJURIES

1. Open and maintain the upper airway.
2. Give rescue breathing, if needed.
3. Give oxygen in high concentration.
4. The patient usually prefers to sit up.
5. Cover a sucking chest wound with an airtight dressing.
6. Stabilize a flail chest.
7. Control external bleeding.
8. Stabilize an impaled object in place.
9. Monitor vital signs.
10. Splint simple rib fractures for comfort.

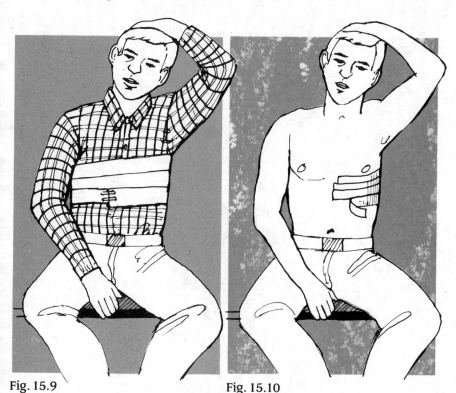

Fig. 15.9   Fig. 15.10

16

Injuries to the Abdomen, Pelvis, and Genitalia

Certainly, it is by their signs and symptoms, that internal diseases are revealed to the physician. But daily observation shows, that there is no uniform and invariable relationship between the extent and intensity of disease, and its external signs. The prominence, the number, and the combination, of these, depend upon many circumstances beside the disease with which they are connected.

—*Elisha Bartlett*
  Philosophy of Medical Science

INJURIES TO THE ABDOMEN

Abdominal injuries can be either **open** or **closed**. **Open injuries** are caused by sharp or high-velocity objects that create an opening between the peritoneal cavity and the outside, sometimes puncturing or lacerating abdominal organs. **Closed injuries**, which include contusions of the abdominal wall and crushing injuries or lacerations of internal organs, usually are caused by blunt trauma.

The abdomen contains both hollow and solid organs. Hollow organs such as the gallbladder, stomach, and intestines contain liquid or semisolid material composed of digested food, bacteria, enzymes, emulsifying agents, and hydrochloric acid. When these hollow organs rupture, their highly irritating and infectious contents may spill into the peritoneal cavity, producing an inflammatory reaction called **peritonitis.**

During the hour or more after organ rupture, localized pain and tenderness at the injury site spread to involve the rest of the abdomen. The abdomen becomes rigid and distended, the pulse faster and weaker, and normal bowel sounds–as heard by listening with a stethoscope or ear placed against the abdomen – disappear as the intestines become paralyzed. The patient may vomit and will appear progressively sicker. The patient may prefer to lie quietly on the back or side with the knees flexed. Abdominal pain is increased by moving, straightening the knees, or taking a deep breath.

Solid organs such as the liver, spleen, kidneys, and pancreas have a rich blood supply. Damage to these organs by blunt or penetrating trauma usually causes severe bleeding. Blood in the peritoneal cavity is less irritating than bowel contents; thus, the major signs and symptoms tend to be those of shock rather than peritonitis, although the abdomen may become distended, tender and rigid, and bowel sounds may disappear.

Abdominal trauma also may injure the aorta, inferior vena cava, or large arteries and veins, resulting in severe or fatal hemorrhage.

Abdominal injuries may be obvious, such as a large, open wound with protruding bowel, or quite subtle, such as a blow to the flank that initially causes little pain but has lacerated the spleen or liver. Suspect serious internal injuries in any patient who has suffered blunt trauma to the abdomen.

Steps in Assessment of Abdominal and Pelvic Injuries

1. Note the mechanism of injury and consider whether it might be expected to produce a significant abdominal injury.
2. Perform a primary survey and give basic life support, as needed.
3. During the secondary survey, question the patient to determine the circumstances of the accident and any symptoms. Determine and record the characteristics of abdominal pain, including time of onset, location at onset, change in position or severity with time, radiation, character (dull, aching, crushing, sharp, burning, stabbing, crampy, constant, intermittent), severity, and relationship to position or motion (including breathing and coughing).
4. Check and record vital signs. Note the character and rate of breathing, the patient's position, and whether the patient resists moving or changing position.

Table 16.1

SUMMARY OF ASSESSMENT OF A PATIENT WITH ABDOMINAL AND PELVIC INJURIES

1. First impression. Determine the mechanism of injury.
2. Primary survey. Give basic life support, as needed.
3. Secondary survey
   a. Ask specific questions, especially about pain.
   b. Monitor vital signs.
   c. Examine the abdomen.
4. Anticipate vomiting and prevent the patient from aspirating vomitus.
5. Inspect vomitus or urine, if either are obtained.

Table 16.2

SUMMARY OF EMERGENCY CARE OF A PATIENT WITH ABDOMINAL INJURIES

1. Keep the patient warm and supine.
2. Keep the patient in the most comfortable position.
3. Give the patient nothing by mouth.
4. Maintain the airway and avoid aspiration of vomitus by the patient.
5. Use suction, if necessary.
6. Control external bleeding.
7. Cover wounds.
8. Protect eviscerated organs with an occlusive dressing.
9. Stabilize an impaled object in place.
10. Monitor and record vital signs.
11. Anticipate and treat shock.

5. Have the patient lie with the knees bent. Expose and examine the abdomen. If there are obvious wounds, inspect them for protruding fat or intestines. Also look for bruises, bleeding, tenderness, muscle rigidity, and abdominal distention. If the wound was made by a bullet or long, sharp object, search for an exit wound. Stabilize impaled objects in place. The locations of tenderness, wounds, or bruises are significant because they may indicate injury of underlying internal organs.
6. Nausea and vomiting usually will develop and should be anticipated. Keep a receptacle at hand and help the patient turn the head to one side to avoid aspiration. Inspect vomitus for the presence of blood, bile, undigested food, etc.
7. Collect any voided urine and inspect it for the presence of blood.

Emergency Care of Abdominal Injuries

1. Keep the patient warm and lying down in the most comfortable position, usually on the back or side with the knees flexed.
2. Do not give the patient anything by mouth and watch for vomiting. If vomiting occurs, monitor and clear the upper airway as necessary.
3. Control external bleeding by direct pressure.
4. If abdominal wounds are seen, the injury is considered to be an *open* abdominal injury, even if the abdominal wall has not been completely penetrated. The rescuer has no way of knowing whether underlying organs have been injured. Apply a dry sterile dressing to the wound and watch the patient for signs of internal bleeding, shock, or the development of peritonitis.
5. If abdominal organs are protruding from open wounds, cover them with an occlusive dressing (Fig. 16.1) consisting of a universal dressing or several layers of sterile compresses moistened with sterile physiological saline solution or, in a pinch, with clean water. Cover the dressing with a layer of clean, preferably sterile, airtight material (such as foil, plastic wrap, or a plastic bag) to keep the organs from drying out.
6. Stabilize impaled objects in place using large bulky dressings held firmly with tape or roller bandages.
7. Regularly monitor and record the vital signs, particularly the pulse, respirations, and blood pressure.
8. Shock should be anticipated; if it occurs, raise the patient's legs 12 inches (see Chapter 7).
9. Transport the patient lying down in the most comfortable position to a hospital as soon as possible.

INJURIES TO THE PELVIS AND GENITOURINARY SYSTEM

Kidney Injuries

The kidneys lie against the posterior abdominal wall on either side of the spine and are partly protected by the ribs. Because a kidney injury usually is

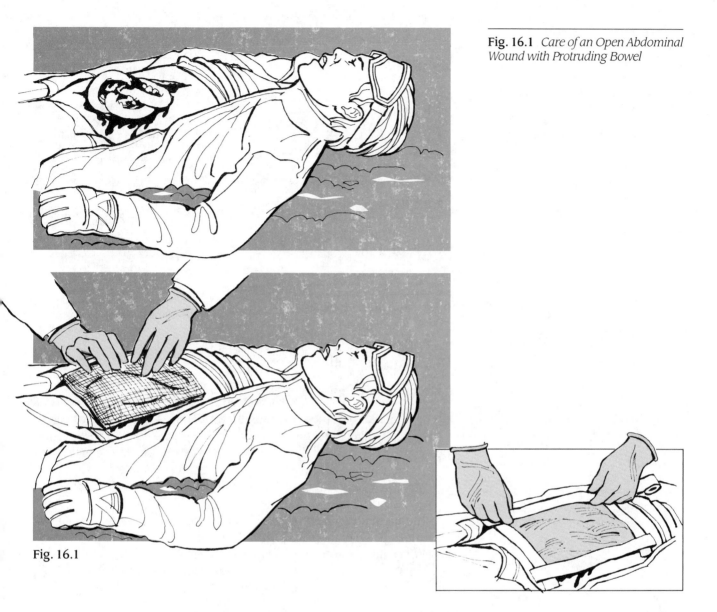

Fig. 16.1 *Care of an Open Abdominal Wound with Protruding Bowel*

Fig. 16.1

associated with fractures of the overlying ribs or adjacent vertebrae, suspect a kidney injury when such fractures occur. The patient usually develops tenderness, swelling, and ecchymosis in the costovertebral angle or the flank. Injured kidneys may bleed severely, resulting in shock. There may be blood in the patient's urine.

Bladder Injuries

The bladder is a hollow organ that serves as a reservoir for the urine. A full bladder is more easily injured than an empty one; therefore, the bladder should be emptied before any type of hazardous exertion. Pelvic fractures frequently lacerate the bladder or tear the urethra (Fig. 16.2). The assessment of injuries to the lower abdomen and genital area should include a search for open wounds, evidence of blunt trauma, and pelvic fractures. Inspect the opening of the urethra for bleeding. Collect voided urine and examine it for blood. Pelvic fractures and damage to pelvic organs can result in shock. The

Fig. 16.2 *The sharp fragments of a fractured pelvis can lacerate the bladder.*

Fig. 16.3 *Diaper-like Bandage for a Wound of the Perineum*

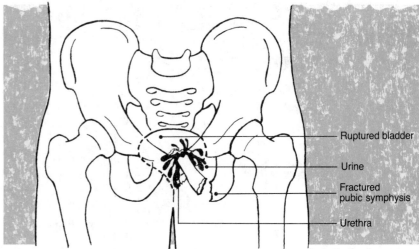

Fig. 16.2

emergency care of injuries to the kidney and bladder is similar to that for abdominal injuries in general.

The Male Genitalia

Injuries to the male genitalia are extremely painful and generally cause the patient considerable anxiety and concern. Any type of soft-tissue injury can occur. Amputation of the penis causes considerable bleeding, which can be controlled by direct pressure. The amputated part should be preserved as described in Chapter 8 and sent to the hospital along with the patient.

The foreskin of the penis occasionally gets caught in a trouser zipper, causing a very painful injury. If the zipper is stuck, cut it out of the trousers to make transport more comfortable.

The urethra can be bruised by blunt trauma from sharp fragments of a fractured pelvis or from a fall when the patient lands in a straddle position. A patient with a bruised urethra frequently is unable to void.

A testicle contusion is very painful and should be treated by applying a cold pack and stabilizing the area with an athletic supporter.

The Female Genitalia

The internal organs of the female reproductive tract are seldom injured because they are well protected by the pelvis. Although female reproductive organs lie within the pelvis, they are located away from the pelvic walls and rarely are lacerated by a fractured pelvis. However, the uterus of a pregnant woman is susceptible to injury by abdominal or pelvic trauma. Such injury can cause severe internal bleeding or precipitate a miscarriage or premature labor. The emergency care is the same as for patients with abdominal injuries.

Soft-tissue injuries to the external female genitalia, particularly straddle injuries, are very painful. These injuries may cause severe bleeding, usually controllable by local pressure. Anchor dressings with a diaper-like arrangement made from triangular bandages (Fig. 16.3), or use tight-fitting underpants. Never insert dressings or packs into the vagina.

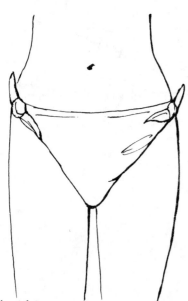

Fig. 16.3

17

Assessment of the Patient with a Medical Illness, Common Medical Problems

I hav finally kum to the konklusion, that a good reliable sett ov bowels is wurth more tu a man, than enny quantity ov brains.

—Josh Billings (Henry Wheeler Shaw)

The preceding chapters of this textbook, which are mostly concerned with the effects of trauma, describe assessment techniques designed primarily to discover the effects of *injury* on the organ systems. The strong emphasis on trauma is deliberate. Each year in the United States one person in three suffers a nonfatal injury, and trauma is the leading cause of death and disability in children and young adults, killing more Americans under the age of 35 than all diseases combined. Nevertheless, nontraumatic illness also is a major public health problem, particularly in older Americans.

A few years ago, it was accurate to say that advances in medical care had controlled or eliminated the major infectious diseases, leaving malignancy and degenerative diseases of the circulatory and respiratory systems as the major causes of death. However, since the AIDS pandemic began in the United States in the early 1980s, AIDS has become the major cause of death in men aged 20 to 40 in a number of major metropolitan areas. By the end of this century, AIDS is predicted to be the major cause of death in young to middle-aged men throughout the United States.

This chapter discusses the assessment of a patient with a medical illness and the causes and significance of common medical complaints, with emphasis on *acute* medical illnesses and those of concern in the outdoor environment.

ASSESSMENT OF A PATIENT WITH A MEDICAL ILLNESS

The first part of the **medical assessment** consists of the first impression and the primary survey, which are performed the same as when assessing an injured patient. If the patient appears to have a medical illness rather than an injury, the important symptoms to elicit and/or pursue during the secondary survey are fever, pain (including headache), weakness, respiratory distress, and variations from the normal functions of the respiratory, gastrointestinal, and genitourinary systems.

If the patient has a fever, and/or an acute infection is suspected, ask about symptoms of head cold, headache, earache, sore throat, cough, sputum production, chest pain, abdominal pain, nausea, vomiting, diarrhea, backache, and pain on urination. Inquire about possible infected wounds.

Further investigate each positive response to determine major characteristics of the symptom such as the time, manner, and circumstances of onset; duration; change in type or location; whether it is improving or worsening, constant or intermittent; whether it is associated with body position or activity (such as walking, breathing, coughing, or eating); whether anything makes it better or worse; and whether the patient has had similar symptoms in the past.

Suggestions of Questions to Ask in Different Situations

1. If the patient complains of headache, ask about the location and duration of the pain, whether it changes with a change in body position, and whether it is steady or throbbing. Determine whether the headache is accompanied by nausea or abnormal visual symptoms,

Table 17.1

IMPORTANT MEDICAL SIGNS AND SYMPTOMS

Fever
Pain
Respiratory distress
Variations from the normal
  functions of the:
    Respiratory system
    Gastrointestinal system
    Genitourinary system

Table 17.2

IMPORTANT SIGNS AND SYMPTOMS OF FEVER OR INFECTION

Head cold	Abdominal pain
Headache	Nausea
Earache	Vomiting
Sore throat	Diarrhea
Cough	Backache
Sputum production	Pain on urination
Chest pain	Wounds

Table 17.3

IMPORTANT CHARACTERISTICS OF POSITIVE SIGNS OR SYMPTOMS

Duration	Change in type or location with time?
Time, manner, and circumstances of onset.	Does anything make it better or worse?
Associated with body position?	Constant or intermittent?
Associated with activity (walking, eating, etc.)?	Similar signs or symptoms in the past?

---

whether the neck is stiff, whether the patient is subject to headaches, and what the patient thinks may have caused the current headache. Take the patient's blood pressure.

2. If the patient complains of a stiff or sore neck, ask whether he or she has suffered a sprain or other injury, and whether he or she has arthritis of the neck. Ask the patient to touch the chin to the chest (inability to do so may indicate meningitis).

3. If the patient has abdominal pain, ask about the location of the pain at onset, its duration, whether it has moved, the type of pain (constant, intermittent, crampy, sharp, dull), whether the pain has changed in type or intensity, and the relationship of the pain to eating, passing flatus, or moving the bowels. It also is important to ask whether the patient has discovered any activity that makes the pain better or worse.

   If the patient has nausea or vomiting, ask about frequency, characteristics of the vomitus, the presence of blood or "coffee grounds" material (digested blood) in the vomitus, the relationship to abdominal pain—particularly whether the pain gets better or worse before or after vomiting—and how long it has been since the patient has been able to keep anything down.

   If the patient has diarrhea, ask about the number and type of bowel movements, whether they contain pus or blood, and the relationship of abdominal pain to moving the bowels.

4. If the patient has chest pain, ask about the type of pain (sharp, squeezing, dull, pressure), duration, location (beneath the sternum, over the lower ribs, over the heart, etc.), whether the pain worsens with coughing or deep breathing or is brought on by exertion, and whether it radiates to the neck, back, jaw, shoulder, or arm. It also is important to know whether the patient has had such chest pain before and whether the patient has known chronic heart or lung disease, particularly coronary artery disease.

5. If the complaint is about weakness, ask the patient to explain what he or she means by weakness. Ask if the patient is actually tired rather than weak, whether the weakness is chronic or of recent onset, and whether it is general or confined to an arm, a leg, or one side of the body. It is important to know if the patient is capable of normal activi-

ties or if the weakness prevents sitting, standing, or walking. Ask if sleeping habits have been normal or have changed and whether the onset of the weakness coincided with the onset of a febrile illness (illness with fever), an injury, or a disease of the respiratory, gastrointestinal, or urinary system.

Do the best possible examination of the symptomatic areas. Using a flashlight and tongue blade or spoon handle, check the throat and tonsils by pressing down on the tongue and asking the patient to say "Ah." Palpate the upper neck under the sides of the jaw to check for tender and/or enlarged lymph nodes. The rattles of bronchitis, the wheezes of asthma, the bubbles of pulmonary edema, and the gurgles of gastroenteritis frequently can be heard by the unaided ear, but the sounds are better heard when the ear or a stethoscope is placed directly against the patient's skin.

Examine the abdomen for distention, tenderness, rigidity, and scars of previous operations or injuries (Fig. 17.1). If a urinary infection is suspected, palpate the costovertebral angles for kidney tenderness. Inspect wounds for swelling, redness, tenderness, or discharge. Inspect the ankles for swelling, particularly **pitting edema**, a type of swelling characterized by a depression or pit that remains after a finger is pressed into a swollen area. If the patient complains that an extremity is weak, compare its strength with that of the opposite, normal extremity by having the patient squeeze both your hands or push the feet or bend the ankles against the pressure of your hands.

It is important to inquire specifically about any medications (or illegal drugs) the patient has been taking and about preexisting conditions such as known gallbladder disease, heart disease, epilepsy, or diabetes that may have contributed to the current problem. Also ask about any previous surgeries and drug allergies. Finally, ask, "Is there anything else about you that we should know?"

Fig. 17.1 *It is important to assess a patient's symptomatic areas.*

Table 17.4

IMPORTANT FACTS ABOUT A PATIENT'S MEDICAL HISTORY

Medicines or illegal drugs being taken.
Preexisting medical conditions.
Previous operations.
Allergies.
Ask: "Is there anything else about you we should know?"

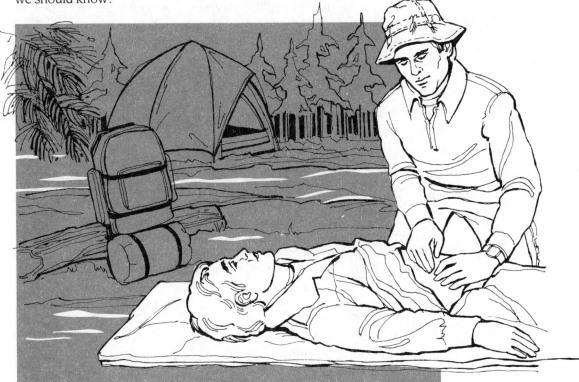

Fig. 17.1

In any seriously ill patient, the patient's condition changes over time. Prepare a written record of serial vital signs and major events such as a change in the location or quality of pain, and record the time of each observation. As with injured patients, any patient with a medical illness other than the most trivial should see a physician.

COMMON MEDICAL COMPLAINTS

The following medical complaints are common in patients with a wide variety of illnesses and injuries. It is important that the rescuer know the possible causes of each complaint, its significance, and its emergency care. The emergency care of a complaint frequently is the same regardless of the underlying cause.

(In medical care, the ending "itis" added to an anatomical term implies infection or inflammation of that anatomical part. For example, appendicitis is an infection of the appendix, and bronchitis is an infection of the bronchi.)

Respiratory Complaints

Respiratory Distress

Respiratory distress includes dyspnea, tachypnea, and hyperpnea—medical terms for breathing that is difficult, abnormally rapid, or abnormally deep. In particular, respiratory distress refers to the patient's awareness of the need for extra efforts to obtain enough air. Respiratory distress occurs in response to lung changes such as narrowed bronchi in patients with asthma or emphysema, stiffness of lung segments in patients with pneumonia, pulmonary edema in patients with heart failure or high altitude illness, and increased fibrous tissue in patients with pulmonary fibrosis; air, blood, or fluid within the pleural cavities, displacing the lung; and changes in blood gases, such as excess carbon dioxide or insufficient oxygen.

Common medical causes of respiratory distress include respiratory infections, pulmonary edema from heart failure or high altitude illness, emphysema, asthma, airway obstruction, lung cancer, pulmonary embolism, and hyperventilation.

Coughing

A **cough** is a short, harsh sound produced by air suddenly rushing out through the larynx. Coughing rids the body of material that irritates the lungs or respiratory passages. The act of coughing consists of a short inhalation followed immediately by closing of the glottis, which is the part of the larynx around the vocal cords. Next, the chest wall muscles contract, building pressure within the chest. The glottis then opens suddenly, and the air rushes out, moving the offending material along with it. Coughing continues until the material is either expelled completely or is moved to a less sensitive part of the airway. The most sensitive areas are the trachea and the larynx, but irritation of the smaller air passages, the lungs, and the pleura also can cause coughing.

Coughing can result from irritation caused by infection, injury, excessive dryness or wetness of the airway lining, a mucus plug, or a foreign body. The medical causes of cough are the same as those of respiratory distress (see above).

Wheezes, Rhonchi and Stridor

Wheezes are high-pitched sounds produced by exhaled air traveling through small air passages narrowed by swelling or spasm. **Rhonchi** are coarser sounds produced by air moving through larger air passages partly blocked by sputum or other secretions. **Stridor** is a high-pitched sound on inhalation produced by air moving through a narrowed larynx. These sounds often can be heard with the unaided ear.

Wheezes are characteristic of conditions involving the smaller passages of the lungs, including asthma, emphysema, and certain infections (bronchiolitis and bronchitis). Rhonchi typically are heard in patients with diseases of the larger air passages, such as bronchitis and tracheitis. Stridor is heard in patients with irritation, infection or a growth that causes swelling or obstruction of the upper part of the respiratory tract, particularly the larynx.

Respiratory Infections

Patients with an upper **respiratory tract infection**, such as a head cold, usually complain of shortness of breath when they actually mean nasal stuffiness caused by swelling of the nasal passages. Hay fever, an allergic condition of the upper respiratory tract, can cause similar symptoms.

Infections of the epiglottis and larynx occasionally cause enough swelling to obstruct the upper respiratory tract, especially in children whose respiratory passages are relatively smaller than those of adults. Stridor and cough are characteristic of these infections.

Pneumonia is caused by a viral or bacterial infection that results in consolidation (stiffening) of segments of the lung as the alveoli and their intervening spaces become filled with blood and pus (Fig. 17.2). Patients with pneumonia are short of breath because of this stiffness and the lowered level of oxygen in their arterial blood. Patients with pneumonia or bronchitis usually have a severe cough and produce greenish or yellowish sputum; the sputum produced by patients with pneumonia may contain blood.

Pulmonary Edema

In patients with **pulmonary edema**, the fluid portion of the blood leaves the capillaries and collects in the alveoli, stiffening them and interfering with oxygenation of the blood (Fig. 17.3). Among the causes are increased capillary pressure and leaking capillaries damaged by inhalation of smoke or toxic fumes.

Increased capillary pressure can be caused by back pressure from a failing heart or by transmission of high arterial pressure to the capillaries by abnormal high-pressure bypasses that develop in the lungs at high altitude. Bubbly sounds, wheezes, and rattles frequently can be heard with the unaided ear. The patient is short of breath, coughs frequently, and finds it easier to breathe in a sitting position. Patients with severe pulmonary edema produce frothy pink sputum because the capillaries are so damaged that they allow leakage of red cells as well as plasma.

Emphysema

Emphysema, a chronic degenerative lung disease most commonly caused by cigarette smoking, is a serious problem in modern society. The cause is progressive lung damage resulting from years of exposure to pulmonary irritants and repeated infections. Repeated irritation of the lungs causes scarring, narrowing and chronic inflammation of the bronchi, and obstruction

Fig. 17.2 *Microscopic Appearance of a Normal Lung and Appearance of a Lung with Pneumonia*

Fig. 17.3 *Microscopic Appearance of Pulmonary Edema*

Fig. 17.4 *Microscopic Appearance of Emphysema*

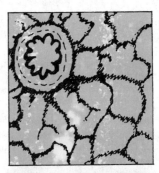

a

Normal Lung

b

Lung with Pneumonia

Fig. 17.2

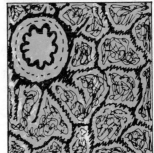

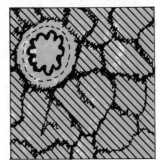

Pulmonary Edema

Fig. 17.3

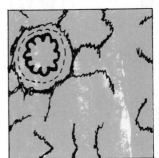

Emphysema

Fig. 17.4

Fig. 17.5 *Emphysema Patient with Enlarged Chest*

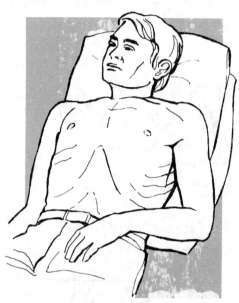

Fig. 17.5

of the alveoli. The walls between the alveoli break down, creating fewer, larger alveoli (Fig. 17.4). As the patient's lungs become larger and less efficient, the chest enlarges, giving the patient a characteristic, barrel-chested appearance (Fig. 17.5).

Breath sounds heard with a stethoscope typically are quieter than normal; exhalations are prolonged because it takes longer to exhale through the narrowed bronchi. Eventually, the oxygen level in the blood drops and the carbon dioxide level in the blood rises. Shortness of breath is caused by the increased work required to breathe and the altered blood levels of carbon dioxide and oxygen. Coughing, wheezing, and rhonchi are commonly noted. Patients with severe emphysema cannot exert themselves enough to walk even a few steps without supplemental oxygen from a portable tank. Because of their disability, patients with emphysema are unlikely to ski or travel on foot in the outdoors.

Asthma

Asthma is a condition in which periodic attacks of coughing, wheezing, and dyspnea occur. Some asthmatics suffer attacks when they inhale substances, such as pollen, that they are allergic to; in others, attacks are precipitated by irritation caused by infection, air pollution, cold air, or exercise.

During an asthma attack, the patient is short of breath, prefers to sit upright, and wheezes audibly. Shortness of breath is caused by the increased work required to move the air in and out of the narrowed bronchi.

Airway Obstruction

Most of the important causes of **airway obstruction** are related to trauma or unconsciousness and are discussed in Chapters 5, 13, and 14. Medical conditions such as infections of the larynx and epiglottis and malignant disease can cause upper-airway obstruction. The accidental inhalation of food or small foreign bodies such as peanuts and beads is an important cause of obstruction, particularly in infants and small children. A characteristic sign of upper-airway obstruction is a crowing type of stridor.

Malignant Disease

Respiratory distress, rhonchi, and cough are common manifestations of **malignant disease** of the upper or lower respiratory tract, especially cancer of the lung, which has long been the most common cancer in men and recently replaced breast cancer as the most common cancer in women. In patients with lung cancer, respiratory distress occurs when cancer replaces normal lung tissue, a process that causes irritation and obstruction of the respiratory tract, and decreased oxygenation of the blood. Common warning signs of respiratory tract cancer are chronic cough, blood in the sputum, progressive shortness of breath, weight loss, and chronic hoarseness.

Pulmonary Embolism

Blood clots that form in the veins of other parts of the body may be carried by the venous blood flow into the lungs, where they are eventually trapped as the branches of the pulmonary arteries become smaller and smaller, causing **pulmonary embolism**. Blockage of a pulmonary artery cuts off blood flow through the segment of the lung it supplies, producing an infarct, an area where the alveoli and their walls become filled with blood and edema fluid.

Symptoms of pulmonary infarct include respiratory distress, cough, spitting up blood (hemoptysis), and chest pain that worsens with breathing and coughing. The location of the chest pain is a reliable indicator of the location of the infarct. Large pulmonary emboli may block larger vessels and interfere significantly with the flow of blood through the lung, causing shock.

Pulmonary emboli most commonly originate from clots in the deep veins of the legs and pelvis. Deep clots of the lower extremity may cause no signs and symptoms, or they may produce slight swelling and tenderness of the calf, with pain if the ankle is dorsiflexed (Fig. 17.6).

Pulmonary emboli usually develop in people who are forced to be inactive because of illness or during recovery from surgery. They also can develop following trauma, particularly in patients with fractures of the pelvis or extremities. The blood thickening that results from increased production of red blood cells during acclimatization to high altitude predisposes climbers to clotting, especially if they are confined in a tent or snow cave by long periods of bad weather.

Hyperventilation

Hyperventilation is a common and benign form of respiratory distress that involves a progressive and predictable series of events leading to frightening signs and symptoms in the affected individual and considerable alarm in family and friends. The respiratory distress of a patient who hyperventilates is rarely caused by respiratory system disease.

The episode usually starts with an increase in the rate and depth of breathing caused by altitude, nausea, an emotional reaction such as anxiety or fright, or chest pain from gas in the digestive tract or some other equally harmless condition. These breathing changes cause excessive loss of carbon dioxide from the blood. Because carbon dioxide is acidic, its loss makes the blood more alkaline. This alkalinity interferes with the normal function of muscles and nerves, causing coldness, numbness, and tingling of the hands, feet and mouth, as well as a feeling of lightheadedness and increased shortness of breath.

These symptoms alarm the patient, who may fear that a stroke, heart attack or other catastrophe is occurring, and cause him or her to breathe

Fig. 17.6 *Test for a deep blood clot in the leg by bending the foot toward the head.*

Fig. 17.7 *A patient who hyperventilates may develop flexor spasms in the hands.*

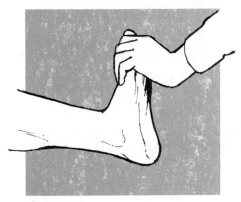

Fig. 17.6

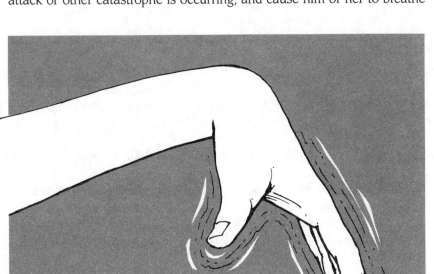

Fig. 17.7

even harder. As the alkalinity of the blood increases further, the patient's hands and feet turn blue and go into flexor spasms (Fig. 17.7). This series of events ultimately leads to unconsciousness, which returns the breathing to normal, allowing the patient to recover.

Emergency Care of a Patient with a Respiratory Complaint

1. Try to determine the most likely cause of the complaint (see the section on assessment, above).

2. Oxygen is indicated for patients with moderate to severe respiratory distress, especially cyanotic patients. An exception is the patient who is obviously hyperventilating. Unless the patient has emphysema, give oxygen in high concentration and at a high flow rate. Patients with emphysema should receive oxygen at a rate of 2 liters per minute. The lower rate is used because the main stimulus driving the emphysema patient's respiratory center is oxygen lack rather than an excess of carbon dioxide, which stimulates the respiratory center in normal individuals. Giving high-concentration oxygen to a patient with severe emphysema may raise the blood oxygen level high enough to remove this stimulus, causing breathing to stop.

3. People with upper-respiratory infections who experience dyspnea caused by nasal congestion can improve the condition by using non-prescription decongestant tablets. Adults with high blood pressure and children should use decongestants with caution, and people with earaches should not use decongestants at all. General body discomfort and an irritating cough can be controlled with nonprescription analgesics and cough suppressants. Patients with upper-respiratory infections who are producing yellow or green secretions from the nose or chest should be encouraged to see a physician. Children with infections of the larynx and epiglottis may develop dangerous upper-airway obstructions and should be taken to an emergency room.

4. Patients who are suspected of having pneumonia or severe bronchitis should see a physician.

5. Patients with respiratory distress who are producing large amounts of lung secretions may require suctioning.

6. Asthmatic patients may carry tablets or inhalers that relax bronchial spasms. They may need assistance in using these medicines.

7. The emergency care of airway obstruction is discussed in Chapter 5.

8. Other than giving oxygen, there is no effective emergency care for patients with pulmonary embolism. Climbers confined to cramped shelters can reduce their risk of developing blood clots by periodically exercising their extremities.

9. Hyperventilation should be managed by talking calmly to the patient and encouraging him or her to breathe in and out of a paper bag for five to 10 minutes.

Table 17.5

SUMMARY OF EMERGENCY CARE OF A PATIENT WITH A RESPIRATORY COMPLAINT
1. Assess the patient and determine the most likely cause.
2. Allow the patient to assume the most comfortable position.
3. Give oxygen, if indicated.
4. Assist an asthmatic in taking his or her own medications.
5. Relieve airway obstruction, if present (see Chapter 5).
6. Manage hyperventilation by calming the patient and having him or her breathe into a paper bag.
7. Symptomatic relief:
    a. For nasal congestion, take nonprescription decongestants (cautions for use by patients with high blood pressure or earache).
    b. For cough, take nonprescription cough suppressants.
    c. For discomfort, take nonprescription analgesics.
8. The patient should see a physician if he or she has:
    a. Pneumonia or severe bronchitis.
    b. Earache.
    c. Yellow or green sputum coming from the nose or chest.
    d. An infection of the upper airway with stridor.

Gastrointestinal Complaints

Indigestion

Indigestion is a sign that the normal function of the stomach is disturbed. Symptoms include heartburn, pain, and nausea and vomiting.

Heartburn is a burning feeling in the epigastric area or beneath the sternum. It usually follows a rich or spicy meal and often is accompanied by increased saliva production. Heartburn can be relieved by antacids.

The pain associated with indigestion can be a dull discomfort or cramp in the epigastric area, or a feeling of fullness or pressure.

Nausea or vomiting are discussed below.

Indigestion usually results from a mild to severe stomach inflammation triggered by causes such as stress, a viral infection, excessive alcohol intake, or a meal that is too large, too rich, or too spicy. It also can be an early symptom of an ulcer or stomach cancer. Persistent indigestion should be investigated by a physician.

Difficulty in Swallowing

Difficulty in swallowing (dysphagia) is caused by abnormal function of the esophageal muscles, which move food and liquids from the mouth and pharynx toward the stomach, or obstruction of the esophagus by scar tissue, tumor, or a swallowed foreign body.

Dysphagia may be acute, chronic, or intermittent. The most common cause is a temporary spasm of the esophageal muscles. The most serious cause is a malignant neoplasm (new tissue growth), which usually causes slowly progressive dysphagia with difficulty in swallowing solids at first, followed by difficulty in swallowing both solids and liquids. All causes of dysphagia should be investigated by a physician.

Nausea and Vomiting

Nausea and vomiting are common symptoms that reflect the stomach's tendency to react to any noxious stimulus by emptying its contents. These stimuli can act directly on the stomach or indirectly through nerve pathways. Direct stimuli include gastroenteritis caused by infection, overuse of alcohol, food poisoning, irritating drugs such as aspirin, or stress (nervous stomach); peritonitis; abdominal trauma; and ulcer or tumor of the stomach.

Indirect stimuli including effects of high altitude, severe headache, motion sickness, psychosomatic illness, and severe medical illness or injury of any type.

Vomiting may be mild or severe, acute or chronic. The major serious effects of vomiting are inability to eat and loss of fluids and electrolytes, leading to starvation, dehydration, and metabolic abnormalities; and aspiration of vomitus, causing airway obstruction and severe lung infection. In the outdoor setting, vomiting usually is caused by gastroenteritis, food poisoning, or the effects of altitude, and is self-limited. However, if vomiting continues, the patient must be taken to a hospital.

Vomiting of blood is always serious. It can be caused by swallowing blood from a nosebleed, but the usual cause is disease of the stomach or esophagus. The most common causes are bleeding from inflammation of the stomach, a stomach or duodenal ulcer, or esophageal varices (large, fragile veins in the lower esophagus that accompany cirrhosis and other chronic liver diseases).

Vomited blood can be bright red or, if partly digested, can resemble coffee grounds. A patient who is vomiting blood should be taken to the hospital as soon as possible.

Diarrhea

The passage of soft or liquid stools with abnormal high frequency is called **diarrhea**. In severe cases, there may be pus or blood in the stools. Prolonged, severe diarrhea can lead to dehydration and starvation because food and liquid is lost through the stools. Diarrhea may be accompanied by nausea and vomiting. The most common cause of diarrhea is a viral infection of the bowel. Bowel infections such as cholera and dysentery are caused by bacteria. A protozoan, *Giardia lamblia*, causes many cases of diarrhea contracted in the wilderness. Chronic, mild diarrhea usually is brought on by emotional stress.

Many cases of diarrhea are caused by contaminated food or water. Staphylococci grow easily in bland, creamy foods left at room temperature for a few hours. Staphylococci produce a toxin that causes violent vomiting, diarrhea, and cramps. This toxin is not destroyed by reheating the contaminated food.

Food prepared with dirty hands may be contaminated by staphylococci or other organisms. Giardia is carried by beavers and many other wild animals and is transmitted to man through contaminated water.

Mild diarrhea can be controlled by a light diet containing broth, bouillon, tea, toast, gelatin, citrus soft drinks such as 7-Up or Sprite, and water. Rich or spicy foods, milk, and fruit juice should be avoided at first. Electrolyte-containing preparations, such as half-strength Gatorade, can be used to help replenish lost electrolytes. More severe diarrhea may be controlled by a nonprescription preparation such as Pepto-Bismol or Kaopectate. A patient in a remote area who develops severe diarrhea accompanied by chills, fever, pus and/or blood in the stools should be evacuated for medical care.

Diarrhea is prevented by scrupulous attention to personal cleanliness, by protecting food from contamination and spoilage, and by boiling, filtering, or chemically disinfecting water (see Chapter 1).

Blood in the Stools

Bright red **blood in the stools** usually means either bleeding from the lower bowel or bleeding higher in the gastrointestinal tract with very rapid passage of blood through the bowel. The most common cause is bleeding from hemorrhoids or a fissure (crack or small ulcer) of the anus. Maroon or black blood comes from higher up, usually from a bleeding ulcer. The dark color is caused by partial digestion of the blood as it passes through the gastrointestinal tract. About 60 milliliters (2 ounces) of blood are required to produce a black stool. Bismuth preparations such as Pepto-Bismol and vitamin-mineral supplements containing iron also can turn the stool black.

Dark-colored or black blood in the stool always signifies a serious condition, and the patient should see a physician as soon as possible. Bright red blood accompanied by pain on moving the bowels is almost always caused by bleeding from hemorrhoids, a fissure, or abrasion from a hard stool; these situations represent an emergency only if bleeding is profuse or long lasting.

Jaundice

Jaundice is a yellow discoloration of the skin, mucous membranes, and the whites of the eyes caused by an abnormal buildup of **bilirubin** in the blood. Bilirubin, a byproduct of the normal breakdown of the red blood cells, accumulates if red cell breakdown is accelerated or if the normal bilirubin excretion pathways become blocked or function abnormally. The most common causes of jaundice are liver disease (such as hepatitis) and obstruction of the bile ducts by a gallstone or tumor. Jaundice is always the sign of a serious condition; the patient should see a physician promptly.

Colic

Colic is intermittent, severe abdominal pain caused by obstruction of a hollow, muscular organ such as the bowel or ureter. The pain is caused by the strong contractions of the muscles behind the obstruction as they try to force the contents of the organ past the obstruction. Pain resembling colic also occurs with severe gastroenteritis because of irritation and spasm of the bowel muscles.

Common causes of colic are stones in the gallbladder or bile ducts, stones in the ureter, and intestinal obstruction caused by adhesions or a tumor. Gallbladder or bile duct colic usually is felt in the right upper abdominal quadrant and in the back, near the lower angle of the scapula; ureteral colic is felt in the flank; and intestinal colic, around the navel. Colic frequently is a symptom of serious disease and is so painful that medical assistance is required.

Constipation

Constipation, the passage of hard, dry stools at less than normal intervals, can be caused by inadequate physical activity, partial dehydration, chronic anxiety, or inadequate bulk in the diet. Constipation must be distinguished from the infrequent passage of stools of normal consistency, a situation that is normal in many people. Excessive bowel-consciousness is a common preoccupation encouraged by laxative peddlers. The elderly, who may be inactive and subsist on a bulk-poor diet, are more likely to be afflicted with constipation than younger, more athletic people. Persistent constipation or other changes in bowel habits without apparent cause should be investigated; they may be early symptoms of bowel cancer.

Table 17.6

SUMMARY OF EMERGENCY CARE OF GASTROINTESTINAL COMPLAINTS

1. Mild indigestion: Try antacids such as Rolaids or Maalox.
2. Dehydration caused by diarrhea or vomiting: Give liquids by mouth. Electrolytic liquids such as broth, bouillon or half-strength Gatorade are best. If the patient cannot keep liquids down, he or she will likely require evacuation and intravenous therapy. Later, the patient can try bland foods such as tea, toast, broth, and gelatin.
3. Vomiting related to altitude diseases: Descent.
4. Diarrhea: Try nonprescription medicines such as Pepto-Bismol.
5. Constipation: Eat cooked fruits and vegetables, increase water intake (especially hot water), take mild laxatives (milk of magnesia, etc.), if necessary.
6. Colic: Apply heat to the abdomen.
7. There is no field treatment for dysphagia, severe vomiting or diarrhea, vomiting of blood, abdominal injury, peritonitis, jaundice, severe rectal bleeding, or a severe illness of any type with gastrointestinal symptoms.

Genitourinary Complaints

Painful Urination

Painful urination (dysuria), usually accompanied by the passage of small amounts of urine at frequent intervals, is a symptom of infection or irritation of the bladder or urethra. Patients with serious urinary tract infections may develop chills, fever, weakness, and pain over a kidney. Occasionally, blood may be found in the urine. The emergency care for painful urination is to encourage the patient to drink adequate fluids and consult a physician.

Blood in the Urine

Blood in the urine (hematuria) can be caused by a urinary infection or a tumor or stone in the urinary tract. The condition may be painless or may be accompanied by dysuria or colic. All patients with hematuria should consult a physician.

Frequent Voiding

Frequent urination (frequency) may be associated with a urinary infection. However, frequency without dysuria, especially when small amounts of urine are voided each time, usually means obstruction of the outflow of the bladder. This condition commonly occurs in elderly men as a result of enlargement of the prostate gland. Frequent voiding of large amounts of urine can be a symptom of diabetes; it also can occur with excessive water consumption and as blood volume is reduced during acclimatization from hot to cold weather.

Incontinence

Incontinence is the uncontrolled passage of urine or feces which soils the patient's clothing. It can occur in cases of urinary tract infections, diarrhea, unconsciousness, epileptic seizures, senility, overuse of drugs or alcohol, loss of bowel and bladder control following a spinal cord injury, or severe illness or injury in general. Incontinence is always of concern and may cause the patient considerable embarrassment. The cause may be obvious and require no specific treatment. However, patients with persistent incontinence or newly developed incontinence should see a physician.

Inability to Urinate

Inability to urinate can occur in anyone with severe pain, particularly patients with multiple injuries immobilized on a spine board. Rescue groups should carry lightweight urinals or wide-mouth plastic bottles to aid such patients in emptying their bladders. Some normal people are unable to urinate unless allowed to sit or stand. Bladder distention can be very painful, making it even more difficult to void. Urinary retention in elderly men usually is related to urethral obstruction from an enlarged prostate.

The emergency care for inability to urinate is to transport the patient to a hospital or physician so that a bladder catheter can be inserted.

Abnormal Menstrual Flow

Although the average menstrual period occurs at intervals of about 28 days and lasts five to seven days, there can be considerable variation in interval, quantity, and duration of menstrual flow in normal women. Any vaginal bleeding aside from the regular menstrual flow is considered **abnormal** and should be investigated by a physician, although spotting between periods and periods with excessive flow and length are fairly common and usually benign.

The most serious types of abnormal bleeding are associated with pregnancy and can be divided into abnormalities of early and late pregnancy. If a woman who has missed several periods and possibly has noticed some morning nausea or breast tenderness has vaginal bleeding, she may be having a **miscarriage**. If she also develops abdominal pain and tenderness, she may be bleeding internally because of an **ectopic pregnancy** (a pregnancy in which the fetus implants outside of the uterus). A woman who bleeds during the last few months of pregnancy may be entering premature labor or developing another complication of late pregnancy. All of these conditions are potentially serious because of the danger of fetal loss and of severe bleeding and shock. Any pregnant woman with vaginal bleeding should be taken to a hospital.

Urethral and Vaginal Discharge

Urethral discharge in both females and males is always abnormal and usually is caused by infection. The patient usually is concerned because of the discomfort and the possibility of having contracted a sexually transmitted infection. There is no emergency care other than to recommend consultation with a physician.

A certain amount of **vaginal discharge** is normal for most women, especially before and after the menstrual period. A physician should be consulted about a vaginal discharge that is abnormally profuse, irritating, discolored, bloody, or foul-smelling.

MISCELLANEOUS COMPLAINTS

Vertigo

A patient who complains of **vertigo** should be questioned to distinguish true vertigo, which means a sensation of whirling ("the room spins around"), from mere lightheadedness. Severe vertigo frequently is accompanied by vomiting.

Vertigo is quite common in the elderly, who usually develop the condition because of impaired circulation. If vertigo is accompanied by deafness or ringing in the ears, the rescuer should suspect chronic ear disease. Younger people can develop vertigo from viral infections and other disturbances of the balancing organ in the inner ear. Vertigo can be so severe that the patient is unable to turn over in bed or sit up without vomiting. Hospitalization may be required. Vertigo also can be a symptom of head injury (see Chapter 13) or high altitude cerebral edema (see Chapter 19). Persistent vertigo may be an early symptom of a brain tumor. Severe or persistent vertigo should always be investigated by a physician.

Headache

Five to 10 percent of Americans suffer from recurrent **headaches**, mostly of the vascular (migraine) or muscle tension variety. The vast majority of headaches are uncomfortable but harmless; occasionally a headache is a sign of serious illness or injury such as meningitis, severe high blood pressure, or brain tumor. Common causes of benign headaches are emotional upsets, lack of sleep, eyestrain, the effects of altitude, a respiratory infection, or a hangover. Causes of headaches in outdoor enthusiasts include a hard fall while skiing and traction on the neck muscles caused by the weight of a heavy pack.

Migraine headaches usually are recurrent, throbbing, one-sided, accompanied by nausea, and preceded by some type of abnormal visual phenomena such as blurred vision or bright, moving lights. Muscle tension headaches usually are bilateral, involve both the forehead and the occiput, and radiate into the neck and shoulders.

People who are susceptible to headaches should be encouraged to take their regular medication if they have it with them. Common, nonprescription medicines such as aspirin and acetaminophen usually will control mild headaches; patients with severe or unrelenting headaches should see a physician.

18

Medical Emergencies

A man is as old as his arteries.

—*Pierre J. G. Cabanis*

Because the body can respond to illness and injury in only a limited number of ways, different conditions can produce similar signs and symptoms. Emergency care can be directed at either signs and symptoms or at specific illnesses and injuries. This chapter examines in detail selected important **medical illnesses** that may be encountered in the outdoors. The causes and emergency care of the most common *symptoms* of medical illness are presented in Chapter 17.

HEART DISEASE

Heart disease continues to be the most common cause of death in the middle-aged and elderly and can affect younger individuals as well. The function of the heart, its sensitivity to lack of oxygen, and the importance of a normal myocardial blood supply already have been emphasized. The most common cause of heart disease is reduction of blood flow to the heart muscle by **arteriosclerosis**, the gradual stiffening and narrowing of the coronary arteries caused by fatty material deposits and scar tissue within the arterial walls (Fig. 18.1). When the heart does not receive enough oxygen and nutrients, a condition called coronary artery disease develops. Other less common types of heart disease are caused by congenital abnormalities of the heart or by damage from infection, toxins, or injury.

In the early stages of coronary artery disease, the heart may function normally, and symptoms may develop only when the heart is stressed by high altitude, unaccustomed physical activity, or strong emotion. Unfortunately, these stresses are not rare in sedentary individuals who undertake a hunting, hiking, or skiing trip. Ski patrollers, outdoor group leaders, and wilderness rescuers can expect to encounter patients with coronary artery disease. As coronary artery disease progresses, symptoms occur when the patient is at rest; eventually, symptoms may be present constantly, and the patient may enter a state of chronic heart failure that markedly restricts activity.

Fig. 18.1 *Arteriosclerosis in the Wall of a Coronary Artery*
  a. *Cross-section of a Normal Coronary Artery*
  b. *Artery Narrowed by a Plaque*

Fig. 18.2 *Most Common Locations of Anginal Pain (shaded area)*

Fig. 18.3 *A blocked coronary artery (a.) causes injury or death to the part of the heart muscle it supplies (shaded area, b.).*

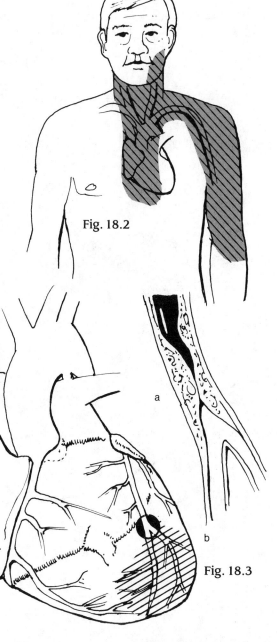

Fig. 18.2

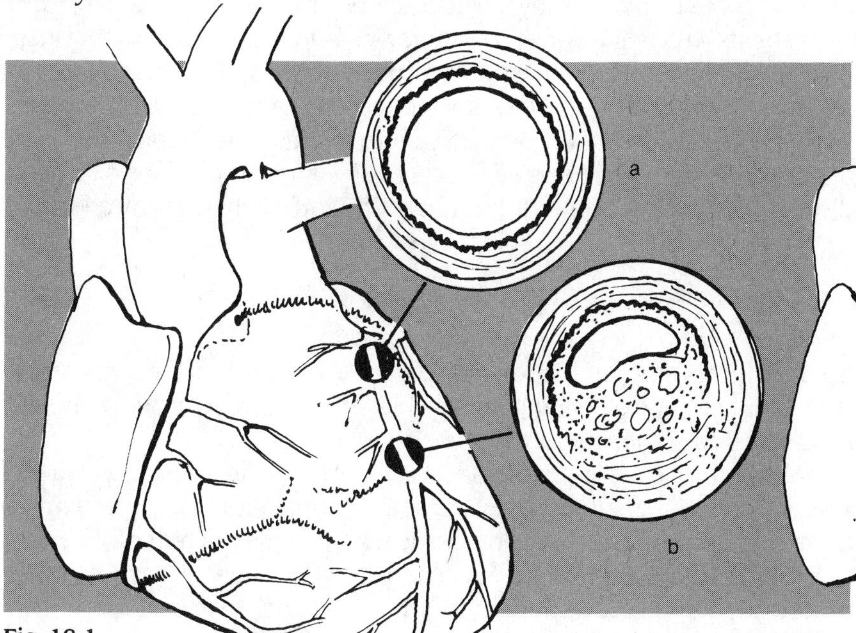

Fig. 18.3

Fig. 18.1

Fig. 18.4 *The Rothberg position is used in the emergency care of a heart-attack patient.*

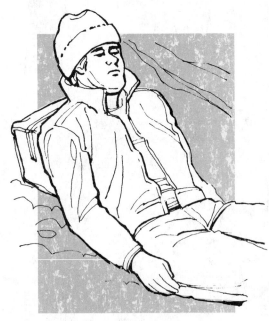

Fig. 18.4

The most common manifestations of coronary artery disease likely to be seen by the rescuer are **angina pectoris** and **acute myocardial infarction.**

Angina Pectoris

Angina pectoris (usually called angina) is a characteristic type of pain that occurs when the heart muscle is temporarily starved for oxygen. It usually appears during emotional stress or physical exertion, when the heart requires a larger blood supply than the narrowed coronary arteries can deliver. Angina can be relieved by measures that reduce the heart's need for oxygen, such as rest. As the coronary arteries progressively narrow, angina may occur at rest or even during sleep.

Anginal pain is felt beneath the sternum in the midline of the anterior chest or, less commonly, in the throat. It frequently radiates from the chest to the neck or jaw, one or both shoulders (usually the left), the left arm, or, in rare cases, to the upper abdomen (Fig. 18.2). The patient describes the pain as squeezing, crushing, vise-like, or burning; angina is almost never characterized as sharp, sticking, or aching. The pain rarely lasts longer than 15 minutes. Angina may be mistaken for indigestion, pleurisy, and other types of upper-abdomen and chest pain. Occasionally, the patient's first attack of angina pectoris occurs under the stress of an outdoor recreational experience. However, most patients have been diagnosed as having angina and carry medication to use in case of an attack.

Most drugs used to treat angina either enlarge (dilate) the coronary arteries or slow the heart rate and the strength of its contractions, either of which tends to improve the mismatch between the heart's need for more blood and the ability of the coronary arteries to supply it. The most common medication carried by patients with angina is **nitroglycerin.** Nitroglycerin is dispensed as small white tablets, which are placed under the tongue and absorbed into the bloodstream through the mucous membranes of the mouth. Nitroglycerin should relieve anginal pain within three to five minutes.

The emergency care of a patient with angina is to encourage the patient to sit down, rest, and take any medicine carried for the pain.

Patients with angina are able to enjoy less-strenuous outdoor activities, but they should be discouraged from attempting strenuous activities in remote locations because of their limited capacity for exercise. A patient with angina pectoris also is a candidate for more serious heart problems such as abnormal rhythms and heart attacks. A mild heart attack may be difficult to distinguish from a severe attack of angina pectoris. If there is any question, the patient should be taken promptly to a hospital.

Heart Attack

Because increasing numbers of middle-aged and elderly persons are participating in skiing and other outdoor activities, the incidences of **heart attacks** at ski areas and other outdoor locations will continue to increase.

Although the term heart attack is commonly used for any sudden episode caused by malfunction of the heart, it usually is reserved for a **myocardial infarction,** which means the death (infarction) of part of the heart muscle (myocardium). It usually occurs when a blood clot or some other process blocks or narrows a coronary artery in a patient with coronary artery disease. The left side of the heart is most commonly involved (Fig. 18.3).

Other types of heart attacks are caused by the sudden onset of a rapid or irregular heartbeat or by sudden failure of the heart muscle in patients with certain types of disease of the heart valves.

Signs and Symptoms of a Heart Attack

1. Sudden death may be the first sign.
2. Pain similar to that of angina pectoris (see above) but usually more severe and longer lasting. The patient may have had a previous heart attack or previous episodes of angina. Pain caused by a heart attack is unrelated to exertion and is not relieved by rest or nitroglycerin.
3. Anxiety and fear of death.
4. Cold, clammy, pale, occasionally cyanotic skin.
5. Respiratory distress.
6. The pulse may be normal or abnormal. Common abnormalities include a rapid and/or irregular pulse, a slow regular pulse, or a weak pulse.
7. The blood pressure may be high, low, or normal.
8. The patient usually prefers to sit up or lie with the chest elevated. In rare cases the patient may want to walk around.

Complications of Heart Attack

1. **Cardiac arrest**. Cardiac arrest occurs when the heart ceases to pump blood because of either a sudden, rapid, irregular, worm-like twitching of the heart muscle (**ventricular fibrillation**) or a complete cessation of heart contractions.
2. **Cardiogenic shock**. Damage to heart muscle may reduce the cardiac output to the point that the blood pressure can no longer be maintained. The signs and symptoms of cardiogenic shock are those of shock, in addition to those of a heart attack.
3. **Pulmonary edema**. In patients with pulmonary edema, the undamaged right side of the heart continues to pump blood into the lungs while the damaged left side is too weak to handle even a normal volume of blood coming from the lungs. Blood builds up in the lungs, increasing the hydrostatic pressure, which forces the fluid part of the blood out into the alveoli. The signs and symptoms of pulmonary edema are discussed in Chapter 17.

Emergency Care of a Heart-Attack Patient

1. The patient should find the most comfortable position and stay still. Maintain body temperature in the normal range. The patient usually will want to sit up, especially if short of breath.
2. Give oxygen in high concentration, preferably by mask.
3. The patient should be kept in a quiet area and shielded from bystanders. Reassure and calm the patient. Watch for the development of complications.
4. If shock develops, it may have to be treated with the patient's head and chest raised (the Rothberg position, Fig. 18.4) because of shortness of breath.
5. If cardiac arrest occurs, administer CPR.

Table 18.1

SUMMARY OF SIGNS AND SYMPTOMS OF A HEART ATTACK

1. Pain, described as squeezing, crushing, or a sensation of pressure.
2. Pain beneath the sternum, typically radiating to the throat, jaw, left shoulder, and left arm. The pain occasionally radiates to both shoulders, both arms, and the epigastrium.
3. Anxiety and fear of death.
4. Respiratory distress.
5. Pale, cold, clammy skin.
6. The pulse can be normal or subnormal.
7. Blood pressure can be normal or abnormal.
8. The patient usually prefers to sit up.
9. Complications:
   a. Cardiac arrest.
   b. Cardiogenic shock.
   c. Pulmonary edema.

Table 18.2

SUMMARY OF EMERGENCY CARE OF A HEART-ATTACK PATIENT

1. Keep the patient in the most comfortable position.
2. Give oxygen in high concentration.
3. Calm and reassure the patient.
4. Shield the patient from bystanders.
5. Watch for complications.
6. Monitor and record vital signs.
7. Give CPR, if necessary.
8. Provide rapid access to an ACLS team.

6. Treat pulmonary edema by propping up the patient in a seated position and administering oxygen.
7. The greatest risk of death is in the first few hours or days after a heart attack when the risk of cardiac arrest, usually caused by ventricular fibrillation, is highest.

Many people have died of cardiac arrest when, with proper treatment, they could have lived normal lives for many years. Therefore, the *most important emergency care* for a heart-attack patient is rapid access to an advanced cardiac life support team equipped with a heart monitor, defibrillator and appropriate medication, and in contact by radio with a hospital emergency department. The ACLS team will rapidly transport the patient by ambulance or helicopter to a hospital with an intensive care unit. These resources may not be readily available in every outdoor situation and may be totally unavailable in the wilderness.

A patient who suffers a heart attack at an alpine ski area should be evacuated to the first aid room in an oversnow vehicle with a large bed so CPR can be administered if needed. The patient should be accompanied by at least two patrollers. Some patrols have devised techniques for administering CPR to a patient being transported in a toboggan. More experience with these techniques is needed to judge their effectiveness. Radio ahead so that an ambulance or helicopter can be summoned promptly.

Vehicles other than ambulances or helicopters should be used to transport heart-attack patients to a hospital only as a last resort. If an alternate vehicle must be used, it should be a station wagon or van. Oxygen, airways, and suction equipment should be taken along, and two or more patrollers should accompany the patient and driver.

Some ski areas have paramedics or physicians on roster and are equipped with intravenous fluids, drugs, and cardiac monitor-defibrillators. While this equipment can buy time, its availability should not be used as an excuse to delay summoning the ACLS team.

Conditions that may be hard to distinguish from a heart attack include pulmonary embolus, spontaneous pneumothorax, inflammation of the sac around the heart (pericarditis), a perforated peptic ulcer, disease of the pancreas or gallbladder, hyperventilation, certain types of indigestion (particularly a gas bubble in the stomach or intestines under the left lower ribs), and inflammation of the muscles or joints of the chest wall. Differentiating these conditions from a heart attack may require the expertise of a physician and the facilities of a hospital.

Because a patient with a severe heart attack may die even in the best-equipped hospital intensive care unit, rescuers should be realistic about their ability to resuscitate such patients. The fatality rate for patients who suffer heart attacks under nonurban conditions may be as high as 50 percent; the rate may climb to 100 percent for patients who develop cardiac arrest.

STROKE

Strokes, frequently called **cerebrovascular accidents**, are caused by interference with the blood supply to a part of the brain, usually because of an artery clot or rupture with hemorrhage into the brain substance (Fig. 18.5). Strokes occasionally occur when a blood clot travels to the brain from another part of the body.

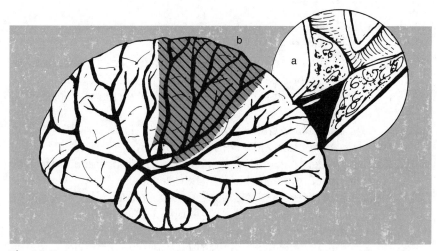

Fig. 18.5

Fig. 18.5 *A blocked cerebral artery (a.) causes injury or death to the part of the brain it supplies (shaded area, b.).*

Minor transient strokes, called **transient ischemic attacks** or TIAs, occur when blood flow through a narrowed brain artery is temporarily inadequate to support the function of the brain area supplied. TIAs are analogous to angina pectoris in patients with coronary artery disease. The underlying cause of most strokes is arteriosclerosis of the arteries that supply the brain— principally the carotid arteries – and their branches. Strokes are most common in the elderly and in people with hypertension and diabetes.

The onset of a stroke may be sudden or progress slowly over hours or days, and may be accompanied or preceded by headache or dizziness. Strokes usually are spontaneous, although they may follow a head injury. The location of the damage in the brain frequently can be suspected from signs and symptoms, particularly the type and location of impaired sensation and motion.

Signs and Symptoms of Stroke

1. The patient may have impaired consciousness, ranging from slight confusion to deep coma.
2. One side of the body may be weak or paralyzed. In an unconscious patient, one side is more limp than the other. The patient frequently suffers facial muscle weakness, which causes loss of expression and drooping of the involved side of the face.
3. The patient may drool, have difficulty swallowing, or develop slurred speech.
4. Breathing may be noisy because the tongue and throat muscles have weakened. Dyspnea may occur as a consequence of partial obstruction of the upper respiratory tract.
5. The patient's head and eyes may be turned to one side.
6. Convulsions, dizziness, and headache occasionally occur.
7. The patient's blood pressure may be normal or elevated.
8. Patients who have suffered stroke may develop a characteristic speech impairment marked by ability to understand what is said to them but inability to choose the right words to reply (**expressive aphasia**). With severe aphasia, the patient repeats one or two words, such as ''No!'', no matter what is asked; with milder aphasia, the patient chooses the wrong word or has a memory lapse when searching for certain words.

Table 18.3

SUMMARY OF SIGNS AND SYMPTOMS OF STROKE

1. Impairment of consciousness.
2. Weakness or paralysis, usually of one side of the body.
3. Drooling, difficulty in swallowing, slurred speech.
4. Upper airway obstruction may occur.
5. The patient's head and eyes may be turned to one side.
6. Occasionally, convulsions may occur.
7. Headache and dizziness ·may occur.
8. Blood pressure can be normal or high.
9. Aphasia.

Table 18.4

SUMMARY OF EMERGENCY CARE OF A STROKE PATIENT

1. Give general care for unconsciousness, as appropriate.
2. Maintain the upper airway.
3. Use suction, if necessary.
4. Give oxygen in high concentration.
5. Monitor and record vital signs, particularly the level of consciousness.
6. Keep the patient lying down with the head and upper body slightly elevated. Do not use a pillow.
7. Avoid casual conversation within the patient's hearing.
8. Give nothing by mouth.
9. Evacuate the patient to a hospital.

Fig. 18.6 *Islet Cells of the Pancreas*

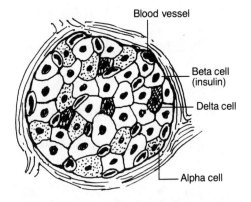

Fig. 18.6

Emergency Care of a Stroke Patient

1. Give general care for unconsciousness, if needed (see Chapter 13).
2. Pay strict attention to the upper airway. Even if conscious, stroke patients may be unable to rid their airways of secretions. Suctioning may be required.
3. Give oxygen in high concentration.
4. Periodically monitor and record vital signs.
5. Keep the patient lying in the semiprone or NATO position, preferably with the upper trunk and head slightly elevated.
6. A patient with stroke who is aphasic or unable to speak may still be able to hear and understand almost normally. Be careful about casual conversation near the patient.
7. Give nothing by mouth initially. If evacuation will be delayed, the patient may be given small amounts of liquid. This should be done slowly and cautiously to prevent choking.

DIABETES

Diabetes is a disease characterized by an absolute or relative deficiency of **insulin**, a hormone that controls the use of glucose. Insulin is formed by the islet cells of the pancreas (Fig. 18.6). Because all cells require glucose to function properly, lack of insulin causes serious disruption of cellular metabolism.

When the body is unable to use glucose for fuel, it is forced to burn fat. As discussed in Chapters 1 and 2, fat is initially broken down into acidic compounds (ketone bodies). When these compounds are produced faster than they can be burned, they accumulate, causing the blood to become more acidic, a condition called **acidosis**. In addition, the unused glucose accumulates in the blood and is excreted through the kidneys along with large amounts of water and electrolytes. This accounts for the dehydration, loss of weight, increased urination, and increased thirst seen in patients with uncontrolled diabetes. Severe uncontrolled diabetes may progress to **diabetic ketoacidosis**, a serious condition accompanied by weakness, confusion, stupor, nausea, vomiting, and abdominal pain. Severe acidosis causes rapid, deep respirations. If untreated, diabetic ketoacidosis will progress to **diabetic coma** and death.

There are two types of diabetes: **juvenile diabetes**, also known as labile, Type I, or insulin-dependent diabetes mellitus (IDDM); and **adult-onset**, also known as stable, Type II, or non-insulin-dependent diabetes mellitus (NIDDM). Patients with juvenile diabetes produce little or no insulin and require daily injections of insulin. Juvenile diabetes is more difficult to control, and these patients are more prone to developing ketoacidosis than are patients with adult-onset diabetes. Patients with adult-onset diabetes are able to make insulin, but the amount is insufficient for their needs. Patients with adult-onset diabetes usually are overweight, and although their diabetes frequently can be controlled by diet and weight loss, they may require insulin as well. In mild cases, oral medication that stimulates insulin production can be used instead of insulin.

All diabetics are subject to premature development of such complications as arteriosclerosis, impaired vision, high blood pressure, and kidney disease. Because these complications occur sooner in poorly regulated diabetics, most diabetics routinely monitor their blood or urine glucose levels to aid in maintaining strict control of their disease. New techniques that measure blood glucose level from a drop of blood obtained from a finger-stick have helped many diabetics achieve better control of blood glucose levels.

Patients with well-regulated diabetes are able to lead almost normal lives and can participate in skiing and other outdoor sports. Diabetics who require emergency care for their disease usually are suffering from either **hypoglycemia** (insulin shock) or **diabetic coma**; hypoglycemia is much more common.

Hypoglycemia

When blood glucose falls to abnormally low levels, diabetics may develop **hypoglycemia** (insulin shock). Insulin shock can occur when a patient who has taken a normal dose of insulin or an oral antidiabetic agent exercises more than usual or eats too little. Because the brain is very sensitive to a low blood glucose level, the first sign of insulin shock usually is an alteration of the patient's normal mental state.

Signs and Symptoms of Hypoglycemia

1. Personality changes, confusion, stupor, or coma.
2. Signs of sympathetic nervous overactivity such as pale, moist skin and a rapid pulse.
3. Headache.
4. Hunger.
5. Convulsions occasionally occur.
6. The patient usually is wearing a medical-alert tag or bracelet or has a wallet card indicating the presence of diabetes.

Emergency Care of Hypoglycemia

1. The most important step is to give the patient sugar while he or she can still swallow. The source can be a sugary liquid such as orange juice or a soft drink, candy, or a spoonful of table sugar. Commercially available tubes or squeeze bottles of concentrated glucose solution can be carried in a rescuer's first aid kit or a ski patroller's fanny pack. This glucose preparation can help revive even a semi-stuporous patient because, when squeezed into the pocket between the patient's cheek and teeth, it is swallowed by reflex action. A patient in insulin shock should improve within a few minutes after being given sugar. As soon as the patient is sufficiently alert, give him or her additional sugar, followed by a sandwich or other solid food.
2. General care for unconsciousness should be given as necessary (see Chapter 13).
3. A diabetic who recovers from hypoglycemia after being given sugar and food should be encouraged to rest a few hours before resuming

normal activity. Because permanent brain damage can result from prolonged low blood glucose levels, a patient who is unconscious or does not recover rapidly should be taken to a hospital as soon as possible.

Diabetic Coma

Diabetic coma occurs in people with previously undiagnosed diabetes and in known diabetics who have taken insufficient insulin or whose insulin requirement is increased because they are acutely ill.

Table 18.5

SUMMARY OF COMPARISON BETWEEN DIABETIC COMA AND HYPOGLYCEMIA

Category	Coma	Hypoglycemia
Onset	Gradual	Rapid
Sensorium	Confusion, stupor, coma	Same
Respirations	Rapid, deep	Usually normal
Pulse	Rapid, weak	Rapid
Blood pressure	Low	Normal
Skin	Flushed, dry, warm	Pale, moist
Breath	Fruity odor	Normal
Weakness, fatigue	Present	Present
Headache	May be present	Frequent
Hunger	No	Yes
Thirst	Yes	No
Convulsions	Rare	Not rare
Shock	May occur	Rare
Treatment		
General care for unconsciousness	As needed	As needed
Sugar	If in doubt about diagnosis	Yes—urgent
Response	Slow (in hospital)	Rapid, to sugar

Signs and Symptoms of Diabetic Coma

1. Confusion, stupor, or coma.
2. Rapid, deep respirations.
3. The skin usually is flushed, dry, and warm. The patient may have poor tissue turgor (dry, shrunken, less elastic skin) caused by dehydration.
4. A fruity breath odor.
5. Weakness and fatigue.
6. In some cases, signs of shock may develop.
7. The patient usually wears a medical-alert tag or bracelet or has a wallet card indicating that he or she has diabetes.

Diabetic coma is a medical emergency. There is no satisfactory emergency care in the field for a patient in diabetic coma, even if insulin is available. The patient must be taken rapidly to a hospital. Give general care for unconsciousness, if needed (see Chapter 13).

Consider the possibility of diabetes in every unconscious or semiconscious person. If the cause of unconsciousness is not obvious, look for medical-alert tags and wallet cards. At times, it may be difficult for even a physician to be sure whether a diabetic is suffering from diabetic coma or hypoglycemia; when there is any doubt, *always* give sugar. Sugar provides quick relief if the problem is hypoglycemia; if the problem is diabetic coma, extra sugar does no harm.

SEIZURE DISORDERS

The term **seizure** is used for any sudden, transient alteration of normal brain function. Seizures usually are accompanied by abnormal sensations or movements and usually include at least a minimal alteration in consciousness. They are thought to result from sudden abnormal electrical discharges. Severe seizures are called **convulsions**. **Epilepsy**, a medical condition characterized by recurrent episodes of seizures, affects about one person in every 200. Although seizures can be caused by stroke, head injury, meningitis and brain tumor, the cause of most seizures is unknown. Seizures in children may be associated with a high fever.

Seizures can be of many types, depending on the brain area involved. They can be roughly classified into two groups: **generalized seizures** and **partial seizures**.

Generalized seizures, also called grand mal seizures, typically are preceded by an **aura**, a peculiar sensation that can be a sound, sight, or smell. The aura, which is always the same sensation, signals the patient that a seizure is about to occur. Next, the body muscles suddenly contract, frequently causing the patient to cry out hoarsely and fall to the ground with bowed back and rigid arms and legs. This stage, called the tonic phase, is followed within a few seconds by violent, rhythmic contractions of the neck, back, and extremities (the clonic phase). During the attack, which usually lasts only a few minutes, the patient may bite his or her tongue, defecate, urinate, or be injured by striking an object. After a seizure, the patient remains unconscious or sleepy for several minutes to an hour or longer.

Partial seizures, sometimes called petit mal seizures, involve smaller areas of the brain. There are many types of partial seizures. They may produce body movements, automatic behavior or strange sensations, and may or may not involve disturbances in consciousness.

Emergency Care of a Patient Suffering a Generalized Seizure

1. Because there is no way an impending convulsion can be stopped or prevented, the rescuer should concentrate on protecting the patient from injury. If the patient feels a seizure is about to occur, help him or her lie down in an open area away from obstacles. If possible, a patient in an exposed or dangerous position, such as in water or on a cliff, should be immediately removed or secured in some way.
2. During a seizure, do not attempt to restrain the patient. In the past, it was popular to force an object between the patient's teeth to prevent

Table 18.6

SUMMARY OF EMERGENCY CARE OF A PATIENT SUFFERING A GENERALIZED SEIZURE

1. Protect the patient from self-injury.
2. Do not restrain the patient.
3. After the seizure is over, open and maintain the airway and give additional care for unconsciousness, as needed.
4. Assess the patient for injuries.
5. Allow the patient to rest until he or she is fully conscious and functional.
6. Ask about seizure medication.
7. Advise the patient to see a physician if there is no history of seizure.
8. Manage aberrant behavior (see Chapter 4).

the person from biting the tongue. Such attempts are no longer advocated because they generally are useless or even dangerous to both patient and rescuer.

3. Breathing may stop temporarily during a seizure but almost always resumes without treatment.
4. After the seizure, the patient may be unconscious, confused, or very sleepy. Open and maintain the airway as necessary. Assess the patient for possible injuries caused by the seizure. Be alert for other problems that may develop in the unconscious state, as discussed in Chapter 13. Allow the patient to rest until he or she is fully conscious and functional.
5. People known to have epilepsy usually take medication to prevent seizures. Ask whether the drug is being taken regularly. It may be appropriate to suggest that the patient see a physician promptly. If the patient has no history of previous seizures, advise him or her to consult a physician as soon as possible.

Partial seizures usually require no emergency care unless the patient is confused and is engaged in some type of clearly dangerous automatic behavior. The patient should not be physically restrained unless absolutely necessary. Handle such patients as recommended in the section on aberrant behavior in Chapter 4.

CARBON MONOXIDE POISONING

Carbon monoxide is a colorless, odorless gas that is produced by incomplete combustion of carbon-containing substances. Dangerously high levels of carbon monoxide can form whenever fuel is burned in a poorly ventilated space. When inhaled, carbon monoxide combines with the hemoglobin in red blood cells and renders the cells incapable of carrying oxygen. Symptoms of tissue anoxia occur when 20 percent of the hemoglobin is combined with carbon monoxide; unconsciousness occurs by the time the hemoglobin is 60 percent saturated. (The hemoglobin of heavy cigarette smokers often is as much as 10 percent saturated.)

Carbon monoxide poisoning is fairly common. In the United States, carbon monoxide poisoning causes several thousand deaths each year, many of them suicides. Carbon monoxide poisoning can be a significant hazard in the outdoor environment, particularly when stoves are used in poorly ventilated shelters such as snow caves and igloos. Tents can be hazardous during blizzards if snowdrifts make it impossible to cook outside. Many famous polar explorers, including Admiral Richard E. Byrd, S.A. Andree and Vilhjalmur Stefannson, were killed or narrowly escaped death from carbon monoxide poisoning caused by operating stoves in tightly closed areas. People stranded in vehicles during blizzards also are at risk if the engine is kept running to warm the occupants.

The signs and symptoms depend on the amount of carbon monoxide the patient has inhaled. In mild cases, the patient may have only dizziness, headache, and confusion; severe cases can cause a deep coma. Sudden respiratory arrest may occur. The classic sign of carbon monoxide poisoning is cherry-red skin color; in practice, the skin may be pale, blue, or red. Carbon monoxide poisoning should be suspected whenever a person in a poorly ventilated area suddenly collapses. Many experts feel that some effects attributed to acute mountain sickness (see Chapter 19) may, in fact, be caused by carbon monoxide. Recognizing this insidious condition may be difficult when all members of the party are affected.

The emergency care of a patient with carbon monoxide poisoning is to immediately remove him or her from the contaminated area. Patients with mild carbon monoxide poisoning who have not lost consciousness need fresh air and bed rest for a minimum of four hours. More severely affected patients may require rescue breathing. They should be given oxygen and be taken to a hospital. Fortunately, carbon monoxide is excreted by the lungs within a few hours.

To prevent carbon monoxide poisoning, avoid cooking in snow caves and igloos whenever possible. When cooking in a snow cave or igloo is necessary, provide adequate ventilation by leaving the entrance open and making a ventilation hole in the roof the diameter of a ski pole basket (3 to 4 inches). Occupants stranded in vehicles should keep the exhaust pipe cleared of snow and should leave a downwind window partly open whenever the engine is running.

SUBSTANCE ABUSE

Substance abuse refers to the use of mind-altering chemicals without a legitimate medical purpose. These chemicals are self-prescribed and self-administered, usually because they alter perception of the environment and cause artificial exhilaration, tranquility, or disorientation. The substance can be a prescription drug used in excessive amounts or in an illegal manner, an illegal drug, or a nonprescription substance such as ethyl alcohol. These substances may cause either dependence or addiction; the substance abuser's life may revolve around obtaining and using the drug to the point that the abuser's career, social functioning, and even simple hygiene are neglected.

Because intravenous drug users often are indifferent to sterile precautions, they are subject to diseases transmitted by dirty needles, including hepatitis and AIDS. Medical personnel find the treatment of addicts and substance abusers to be frustrating and frequently unsuccessful. Much crime in this country is committed to obtain money for the purchase of illegal drugs. However, in terms of misery and cost, the most significant form of substance abuse is **alcoholism**.

Before discussing individual substances, it is necessary to define several commonly used terms:

Drug–Any substance that alters mental or physical function when introduced into the body.

Tolerance–A state in which the body adjusts to the presence of a drug so that increasing amounts are required to produce the desired effect.

Physical dependence – A state in which the drug changes body physiology so that suddenly stopping its use causes well-defined symptoms of withdrawal. Thus, the abuser takes the drug *not* for its mind-altering effects, but to feel *normal*.

Psychological dependence – A state in which the abuser becomes obsessed with taking the drug and continues to take it despite obvious physical, mental, or social harm. Most of the abuser's waking hours may be devoted to obtaining and using the drug.

Addiction – A state that includes tolerance, physical dependence, and psychological dependence. The abuser is forced to spend more and more time obtaining and using the drug, usually in increasingly larger doses. If the addict cannot obtain the drug, severe and sometimes fatal withdrawal reactions may occur.

Polydrug abuse – Abuse involving more than one drug. It may occur as an isolated instance, such as when an abuser tries a substitute for an unavailable substance, or on a regular basis. It may be deliberate or accidental, such as when an abused substance is adulterated or "cut" with other substances. Polydrug abuse has become so prevalent that, when presented with a drug-abuse patient, many emergency physicians will presume polydrug abuse until proven otherwise. A practical problem for the rescuer is that signs and symptoms may be confusing, misleading, and not typical of any drug or class of drugs.

Specific Drugs

Alcohol

Alcohol is the most commonly abused drug in industrial nations. In the United States, more than 10 million people are alcoholics, over 200,000 deaths per year are caused by alcohol, and the economic costs of alcoholism total billions of dollars annually. Over half of our nation's traffic fatalities and drownings involve alcohol. There is no way to measure the social costs of alcohol in breaking up families and wrecking careers.

Alcohol is a legal drug; its sale has few restrictions, and moderate alcohol consumption has the tacit approval of society. Unfortunately, many individuals are unable to use alcohol in moderation since it can cause strong psychological and physical dependence.

Alcohol is a powerful central nervous system depressant that interferes with normal judgment, dulls awareness, and increases reaction time. Its so-called stimulatory effects, which usually occur early during the development of intoxication, are caused by interference with the function of the higher brain centers. Another physiological effect is dilation of the small blood vessels in the skin, which can cause accelerated heat loss in a cold environment and accounts for the ruddy complexion of the chronic drinker.

Acute use of alcohol lowers blood sugar. Chronic use damages the brain, heart, liver, and other important organs. Alcoholics may develop chronic malnutrition and vitamin deficiencies because of poor appetite and improper diet. Alcohol use during pregnancy may cause fetal alcohol syndrome, which is characterized by growth retardation, mental deficiency, small head circumference, and other structural abnormalities.

The signs and symptoms of alcohol intoxication are well-known and fall into two patterns: early intoxication, which is characterized by excitement, talkativeness, aggressiveness, and dilated pupils; and late intoxication, characterized by disorientation, slurred speech, and inability to concentrate. This state may progress to stumbling and falling, drowsiness, stupor, and coma.

Chronic alcoholism is found at all levels of society, affecting business and professional people, homemakers, and other "pillars of the community," as well as the destitute. Early in the disease, the patient may appear normal and may deny having any problem with alcohol. A high index of suspicion and careful questioning of the patient and close family members may be necessary to disclose warning signs and symptoms such as solitary drinking, morning shakes, morning drinking, binge drinking, and blackouts (periods of amnesia).

Later in the disease, the chronic alcoholic may be disheveled and unwashed; he or she may experience memory loss, apathy, tremors, jaundice, chronic indigestion, and chronic diarrhea. Alcohol withdrawal in chronic users produces anxiety, tremors, insomnia, nausea, vomiting, convulsions, agitation, and hallucinations.

Alcoholics with chronic liver disease (cirrhosis) develop large, dilated veins in the upper stomach and lower esophagus (esophageal varices) because the blood is forced to bypass the injured liver. Severe gastrointestinal hemorrhage can occur if these veins rupture.

Narcotics

Narcotics can be made synthetically or produced from the seeds of the opium poppy. A major legitimate medical use is to relieve pain. Commonly used narcotics include morphine (Morphine, Roxanol), meperidine (Demerol), methadone (Dolophine), codeine (contained in many combination products such as Tylenol with codeine), and hydromorphone (Dilaudid). The principal illegal narcotic is heroin.

Narcotics are central nervous system depressants and powerful respiratory depressants. Tolerance develops rapidly so that increasingly large doses are required to produce the same effects. Most narcotics are given by injection, although they can be taken orally, and some—such as opium gum—can be smoked.

The signs and symptoms of narcotic use include lethargy, stupor, slowed pulse and respirations, low blood pressure, and mild hypothermia. Many narcotics cause pinpoint pupils (meperidine is an exception). Chronic use causes nasal stuffiness and constipation. Acute overdose may cause coma and death from respiratory failure.

Withdrawal symptoms may include rapid pulse, anxiety, "gooseflesh," nausea, vomiting, diarrhea, abdominal cramps, frequent sniffling, severe runny nose, and shakiness.

Other Central Nervous System Depressants

Other central nervous system depressants are used legitimately in medicine to produce sleep, for their tranquilizing effects, and occasionally as anticonvulsants. They alter the state of consciousness and relieve anxiety to some extent but do not relieve pain or cause a "high." Common examples of barbiturates include secobarbital (Seconal), amobarbital (Amytal), pentobarbital (Nembutal), and phenobarbital (Luminal). Nonbarbiturates include chloral hydrate (Noctec), glutethimide (Doriden), methaqualone (Quaalude), ethchlorvynol (Placidyl), flurazepam (Dalmane), triazolam (Halcion), alprazolam (Xanax), diazepam (Valium), lorazepam (Ativan), and chlordiazepoxide (Librium).

The signs and symptoms of overdose include impairment of consciousness ranging from drowsiness to coma, slow pulse, low blood pressure, slowed respirations, mild hypothermia and, occasionally, seizures.

Acute withdrawal from depressant drugs may cause insomnia, agitation, disorientation, and hallucinations. Occasionally, shock or seizures may occur.

Central Nervous System Stimulants

Central nervous system stimulants are abused to elevate mood and produce a high. They also may cause seizures, anxiety, hyperactivity, insomnia, agitation, irritability, paranoia, and disorganized behavior. When the drug effects wear off, the user typically becomes depressed, moody, and sleepy. Examples of mild, commonly used stimulants are caffeine, nicotine, some decongestants, and asthma drugs such as theophylline and its derivatives. Illegal stimulants include **cocaine** and **amphetamines**.

Cocaine, the first local anesthetic to be discovered, has since been replaced by better drugs and now has few legitimate medical uses. It is produced from the coca plant, grown in South America. Cocaine is highly addictive and is one of the most widely abused illegal drugs in industrial nations today.

Usually taken by nasal inhalation, inhalation of smoke ("crack") or injection, cocaine induces marked euphoria. Other effects can include symptoms of disturbed mental status such as anxiety, panic, paranoia, confusion, and hallucinations; altered motor activity such as tremors and hyperactivity; seizures; dilated pupils; rapid pulse and respirations; and hyperthermia.

Serious complications such as cardiac arrhythmias, heart attack, stroke, psychotic reactions, shock, and gangrene of the intestine occasionally occur. Chronic use can lead cocaine abusers to neglect jobs, families, proper nutrition, and personal hygiene. Withdrawal may produce symptoms of exhaustion, depression, and anxiety.

Amphetamines were initially introduced into medicine as mood elevators and appetite suppressants. Examples include amphetamine, methamphetamine (Desoxyn), and dextroamphetamine (Dexedrine). Examples of non-amphetamine drugs used as cerebral stimulants or appetite suppressants include methylphenidate (Ritalin) and phenmetrazine (Preludin).

All of these drugs have significant addictive potential and have few legitimate medical uses at present. They are sometimes used by truck drivers on long hauls and students cramming for finals who hope to improve performance and prevent sleepiness.

Abusers take these drugs by mouth or injection. They may cause inability to concentrate, rapid heart rate and respirations, increased blood pressure, and such alterations in mental status as irritability, insomnia, anxiety, hyperexcitement, agitation, confusion, and paranoia. Altered motor activity such as hyperactivity and tremors may occur. Serious reactions such as cardiac arrhythmias, seizures, and coma are seen occasionally. Withdrawal symptoms are similar to those of cocaine.

Cannabis Compounds

Cannabis compounds, probably the most frequently used illegal substances in the United States today, include marijuana, hashish, tetrahydrocannabinol (THC), and oil of hashish. They are made from the Indian hemp plant, *Cannabis sativa*, and are usually introduced into the body by inhaling smoke.

These drugs cause mild euphoria, relaxation, and drowsiness. Side effects include confusion, dream/fantasy states, increased pulse rate, increased appetite, impairment of coordination, short-term memory, capacity to do complex work, and time perception. Occasionally, depression, confusion, acute anxiety, and hallucinations can occur. A common sign of marijuana use is reddening of the whites of the eyes. Heavy marijuana smokers can develop chronic carbon monoxide poisoning. Withdrawal may cause anxiety, loss of appetite, irritability, and nausea.

Inhalants

There are many volatile substances that are abused by being inhaled in an attempt to produce euphoria or mild tranquilization. **Inhalants** include glue, organic solvents such as acetone and toluene, petroleum distillates such as gasoline, nitrous oxide, trichlorethanes (found in typewriter correction fluid), and other halogenated hydrocarbons. Abusers may be overcome by hypoxia while inhaling the vapor with their heads in a plastic bag, a common practice done to increase the concentration of the vapor.

Toxic side effects include dizziness, headache, syncope, respiratory arrest, cardiac arrhythmias, irritation of the lining of the upper respiratory tract, and hallucinations. Chronic use can produce deterioration of the brain and liver.

Hallucinogens

Hallucinogens alter the user's perceptions of the environment, sometimes producing hallucinations or delusions. Hallucinogens are a large and growing group of abused chemicals. New variations are called "designer drugs" since they are designed to be just different enough from existing drugs to keep current drug laws from applying to them.

Commonly used drugs include lysergic acid diethylamide (LSD), psilocybin (derived from *Psilocybe mexicana* or "magic mushrooms"), mescaline and peyote (from the flowering heads of the *Lophophora williamsii* or mescal cactus), "STP," "MDMA," and phencyclidine (PCP). The latter, which is widely abused, is characterized by high potency, unpredictable effects, and frequent accidental ingestion since it may be used to "cut" other drugs.

The acute effects of hallucinogen use are unpredictable but can include euphoria, paranoia, mutism, distorted thought and perception, hyperactivity, gait disturbances, muscular rigidity, decreased pain sensation, and alterations in body temperature. More serious reactions, often called "bad trips," include panic reactions, suicide attempts, violent behavior, psychoses, and other serious psychiatric conditions. Serious accidents can occur when abusers develop misperceptions of their physical abilities and attempt to fly or perform other dangerous actions.

There are no clearly defined withdrawal reactions associated with hallucinogens, although brief recurrences of previous symptoms ("flashbacks") occur occasionally.

Assessment of a Patient with Suspected Substance Abuse

Substance abuse is a widespread problem that is not confined to urban ghettos. Outdoor recreationists may use marijuana and cocaine while professing to abhor pollution of the environment—their own presumably excepted.

Substance abuse should be suspected in anyone whose behavior is inappropriate or whose normal state of consciousness is altered. If the patient does not admit substance abuse, ask pointed questions of any friends or family members who may be present. The major danger lies in not thinking of the possibility of substance abuse or in confusing its effects with those of hypothermia, diabetic coma, insulin shock, epilepsy, psychosis, or a head injury.

Common Signs and Symptoms of Substance Abuse

1. **Central nervous system depression**, including mental dullness, lethargy, inability to concentrate, slurred speech, mental depression, apathy, lack of coordination, stumbling, falling, sleepiness, stupor, or coma.
2. **Central nervous system stimulation**, including excitement, talkativeness, aggressiveness, insomnia, tremors, agitation, aimless activity, disorientation, hallucinations, paranoia, and convulsions.
3. Changes in the **appearance of the eyes**. Opiates produce pinpoint pupils; alcohol, barbiturates and marijuana produce dilated pupils. Unequal pupils suggest a possible associated **head injury**. Alcoholics and marijuana abusers frequently have red eyes caused by engorgement of the blood vessels in the conjunctivae.
4. Changes in the **nose**. Abusers of opiates, cocaine, and other drugs that are taken by sniffing usually have chronic stuffy noses. Opiate abusers develop runny noses and sniffle frequently during early withdrawal. Cocaine abusers may develop perforations of the anterior part of the nasal septum.
5. Changes in the **skin**. Intravenous drug abusers may have multiple scars over accessible veins, usually of the forearms and at the bend of the elbows. Alcoholics frequently have ruddy skin and dilated veins over the nose and cheeks.
6. **Psychiatric changes**. Substance abuse may produce extreme agitation, belligerence, paranoia, hallucinations, delusions, panic reactions, amnesia, and psychosis. Because abusers may lack normal judgment and lose their usual protective instincts and reflexes, they may have to be protected from injuring themselves or others. They may fall, be involved in automobile or machinery accidents, or promote fights and other incidents.

Emergency Care of Substance Abuse Patients

The emergency care of substance abuse patients consists predominantly of caring for the effects of central nervous system depression or stimulation as follows:

1. Open and maintain the upper airway. Treat unconsciousness as necessary, using an oral airway and placing the patient in the semiprone position if he or she vomits.
2. The development of respiratory depression is a definite danger. Monitor the patient closely, and use frequent stimulation such as gentle pinching to keep the patient awake. Give rescue breathing, if necessary.
3. Even though substance abusers rarely go into shock, the patient should be observed for symptoms of shock and treated appropriately if shock occurs.

4. A patient with central nervous system stimulation must be handled calmly. The rescuer should remain patient, reassuring, and nonjudgmental. Refrain from arguing. Do not restrain the patient forcefully, except in an emergency. Remain with the patient until he or she is turned over to the EMS system or another competent authority. Violent patients should be approached very carefully, with several other rescuers close at hand in case assistance is needed.
5. If the patient convulses, follow the treatment outlined for seizure disorders earlier in this chapter.
6. It may be possible to "talk down" a patient who is having a bad trip. The process, which requires considerable patience, is outlined in step 4. above. Aggravating stimuli such as loud voices or music and bright lights should be avoided or removed.
7. Arrange for transport to a hospital. Any vomitus and evidence of drug use such as bottles, tablets, and drug paraphernalia should be collected and sent to the hospital with the patient.

THE ACUTE ABDOMEN

Abdominal pain without diarrhea that lasts more than eight hours is almost always a sign of a serious intra-abdominal condition requiring surgery. Pain may be accompanied by fever, abdominal tenderness, nausea, vomiting, and abdominal distention.

The signs and symptoms of an **acute abdomen** are the same as those of **peritonitis** (see Chapter 16) and include abdominal pain and tenderness which usually spread from a localized area to involve larger areas, increasing abdominal distention and rigidity of the abdominal muscles, loss of appetite, and nausea or vomiting (Fig. 18.7). The patient breathes rapidly and shallowly and lies quietly because it hurts to move or breathe. Later, signs of shock may develop (see Chapter 7), including a rapid pulse, low blood pressure, thirst, anxiety, restlessness, cold and clammy skin, and weakness.

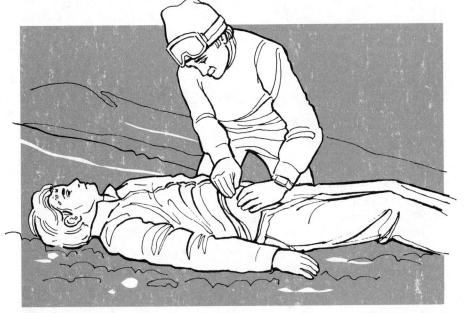

Fig. 18.7

Table 18.7

SUMMARY OF EMERGENCY CARE OF A SUBSTANCE ABUSE PATIENT

1. Open and maintain the airway.
2. Give general care for unconsciousness, as indicated.
3. Monitor and record vital signs.
4. If breathing is depressed, stimulate the patient and give rescue breathing as necessary.
5. Treat shock if it develops.
6. Calm an agitated patient.
7. Do not leave the patient alone until he or she is turned over to the EMS system.
8. Treat convulsions, if present.
9. Preserve vomitus, bottles, pills, and other drug paraphernalia and send the material to the hospital with the patient.

Fig. 18.7 *Assessment of a Patient with a Suspected Acute Abdomen*

Fig. 18.8 *Organs of the Abdominal Cavity*

An acute abdomen is caused by disease of the peritoneum or the organs within the abdominal cavity (Fig. 18.8). The location of pain caused by disease of these organs is discussed in Chapters 3 and 16.

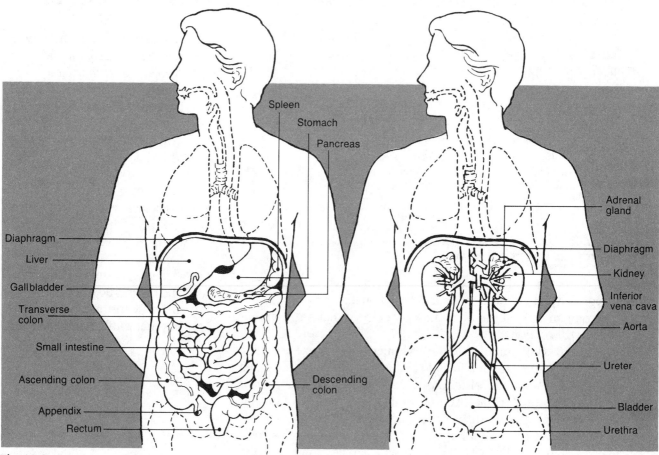

Fig. 18.8   Anterior Organs of Abdominal Cavity   Posterior Organs of Abdominal Cavity

Common Causes of an Acute Abdomen

1. Acute appendicitis.
2. Rupture of a peptic ulcer.
3. Acute cholecystitis (inflammation of the gallbladder).
4. Diverticulitis (inflammation of a finger-like pouch of the lining of the colon).
5. Pancreatitis.
6. Severe kidney infection.
7. Infection of an ovary or fallopian tube.
8. Peritonitis.
9. Acute gastroenteritis in the absence of diarrhea.
10. Intestinal obstruction.

Diabetic ketoacidosis may cause severe abdominal pain which can be mistaken for an acute abdomen.

Assessment of a Patient with an Acute Abdomen

1. First complete the primary survey and begin the secondary survey. The most important parts of the secondary survey are questioning the patient, taking the vital signs, and examining the abdomen. Ask the patient about recent abdominal injury and about the characteristics of the abdominal pain (as outlined in Chapter 17).
2. Inspect the abdominal wall for distention, changes in skin color, scars, and visible peristalsis. Listen for audible bowel sounds and palpate the abdomen to detect areas of tenderness, rigidity, enlarged organs, masses and distention. Tap the costovertebral angles lightly to check for kidney tenderness.

Emergency Care of an Acute Abdomen

1. Keep the patient lying down in the most comfortable position. Most patients will prefer to lie flat or on one side with their knees bent. Maintain the patient's body temperature.
2. Do not give the patient anything by mouth. Watch for vomiting and, if it occurs, monitor and clear the upper airway as necessary.
3. Monitor vital signs and record any new developments or changes in signs and symptoms.
4. If shock occurs, elevate the patient's legs 12 inches.
5. Because there is no effective emergency care for an acute abdomen, arrange for the patient to be taken to a hospital as soon as possible.

Table 18.8

SUMMARY OF EMERGENCY CARE OF AN ACUTE ABDOMEN

1. Keep the patient lying down.
2. Stabilize body temperature.
3. Give the patient nothing by mouth.
4. Watch for vomiting, and maintain the upper airway.
5. Monitor and record vital signs and changes in signs and symptoms, especially the location of pain in the abdomen.
6. Treat shock, if it develops.
7. Take the patient to a hospital as rapidly as possible.

19

Environmental Injuries

The commanding officer should take the utmost care
never to suffer a soldier to sleep, or even to sit down
in his tent with wet clothes, not to be down in a wet blanket
or upon damp straw. The utmost vigilance will be
necessary to guard against this fruitful source
of diseases among soldiers.

> —*Benjamin Rush, M.D.*
> "Directions for Preserving the Health of Soldiers," 1777

There are many hazards in the outdoor environment. Heat, cold, wind, solar radiation, altitude, bodies of water, fire, avalanches, blizzards, and lightning are important causes of injury. Before reading this chapter, review the elements of adaptation to the outdoor environment described in Chapter 1.

FROSTBITE

Frostbite, the actual freezing of a body part, occurs when the heat produced by the shell tissues plus the heat carried to them by the blood is insufficient to counteract the effect of below freezing temperatures. When exposed to cold, the body tends to guard the temperature of core organs by restricting blood flow to the shell.

Certain body areas have a higher risk of developing frostbite than others. The hands, feet, ears, cheeks, and nose are all located far from the heart at the periphery of the body and are subject to rapid heat loss because of their large surface-area-to-volume ratio and their exposed positions.

Other factors that contribute to frostbite include inadequate insulation, wet clothing, fatigue, poor nutrition, alcohol and drug use, restricted peripheral circulation (because of arteriosclerosis or tight clothing), and contact with metal or hydrocarbon liquids such as gasoline. Localized cold injury to tissue occurs in two ways: when intra- and extra-cellular ice crystals form, causing direct cell injury, and when blood circulation is interrupted because of red cell sludging (adhering together because of plasma loss from cold-damaged vessels) and blood clots within small blood vessels.

Frostbite often develops during periods of severe environmental stress when facilities for proper emergency care are nonexistent, and the party's main concern is to escape alive.

Types of Frostbite

Before a frostbitten area has thawed, frostbite can be separated only into **superficial** and **deep** categories. A patient with superficial frostbite (Fig. 19.1) feels a mild tingling or pain followed by numbness. Inspection reveals a grey or yellowish patch of skin, usually on the nose, ear, cheek, finger, or toe. The tissues beneath the area remain soft and pliable. This type of frostbite is common in cold-weather joggers and in skiers riding chairlifts on very cold, windy days.

Deep frostbite is a full- or partial-thickness freezing of a body part that mainly affects the hands and feet. It should be suspected if a painfully cold part suddenly stops hurting when the part obviously is not getting warmer. The affected part is cold, solid and wooden with pale, waxy skin; it resembles a piece of chicken just removed from the freezer.

After a frostbitten part has thawed, it is possible to divide frostbite into four categories of increasing tissue damage, similar to the classification for burns (Fig. 19.2). The first category is superficial frostbite; the other three are degrees of deep frostbite.

Fig. 19.1 Superficial Frostbite

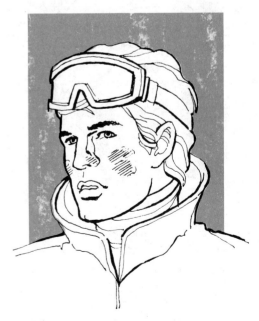

Fig. 19.1

Fig. 19.2 *Second-degree Deep Frostbite*

Fig. 19.3 *Immediate Care of Superficial Frostbite*

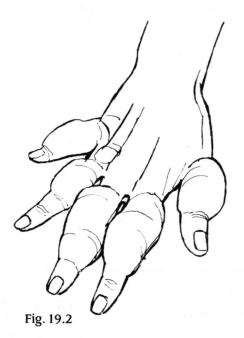

Fig. 19.2

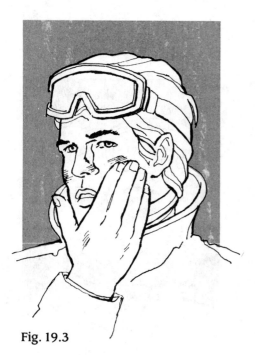

Fig. 19.3

Categories of Frostbite

First-degree frostbite – The affected part is warm, swollen, and tender. Blisters are either absent or are few and small.

Second-degree frostbite – Blisters form within minutes to hours after thawing and enlarge over several days. The blisters typically extend to the tips of the digits and are filled with pink or reddish fluid.

Third-degree frostbite – Blisters are small, contain reddish-blue or purplish fluid, and are situated more proximally on the digits than in second-degree frostbite. The surrounding skin may have a red or blue color and may not blanch when pressure is applied. The part is cool and numb; its joints are stiff.

Fourth-degree frostbite – There are no blisters or swelling. The part remains numb, cold, bloodless, white to dark purple in color, and quickly develops gangrene.

The emergency care of **superficial frostbite** is to apply direct body heat, e.g., by placing a warm hand on a frozen cheek or holding a frozen finger in an armpit (Fig. 19.3). The heat applied should be no warmer than body temperature. The rescuer should consider why frostbite occurred; the patient may need to add clothing or seek shelter.

Deep frostbite is a much more serious injury that poses the danger of tissue loss and permanent damage to surviving tissue. Experiments have shown that the amount of permanent tissue damage depends on both how *low* the temperature is and how *long* the body part is frozen; rapid rewarming causes less damage than slow rewarming.

The proper emergency care for deep frostbite is *rapid rewarming* in a water bath with the water temperature carefully controlled between 102 and 108°F (39 to 42°C). Cooler water rewarms too slowly; warmer water may burn the tissues. Rewarming should be done only in a shelter where the patient's entire body can be kept warm. The rescuer will need a high-registering thermometer and a vessel large enough so that the extremity can be immersed without touching the sides of the vessel. A 20-quart canning kettle is satisfactory for rewarming a foot. As a rule, rewarming continues for 20 to 30 minutes or until the frozen areas turn a deep red or bluish color and the color change has progressed distally as far as it will go. As the water bath cools, *remove the extremity*, add hot water, stir, and retest the water temperature *before* reimmersing the extremity. Rewarming usually causes severe pain.

While the frozen part is being rewarmed, maintain the patient's morale with hot drinks and apply heat to non-frozen body parts to open up circulation to the frozen area. Protect a thawed limb against refreezing, infection, and trauma by applying thick layers of sterile dressings held in place by a loosely applied, self-adhering roller bandage. Leave blisters unopened, separate digits with soft cotton or wool pads, and elevate the part to reduce swelling.

Exercise judgment in deciding whether to rewarm a frozen extremity in the field. Do not attempt rewarming if there is a hospital nearby or if there is any chance that the extremity may *refreeze*. Field rewarming is indicated if there is a good chance that the part will thaw spontaneously during evacuation. However, if the patient cannot be kept warm or cannot be carried out, it is permissible to let the patient walk or ski out on a frozen foot. Care must be taken to keep the foot frozen until it can be rapidly rewarmed under suitable conditions. This has been shown to cause less permanent damage than allowing the part to slowly thaw during transport.

In practice, patients frequently become aware of a frozen part because of the pain that accompanies thawing. Depending on the size and isolation of the party, there may be no alternative to self-evacuation on the thawed foot. If that is the case, refreezing should be prevented at all costs because it inevitably leads to gangrene.

The prevention of frostbite is discussed in Chapter 1.

HYPOTHERMIA

Hypothermia, or "exposure," refers to cooling of the body to a core temperature below 95°F (35°C) as determined by a low-reading rectal thermometer. Hypothermia can occur at temperatures well above freezing; at temperatures below freezing, the patient may suffer frostbite as well. The combination of cold, wind, and water is especially dangerous and can be encountered by people who are stranded in a blizzard at temperatures near 32°F (0°C) or who fall into mountain streams.

During World War II, 30,000 British sailors died of hypothermia; Napoleon is estimated to have lost 500,000 troops because of cold injury during the Russian campaign. Hypothermia is a factor in about one-third of the 8,000 drowning deaths that occur each year in the United States.

When a person's body temperature falls progressively, the initial drop of one to two degrees triggers shivering, followed by clumsiness, stumbling, falling, slow reactions, mental confusion, and difficulty in speaking (Table 19.1). The patient frequently is unaware of what is happening. **Loss of use of the hands** is very serious because it hampers attempts to set up shelter or light a fire. At body temperatures below 90°F (32°C), shivering gradually ceases and the muscles become progressively more rigid. The patient becomes irrational and lapses into a coma. Death may occur at body temperatures below 80°F (27°C). It is important to think of the possibility of hypothermia when dangerous meteorological conditions exist, since hypothermia is an insidious condition and death can occur within two hours of the onset of symptoms. Other members of a party may not recognize hypothermia in their companions because they themselves are becoming hypothermic. When the body is too cold to be capable of shivering, it cannot warm itself without outside help.

Hypothermia is potentially *lethal*. The mortality rate is greater than 50 percent in severe cases and cases complicated by injuries or previous illnesses. The most common cause of death is ventricular fibrillation. However, with proper emergency care the mortality rate should be low in otherwise healthy patients with core (rectal) temperatures at or above 90°F. A patient with severe hypothermia may appear to be dead – the pupils are fixed and dilated, and the patient has no perceptible pulse or visible signs of breathing and has rigidity resembling rigor mortis – but still may be saved with proper emergency care. The motto "No one is dead until warm and dead" emphasizes that *all* patients with hypothermia deserve an attempt at rewarming.

Table 19.1

SIGNS AND SYMPTOMS OF HYPOTHERMIA

(modified from Lathrop)

°F	°C	
99-96	37-35.6	Intense shivering. Impaired ability to perform complex tasks.
95-91	35-32.8	Violent shivering. Difficulty in speaking, sluggish thinking, amnesia.
90-86	32.2-30	Shivering is replaced by muscular rigidity. Exposed skin is blue or puffy. Movements are jerky. Dulled sensorium, but patient still is able to maintain posture and the appearance of contact with surroundings.
85-81	29.4-27.2	Coma, lack of reflexes, atrial fibrillation.
Below 78	Below 25.6	Failure of cardiac and respiratory centers, pulmonary edema, ventricular fibrillation. Death.

Types of Hypothermia

Hypothermia can be divided according to duration of exposure into three categories: **acute** (several minutes to an hour), **subacute** (several hours to a day), and **chronic** (more than a day). These distinctions are significant because there is a large difference between the core and shell temperatures in cases of acute hypothermia, while in subacute and chronic hypothermia the core temperature is closer to the shell temperature. In cases of acute hypothermia, the blood sugar is normal or slightly elevated, and electrolytes and acid base balance are still normal or only slightly disturbed. In cases of chronic hypothermia, the blood glucose level is low, and the patient has developed **acidosis** caused by shivering and starvation.

Hypothermia can be divided according to the patient's core temperature into **mild** (above 90°F or 32°C) and **profound** (below 90°F or 32°C). It also can be divided into **primary**, which occurs in basically healthy individuals who become hypothermic because of inadequate protection or excessively severe environmental conditions, and **secondary**, in which another illness or injury predisposes the patient to developing hypothermia.

Typical Settings in which Hypothermia Occurs

1. **Immersion hypothermia**, which usually is acute or subacute and is caused by immersion in cold water (below 70°F or 21°C). A similar type of hypothermia results from exposure to cold rain and high wind.
2. **Field hypothermia**, which occurs in previously healthy individuals such as skiers, climbers, hikers, and lost hunters. It usually is subacute or chronic and may accompany injuries occurring outdoors in cold weather.
3. **Urban hypothermia**, which occurs in individuals with a physical predisposition, disability, or illness. Predisposing conditions include those that increase heat loss (large surface-area-to-volume ratios in premature infants and newborns, patients with burns, and those with wide-spread skin disorders), those that interfere with heat production or distribution (malnutrition, anemia, old age, endocrine

abnormalities such as hypothyroidism, shock, heart disease, diabetes, arteriosclerosis), those that interfere with temperature regulation (central nervous system disease and injury, certain drugs), and those that interfere with normal judgment (senility, psychosis, drug and alcohol abuse). Many drugs, including sedatives, tranquilizers, Lithium and beta blockers, can accelerate the development of hypothermia. Urban hypothermia usually is subacute or chronic and has a high mortality rate.

4. **Submersion hypothermia** (near drowning in cold water) is acute hypothermia combined with hypoxia. Cooling appears to protect the central nervous system from the effects of hypoxia, but the diving reflex also may play a protective role. This reflex occurs in diving mammals such as the porpoise and consists of holding the breath, slowing the pulse, and shifting blood flow from the shell to the core in response to immersing the body or face in cold water. The diving reflex is present to some extent in man and is more pronounced in children than in adults, which combined with the more rapid cooling that occurs in smaller people, may explain why survival rates following submersion hypothermia are higher in children and infants than in adults. Rare individuals have survived without neurologic damage after being submerged for up to an hour.

Although hypothermia can be suspected from its symptoms, accurate diagnosis depends on documenting a body core temperature below 95°F (35°C), using a low-reading rectal thermometer. In the field, hypothermia should be suspected when a person shivers, appears clumsy, stumbles, drops things, has slurred speech, and lags behind companions. Any person who is found ill or injured outdoors in cold weather or is removed from cold water should be considered hypothermic until proven otherwise.

Emergency Care of a Hypothermic Patient

1. Prevent further heat loss.
2. Rewarm the patient as safely as possible.
3. Rewarm the body core in advance of the shell, if possible.
4. Treat the patient gently to avoid precipitating ventricular fibrillation, which is the major cause of death in hypothermic patients.

The application of these principles depends on the patient's core temperature, the equipment available, and the presence or absence of complicating factors such as other illnesses or injuries.

The first priority is to prevent further heat loss by getting the patient out of the wind or water and into a tent or other shelter. The patient should be given dry clothing and put into a sleeping bag, if available. If a sleeping bag is unavailable, put spare clothing under and over the patient and cover the patient's head. Avoid unnecessary handling and do not allow the patient to sit, stand, or walk until he or she is rewarmed. It may be better to cut off wet clothing than to undress the patient; if no dry clothing is available, wrap the patient in a poncho to reduce evaporative cooling. Meanwhile, build a fire or light a stove.

Further emergency care depends on the patient's measured or estimated core temperature. If a thermometer is unavailable, the patient can be considered to have a core temperature above 90°F (32°C) if he or she is still shivering and capable of appropriate actions such as zipping an open parka and pick-

Fig. 19.4 *High Heat Loss Areas*

Fig. 19.5 *Devices for Delivering Heat to the Body*
  a. *UVIC Heat Treat for Warming Inspired Air*
  b. *Chemical Heating Pad*
  c. *APPLINC Device for Delivering Warmed Air to the Lungs*

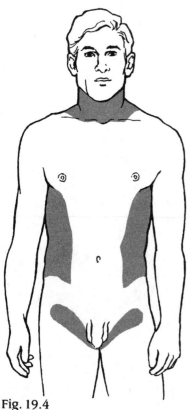

Fig. 19.4

ing up a dropped mitten. The core temperature is very likely below 90°F if the patient is no longer shivering and, especially, if he or she has become stuporous or comatose.

Mild Hypothermia

A hypothermic patient whose rectal temperature is 90°F (32°C) or above can be rewarmed by any means available; these means may be limited under field conditions. Hot rocks or canteens filled with hot water can be wrapped to avoid causing burns, then placed against areas of high heat loss such as the sides of the neck, sides of the chest under the armpits, and the groin (Fig. 19.4). One or two healthy companions can get into a sleeping bag with the patient; all, including the patient, should be stripped to the waist. Shivering is a good self-rewarming method and should be encouraged. Rescue groups can carry chemical heating pads and devices for delivering heated, humidified air or oxygen to the lungs (Fig. 19.5). Several magazine articles have described how a "hydraulic sarong" can be used to warm a patient with hypothermia (Arnold, J.W., M.D., Dayton, L.B., "Hydraulic Sarong: Emergency Treatment for Hypothermic Casualties." *Off Belay*, 21:2, 1975. Arnold, John, M.D., Jenkins, David, "The Hydraulic Sarong: A New Method to Save Hypothermia Victims?" *Summit*, 16:2, March 1970, p. 2.). This method uses a backpacking stove to heat a pot of water, and a bilge pump to circulate the hot water through plastic tubes sewn into a blanket that can be wrapped around the patient's trunk (Fig. 19.6). A newer development is the Heatpac (Fig. 19.7), a small lightweight stove that can deliver 250 watts of heat for several hours using one charcoal cartridge for fuel.

Under more civilized conditions, the rescuer can use a hot tub (at 105 to 110°F or 41 to 43°C) or an electric blanket for rapid rewarming. Heat should be delivered to the trunk alone, with the arms and legs left out. When the patient is able to swallow, he or she can drink hot, sweet liquids. This is mainly to boost the patient's morale since hot drinks produce only minimal increases in body temperature.

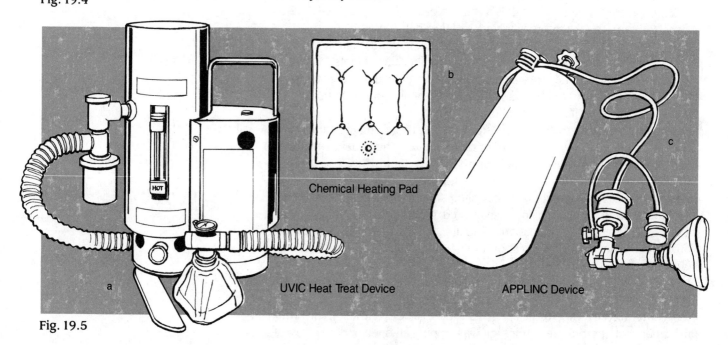

Chemical Heating Pad

UVIC Heat Treat Device

APPLINC Device

Fig. 19.5

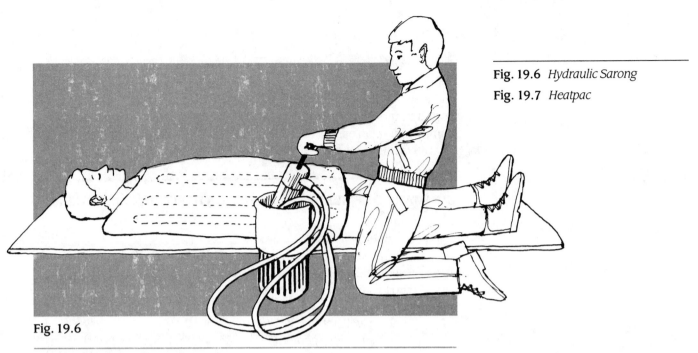

Fig. 19.6

Fig. 19.6 *Hydraulic Sarong*
Fig. 19.7 *Heatpac*

Profound Hypothermia

The mortality rate outside a hospital is high for patients who have a rectal temperature below 90°C (32°C). In-hospital survival is better because personnel can discover, monitor and rapidly treat metabolic and electrolyte problems, and rewarm the patient under controlled conditions with peritoneal dialysis (dripping warm fluid into the peritoneal cavity) or with a heart-lung machine. Thus, the best results are obtained by preventing further heat loss and transporting the patient to medical care rather than attempting field rewarming. Patients with body temperatures this low are in "cold storage" and will be relatively stable for several hours if treated gently.

Before transport, open and monitor the upper airway and stabilize the patient. Prevent heat loss with methods that can be applied during transport. Avoid active methods such as a hot tub or electric blanket.

Because patients with profound hypothermia are dehydrated, warmed intravenous fluids should be given if the expertise and equipment are available. A patient with profound hypothermia will have slow respirations and a low blood pressure. Because these signs are "normal" under these circumstances, rescue breathing and aggressive treatment for shock are rarely indicated. A PASG, which theoretically could cause an auto-transfusion of cold acidic blood from the shell to the core, is contraindicated unless the patient is in shock caused by trauma.

Patients with profound hypothermia may appear to be dead because their pulses and respirations are so difficult to detect. Spend a minute or longer attempting to detect both vital signs before concluding that they are absent. All patients with **submersion hypothermia** should be given CPR immediately. In other types of hypothermia, CPR may actually *precipitate* ventricular fibrillation and should not be given unless careful examination reveals *no* signs of life and ventricular fibrillation is strongly suggested because of a sudden event such as collapse or cessation of a previously detected heartbeat. Once begun, CPR should be continued at the normal rate until the patient is hospitalized. Patients with hypothermia have survived after several hours of CPR. This suggests that patients with hypothermia have a more favorable outlook than those with cardiac arrest from other causes.

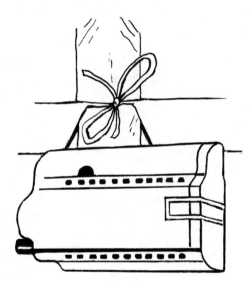

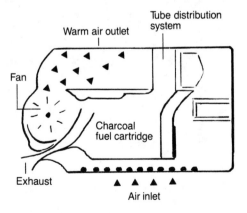

Fig. 19.7

Before transporting the patient, splint fractures and treat other injuries using standard methods. Carry the patient slowly and carefully, avoiding sudden jolts and keeping the head slightly lower than the feet. Rapid transportation methods such as helicopter evacuation are preferable to a long, bumpy, toboggan or snow vehicle ride. If possible, take the patient to a hospital with facilities for open-heart surgery.

Table 19.2

SUMMARY OF EMERGENCY CARE OF A HYPOTHERMIC PATIENT

General

Stop further heat loss:

Get the patient out of the wind and into a tent or shelter.

Build a fire or start a stove.

Add insulation beneath and around the patient. Cover his or her head.

Replace wet clothing with dry clothing.

Treat the patient gently. Do not allow him or her to sit or stand until rewarmed.

Give hot, sweet liquids after the patient is alert, awake, and able to swallow.

Treat any injuries.

Mild Hypothermia (core temperature of 90°F [32°F] or above)

Raise core temperature by whatever means are available:

Hot rocks or canteens can be placed against high heat loss areas.

A rescuer and the patient can lie trunk to trunk in a sleeping bag.

Rescue organizations may use a hydraulic sarong, heating pads, small stove (e.g., Heatpac), or have the patient inhale warmed, humidified air or oxygen.

In "civilized" areas a hot tub (110°F or 43°C) or electric blanket may be available. Leave the patient's arms and legs out.

Severe Hypothermia (core temperature below 90°F or 32°C)

Do not rewarm the patient in the field if he or she can be evacuated within 18 hours. Keep the patient from getting colder:

Use warmed, humidified air, body heat, heat pads, Heatpac or other types of nonactive rewarming that can be maintained during evacuation.

The patient should be given an IV of 5-percent glucose/saline, if suitably trained personnel are available.

Avoid jostling and jolting the patient during transportation.

Avoid CPR unless ventricular fibrillation is highly likely. In cases of near drowning, start CPR immediately.

If the patient cannot be evacuated, use passive, external rewarming (e.g., body-to-body heat in a warm shelter).

If a patient with profound hypothermia cannot be evacuated within 12 to 15 hours, the patient may have to be rewarmed in the field. The best method is passive, external rewarming, e.g., placing one or two companions in a single or double sleeping bag with the patient.

Methods for preventing hypothermia are discussed in Chapter 3. Ski patrollers should watch for the development of hypothermia in persons who lie or stand in the snow for long periods, e.g., accident victims, gatekeepers at races, and skiers stranded on stalled chairlifts. An injury impairs the body's heat conservation mechanisms, making an injured patient more susceptible to cold injury. Cold temperatures and high altitude increase the risk of shock, which predisposes the patient to further chilling, making frostbite and hypothermia more likely. Put insulation beneath and over accident victims and protect them from the wind.

HEAT INJURY

Localized heat injury (burns) is described in Chapter 8. This section discusses **generalized heat injury**, which results when the body's heat loss mechanisms are unable to cope with the combination of heat gain from the environment plus internal heat production. This dangerous situation can cause problems in three ways:

1. The body core temperature may rise to dangerous levels *despite active heat dissipation*. The rise can be caused by excessive environmental heat and humidity or excessive internal heat production.
2. The body core temperature may rise to dangerous levels *because of faulty heat dissipation*.
3. The body core temperature may be normal or slightly elevated, but the stressed heat dissipation mechanisms may cause illness because of *overactivity* or *dysfunction*.

Conditions that increase the risk of heat illness include those that increase heat gain from the environment (large surface-area-to-volume ratios in premature infants and newborns), those that interfere with sweating and the regulation of shell circulation (extensive burns and widespread skin disorders), those that increase heat production (overactive thyroid states, muscular overactivity in hot weather), those that interfere with heat transport from core to shell (old age, heart failure, diabetes, shock, arteriosclerosis, chronic debilitating states, and other causes of poor circulation), and those that interfere with normal judgment (senility, psychosis, drug and alcohol abuse).

Many drugs predispose the user to heat illness by increasing the metabolic rate, or interfering with sweating, skin circulation, or body temperature regulation. These drugs include amphetamines, cocaine, hallucinogens, salicylates (aspirin, etc.), antihistamines, tranquilizers, sedatives, anticholinergics, phenothiazines, antidepressants, and diuretics.

Heat and high humidity are a dangerous combination because heat loss through the evaporation of sweat is less efficient.

There are two types of major heat illness, **heat stroke** and **heat exhaustion**, and two types of minor heat illness, **heat cramps** and **heat syncope**. The division of major heat illness into heat stroke and heat exhaustion is a somewhat arbitrary selection of two points on a continuum; the particular signs and symptoms presented by a given patient ultimately depend on the predominant mechanisms of illness.

Table 19.3

SUMMARY OF THE SIGNS AND SYMPTOMS OF HEAT STROKE

Hot, flushed skin.
Patient may or may not sweat.
Rapid pulse that later becomes thready.
Variable blood pressure.
Confusion, weakness, dizziness, headache.
Patient complains of feeling very hot.
Later complications:
Nervous system: agitation, delirium, stupor, seizures, coma.
Digestive system: nausea, vomiting, diarrhea, blood in stool.
Shock.
Abnormal bleeding.

Table 19.4

SUMMARY OF THE EMERGENCY CARE OF A HEAT STROKE PATIENT

Remove the patient to a cool environment.
Immediately cool the patient by any available means.
Give care for unconsciousness as needed.
Monitor and record vital signs.
Give care for shock as needed.
Give care for convulsions, if needed.
Give oxygen in high concentration.
Transport the patient to a hospital as fast as possible, continuing cooling en route.

Heat Stroke

Heat stroke can be divided into two types: **classic** and **exertional**. Classic heat stroke, seen in the elderly and infirm, is caused by the combination of a hot environment and ineffective mechanisms of heat dissipation. The adverse side effects of the multiple drugs taken by many elderly persons also may be a factor. Exertional heat stroke is caused by excessive internal heat production from physical activity in warm weather. Excess clothing and lack of acclimatization also frequently hinder heat dissipation. Exertional heat stroke has been common in military recruits and football players and now is being seen in long-distance runners.

Suspect heat stroke in anyone who becomes ill in a hot environment, particularly if consciousness is altered.

Signs and Symptoms of Heat Stroke

1. The skin usually is hot and flushed; it occasionally may be pale or blue.
2. The patient may or may not be sweating.
3. The pulse is rapid and initially strong; it may become thready later on.
4. The blood pressure may be high, low, or normal.
5. The patient is confused and complains of weakness, dizziness, headache, and of being very hot.
6. The patient's oral temperature usually is above 105°F (41°C).
7. As the illness progresses, the patient may exhibit:
   a. Signs of injury to the nervous system, such as agitation, delirium, stupor, coma, or seizures.
   b. Signs of injury to the gastrointestinal system, such as nausea, vomiting, diarrhea, or blood in the stool.
   c. Signs and symptoms of shock.
   d. Signs of bleeding, because of damaged blood clotting mechanisms.

Heat stroke is a *true emergency*. The excess heat causes potentially permanent damage to every organ system. The amount of damage is proportional to how high the patient's temperature is and how long it remains elevated.

Emergency Care of a Heat Stroke Patient

1. Immediately cool the patient by whatever means are available. Remove heavy clothing; light cotton clothing can be left in place. The fastest method of cooling is direct application of ice to the skin. In the emergency department, bags of ice from an ice machine are poured over and around the patient (especially between the legs and between the arms and body). Because ice rarely is available in an outdoor situation during hot weather, the most effective cooling method usually is to cover the patient with cloths saturated with cold water and fan the patient to promote evaporative cooling.
   Immediate cooling is extremely important and should be started on the spot. Do not delay, even if a hospital is nearby. Continue cooling the patient during evacuation and transportation. The patient's

temperature usually can be brought back to normal within 45 to 60 minutes. To avoid hypothermia, discontinue cooling when the patient's body temperature is about 1 degree above normal.

2. Provide care for unconsciousness, with particular attention to the airway (see Chapter 13).
3. Frequently check and record vital signs, especially body temperature. Watch the patient for a secondary rise in body temperature after cooling has been discontinued.
4. If shock occurs, elevate the patient's lower extremities 12 inches (see Chapter 7).
5. Convulsions may occur (see Chapter 18).
6. If available, give oxygen in high concentration.

Heat Exhaustion

Heat exhaustion is a form of hypovolemic shock caused by either excessive sweating or the inadequate replacement of water and electrolytes lost by sweating. People who take diuretic medication may develop heat exhaustion during periods of hot weather. Other predisposing factors include lack of acclimatization, diseases of the heart and circulatory system, and wearing heavy clothing. Heat exhaustion should be suspected whenever a person collapses or becomes weak and dizzy in hot weather.

Signs and Symptoms of Heat Exhaustion

1. Thirst, weakness, confusion, cold and clammy skin, a fast or thready pulse, low blood pressure, profuse sweating, restlessness, anxiety, and the other findings typical of hypovolemic shock (see Chapter 7).
2. Normal or slightly elevated body temperature.
3. The blood pressure may be normal when the patient is lying down but may drop when the patient sits up.

Emergency Care of a Heat Exhaustion Patient

1. Move the patient to a cool environment and keep the person lying down until he or she improves.
2. Remove heavy clothing.
3. If the patient is alert and able to swallow, give him or her up to a liter of half-strength Gatorade or a similar commercial solution. A homemade solution of a half teaspoon of table salt dissolved in a liter of cold water can be substituted.
4. If symptoms do not improve within an hour, evacuate the patient to a hospital.

Heat Cramps

People who exercise in hot weather can develop **heat cramps** in active muscles during or after exercise if they replace water without replacing salt lost through sweating. As much as 20 grams of salt per day can be lost by heavy sweating. The muscles of the abdomen, back, and lower extremities are most frequently involved. Heat cramps can be prevented by drinking beverages that contain electrolytes at regular intervals during strenuous exer-

Table 19.5

SUMMARY OF THE SIGNS AND SYMPTOMS OF HEAT EXHAUSTION

Confusion, restlessness, anxiety.
Weakness.
Thirst.
Cold and clammy skin.
Fast and/or thready pulse.
Blood pressure may be normal or low. It may drop when the patient sits up.
Profuse sweating.
Temperature may be normal or slightly elevated.

Table 19.6

SUMMARY OF THE EMERGENCY CARE OF A HEAT EXHAUSTION PATIENT

Move the patient to a cool environment.
Keep the patient lying down.
If the patient is able to swallow, give him or her mildly salted liquids. If improvement is not rapid, evacuate the patient to a hospital.

cise in hot weather. The immediate emergency care for a heat cramp is to massage the muscle and stretch it forcefully in the opposite direction. After the cramp has subsided, the patient should be given full-strength Gatorade or a similar electrolytic beverage.

Heat Syncope

Heat syncope is a mild form of hypovolemic shock that resembles simple fainting (see Chapter 7). It can affect people who sit or stand for long periods in the direct sun or in hot weather. Return of blood to the heart is affected by muscle action; immobility causes blood to pool in the lower extremities so that less blood reaches the heart, the blood pressure falls, and the patient faints.

The signs and symptoms of heat syncope are those of mild, hypovolemic shock (see Chapter 7). Emergency care consists of allowing the patient to lie down and rest in a cool place.

EFFECTS OF ALTITUDE AND SOLAR RADIATION

With ascent from sea level, solar radiation increases and environmental temperature, oxygen partial pressure (PO2) and atmospheric pressure fall. For every 1,000 feet (305 meters) of altitude, the temperature drops about 4°F (2.2°C), the barometric pressure drops 20 mm Hg, and the amount of ultraviolet radiation increases by about 5 percent. The percentage of oxygen in the air remains constant at 21 percent, but the PO2 drops so that at 10,000 feet (3,048 meters) only two-thirds of the sea level value remains, and at 18,000 feet (5,486 meters), only half remains.

Altitude Sickness

Rapid ascent to altitudes of 8,000 feet (2,438 meters) or higher may cause distressing symptoms in unacclimatized individuals, including skiers and hikers who fly from sea level to the mountains. People traveling in vehicles on high mountain roads and in unpressurized aircraft without supplemental oxygen also can experience altitude sickness. Symptoms include fatigue, weakness, headache, loss of appetite, nausea, vomiting, and shortness of breath on exertion. The patient appears pale and ill. Sleep may be difficult for the first few nights. The patient may develop **periodic breathing** (Cheyne-Stokes respirations), a condition characterized by regular periods of increasingly deep breathing followed by periods of no breathing during which the patient may stir or awaken with a sense of suffocation. The patient also may hyperventilate (see Chapter 17), which causes symptoms of light-headedness, dizziness, and tingling of the hands, feet, and mouth.

Altitude sickness is probably part of the syndrome of acute mountain sickness (see below), but there are legitimate reasons for considering it separately. It is important for members of wilderness groups to recognize this common, benign condition to prevent needless evacuations.

The symptoms of altitude sickness develop rapidly and seem to be caused by the *direct* effects of hypoxia on body cells and blood circulation. The effects of hypoxia are aggravated by fatigue and cold, and some people are more susceptible than others. Symptoms of altitude sickness usually disappear after one to two days as the affected individual acclimatizes. Rest and a light diet are helpful. Patients with severe or prolonged altitude sickness should return to a lower altitude. Oxygen is helpful but generally unnecessary. Recent studies have shown that disturbed sleep at high altitude can be improved by taking one 250-milligram tablet of acetazolamide (Diamox) at bedtime. People who have significant difficulty sleeping at high altitude may wish to consult their physicians about obtaining a prescription for this medication.

Acute Mountain Sickness

Acute mountain sickness (AMS) is much less common than altitude sickness. Because it occurs after a lag period and involves a different level of tissue injury, AMS seems to be largely caused by *secondary* changes brought on by the *direct* effects of hypoxia. Although pulmonary edema has been recognized in the Andes for years, it was largely ignored in North America until 1960, when Dr. Charles Houston reported a case in a cross-country skier and suggested that some patients diagnosed as having pneumonia might have pulmonary edema instead. Subsequently, extensive studies were carried out by Indian Army physicians in the Himalayas and by Dr. Houston and others on Mount Logan in Canada. Acute mountain sickness has been reported at altitudes as low as 7,500 feet (2,286 meters); however, in the Western Hemisphere, it is uncommon below 12,000 feet (3,658 meters).

The most significant adverse effects of high altitude hypoxia are seen in the **brain**, where cell membrane damage causes cell swelling, and in the **lungs**, where pulmonary arteries contract unevenly, allowing excessive blood flow through some parts of the lungs and insufficient blood flow through others. After a lag period of six to 96 hours, symptoms of either or both of the major types of AMS begin to appear.

The two types of AMS are **high altitude cerebral edema** (HACE), which is caused by brain cell swelling, and **high altitude pulmonary edema** (HAPE), which occurs when some of the alveoli fill with fluid. Although the incidence of AMS is unknown, following studies on Mount Rainier, Dr. Houston has estimated that up to 5 percent of persons who go to high altitudes (12,000 feet or above) develop a dangerous degree of AMS. HAPE, which occurs with about 10 times the frequency of HACE, is uncommon below 12,000 feet; HACE is uncommon below 14,000 feet (4,267 meters).

Predisposing factors include too rapid ascent, overexertion, and exposure to cold. Children and adolescents seem to be more susceptible to AMS than older individuals, but good physical conditioning does not seem to confer immunity. Individuals who automatically hyperventilate at altitude appear to be less susceptible to AMS; some high altitude symptoms, such as throbbing headache, can be improved by voluntary hyperventilation.

Signs and Symptoms of AMS

    A. High Altitude Cerebral Edema (HACE)
        1. Early signs and symptoms
            a. Headache, which usually is throbbing and may be severe.
            b. Nausea and vomiting.
            c. Insomnia.
            d. Cheyne-Stokes respirations.

Table 19.7

SUMMARY OF THE SIGNS
AND SYMPTOMS
OF HACE AND HAPE

High Altitude Cerebral Edema
  Early signs and symptoms:
    Headache.
    Nausea and vomiting.
    Insomnia.
    Cheynes-Stokes respirations.
  Late signs and symptoms:
    Paralysis.
    Blindness.
    Convulsions.
High Altitude Pulmonary Edema
  Early signs and symptoms:
    Cough.
    Respiratory distress.
    Mild chest pain.
    Weakness.
  Late signs and symptoms:
    Cyanosis.
    Cough that produces sputum.
    Rapid pulse and respirations.
    Audible gurgling sounds
      in the chest.
    Severe respiratory distress.

2. Later signs and symptoms
   a. Ataxia (loss of muscle coordination leading to difficulty maintaining balance).
   b. Confusion, which may progress to stupor, coma, and death without proper care.
   c. Paralysis of one or more extremities, which may resemble the paralysis seen in stroke.
   d. Blindness.
   e. Convulsions.
B. High Altitude Pulmonary Edema (HAPE)
   1. Early signs and symptoms
      a. Dry cough, frequently occurring at night.
      b. Respiratory distress, made worse by exertion.
      c. Mild chest pain, usually perceived as an ache beneath the sternum.
      d. Weakness.
   2. Later signs and symptoms
      a. Cyanosis.
      b. Cough that produces large amounts of frothy, pink sputum.
      c. Rapid pulse and respirations.
      d. Audible, gurgling sounds during breathing. When a stethoscope or the ear is placed on the naked chest, wet crackling sounds can be heard as the patient breathes.
      e. Severe respiratory distress.

Many patients with AMS develop retinal hemorrhages, which can be seen with an ophthalmoscope by suitably trained individuals. The patient usually is not aware of the hemorrhages unless they are present in the parts of the retina responsible for sharpest vision (macula).

The most important impediment to early recognition of AMS is its *insidious onset*. Early signs and symptoms frequently go unrecognized or are ignored by patients and their companions, who also may be suffering some degree of AMS. By the time AMS is suspected, nightfall or bad weather may make evacuation to a lower altitude difficult.

Emergency Care of AMS

1. The most important emergency care measure is *rapid descent to a lower altitude*. Descent should be at least 2,000 feet (610 meters) below the initial altitude and preferably to below 10,000 feet (3,048 meters). Descend early, while the patient can still walk. If the patient can no longer walk, carry him or her in a sitting position.

From a practical point of view, the biggest problem seems to be distinguishing patients with severe altitude sickness or mild AMS who will improve with rest alone from those with severe AMS who require immediate evacuation to a lower altitude. A day or two of rest without evacuation to a lower altitude is appropriate for mildly affected patients *if* their symptoms are mild and not progressive, *if* help is available to carry them down, and *if* they can be carefully observed the entire time, including during the night.

Signs and symptoms that mandate *immediate descent* include ataxia, as tested by the inability to walk a straight line or to get up on the knees without swaying; audible, bubbly sounds in the chest; cyanosis; a rapid pulse or respiratory rate compared to other members of the party, particularly if the sign persists after rest; and a sharp decline in general fitness, which is particularly likely on the afternoon of the second day at altitude.

These guidelines are not absolute. If there is any question, the patient should be evacuated to a lower altitude. The risk of AMS is quite low after the fifth day at the same altitude, but symptoms still can be precipitated by stresses such as swimming in a cold stream, a hard fall, hypothermia, or a respiratory infection.

2. Oxygen in high concentration causes temporary improvement. However, because oxygen supplies are always limited, oxygen use should not delay preparations for descent.
3. Allow the patient to stay in the most comfortable position, usually sitting up.
4. Treat headache with a nonprescription medication such as aspirin or acetaminophen.
5. If the patient loses consciousness, provide care as described in Chapter 13.

The methods of preventing AMS are discussed in Chapter 1.

Table 19.8

SUMMARY OF THE EMERGENCY CARE OF A PATIENT WITH HACE OR HAPE

Recognize the problem and stop further ascent.

Descend rapidly.

Give oxygen in high concentration, if available.

Keep the patient in the most comfortable position. The sitting position is preferable.

Treat headache with mild analgesics.

Give care for unconsciousness, if necessary.

Sunburn, Windburn, and Snowblindness

People are more vulnerable to the harmful effects of solar radiation when they are at higher altitudes, on snow, or on bodies of water because the thin, clear atmosphere at higher altitudes filters out fewer of the harmful, ultraviolet rays, and exposure is increased by reflection off snow or water.

Injury to the skin and eyes is more likely to occur on cloudy days when people often forget to protect themselves and during the longer days of spring and summer.

Sunburn is a first- or second-degree skin burn caused by ultraviolet light in the medium-wave range (UVB), with a wavelength of 290 to 320 nanometers. Repeated sun exposure over many years may lead to chronic degenerative skin changes, such as wrinkling, hyperpigmentation, thickening, and cancer. These changes, which resemble accelerated changes of aging, can be delayed by avoiding excessive sun exposure and using proper skin protection.

The skin is protected by clothing and topical sunscreens. Sunscreen preparations come in two basic types: **physical and chemical**. Physical sunscreens block sunlight. These products consist of opaque greases containing zinc oxide, talc or titanium dioxide, and are particularly suitable for limited areas such as the nose and lips. However, some people find physical sunscreens cosmetically unacceptable. Chemical sunscreens rely on chemical agents to selectively filter out harmful rays. The most effective products now available contain para-amino-benzoic acid (PABA) and its esters, benzophenones, cinnamates, salicylates, and oxybenzone. Some preparations contain both physical and chemical sunscreens.

Skin types can be classified into four groups according to degree of sun sensitivity. People with type I skin burn easily and never tan, while those with type IV skin tan easily and never burn. Types II and III fall in between. Most manufacturers of sunscreen creams, lotions, and lip salves specify the sun protection factor (SPF) on the label. This number, usually between 2 to 39, refers to how much longer skin protected with the product can be exposed to the sun before becoming red compared to unprotected skin. People with type I skin should purchase products with SPF numbers higher than 15; those with type II skin, SPF 6 to 15; those with type III skin, SPF 4 to 6; and those with type IV skin, SPF 2 to 4.

Because sunscreens with a cream or grease base are better at preventing frostbite and windburn than alcohol-based preparations, they are preferable for use by skiers, high-altitude climbers, and others exposed to cold, wind, and strong glare. Apply sunscreens one to two hours before sun exposure and reapply several times during the day, particularly if sweating is heavy.

Treat sunburn the same as any other burn (see Chapter 8), by applying cool compresses. Soothing ointments, which are best avoided if the patient has more than a minimal thermal burn, are useful for sunburn. Consult a physician if the sunburn is extensive or if the skin is blistered.

Windburn is an irritation of the skin that resembles a first-degree sunburn. It can be prevented to some extent by a wearing a face mask or by applying a greasy sunscreen. Treat windburn by applying a greasy sunscreen or other bland grease.

Snowblindness, which is sunburn of the conjunctiva of the eye, can be prevented by wearing suitable dark glasses or goggles. Because radiation can reach the eye by reflection from the snow, glasses should have extensions on each side and below (glacier glasses). Dark grey lenses are best; they should transmit only 10 to 15 percent of light. Goggles should be adequately ventilated and have easily replaceable lenses. A separate set of yellow or red lenses to increase contrast in flat light should be carried.

Symptoms of snowblindness develop six to 12 hours after exposure. The eyes feel irritated ("sand in the eye") and are sensitive to light, the conjunctivae are reddened, and there is excessive tearing, swelling around the eye, and pain on eye motion. Emergency care includes covering the eyes or putting the patient in a dark room, applying cool compresses, and using nonprescription pain relievers. The patient should see a physician; medication may be prescribed to relieve the pain and speed healing.

LIGHTNING AND ELECTRICAL INJURY

High-voltage electrical current represents a significant hazard in modern society because of the large number of electrical appliances and power lines that exist. There are approximately 1,000 deaths from electrocution yearly in the United States and many more cases of severe electrical burns. In the outdoors, people are susceptible to injury from lightning during electrical storms and from high voltage power lines, which can be found even in remote areas. Ski areas use large amounts of electric power, and chairlifts are susceptible to lightning strikes, particularly in late spring.

Rescuers need to know how to protect themselves from the dangers of electricity, especially lightning, and how to care for patients injured by electricity.

Ways in Which Electricity Causes Injury

1. Breathing may stop because of injury to the respiratory control center in the brain.
2. Cardiac arrest or ventricular fibrillation can occur because of a direct effect on the heart.
3. Paralysis, blindness, numbness, loss of hearing or speech, and unconsciousness can occur because of direct effects on the nervous and musculoskeletal systems.
4. Severe, deep burns can occur.
5. Trauma can occur because of falls, frequently caused by strong muscular contractions that throw the patient off balance.
6. Secondary kidney injury may occur because the kidneys are overloaded by the breakdown products of blood and injured muscle.

Lightning is caused by violent vertical air currents associated with the development of cumulonimbus clouds or thunderheads – huge, billowing, vertical clouds with anvil-shaped tops that may tower to 60,000 feet or more. The air currents produce differences of electrical potential between clouds or between a cloud and the earth. Cumulonimbus clouds usually produce large raindrops, huge snowflakes or hail, and tend to develop during the afternoon in warm or hot weather. They also can be part of an advancing cold front.

Lightning causes injury in the same way as any other electric current, except that the duration of the bolt is so short (.0001 to .001 second) that burns are less severe. A person struck by lightning may suffer a characteristic type of superficial skin burn that has a pattern resembling a fern leaf (Fig. 19.8). In addition to direct strikes, people may be injured by ground currents and side flashes from nearby strikes. Strikes often cause a person's clothing to explode off the body by instantly converting sweat or other moisture to steam.

A patient injured by electricity who has not been thrown clear by the jolt must be removed from the source of the current before emergency care can be given. The only safe way to do this is to shut off the power source. The danger to the rescuer is so great that only those with special training and equipment should attempt to remove a *hot* wire directly from a patient.

Because rubber tires provide good insulation, people trapped in a vehicle near a fallen power line are safe as long as they stay inside the car until the electric power is shut off. If the occupants must be evacuated because of a fire or other urgent reason, they should be instructed to jump out, taking care to avoid touching the car and the ground at the same time.

Assessment and Emergency Care of Electrical Injury Patients

1. Because of the danger to the rescuer and the high frequency of pulmonary and cardiopulmonary arrest in patients who have suffered electrical burns, the first impression, primary survey, and basic life support are of special importance (see Chapters 4 and 5). Perform airway management with care because of the chance that the patient could have a neck injury. Because damage to the circulatory and respiratory systems usually is temporary and patients are capable of full recovery, continue CPR as long as possible. CPR and rescue breathing

Fig. 19.8 *Fern Leaf Pattern of a Lightning Burn*

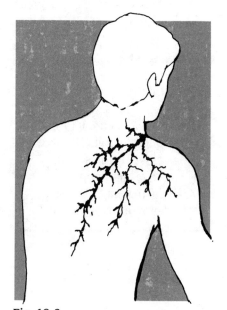

Fig. 19.8

Table 19.9

SUMMARY OF ASSESSMENT AND EMERGENCY CARE OF ELECTRICAL INJURY PATIENTS

Be aware of possible dangers.

Perform a rapid and thorough first impression and primary survey.

Give basic life support.

Consider the possibility of a neck injury.

Give oxygen in high concentration.

Give care for unconsciousness as needed.

Perform the secondary survey and take care of additional injuries, if present.

Monitor and record vital signs at regular intervals.

Do not give up too soon on CPR or rescue breathing.

Take the patient to a hospital as rapidly as possible.

are more successful in victims of electric shock, particularly lightning strike, than in patients with other types of cardiac and respiratory arrest. Breathing may be restored after prolonged respiratory arrest, in particular, so do not give up prematurely.

2. Give oxygen in high concentration.
3. As soon as breathing and heartbeat are restored, examine the patient for burns, wounds, fractures, and other evidence of trauma and damage to peripheral nerves. Dress burns and other wounds and splint fractures.
4. The patient may require care for altered consciousness (see Chapter 13) and shock (see Chapter 7).
5. Recheck and record vital signs and the state of consciousness, motion, and sensation at frequent intervals.
6. Take the patient to a hospital as soon as possible.

Prevention of Electrical Injury

Most substances can be divided into **conductors** and **insulators**. Conductors transmit electric currents; insulators resist the flow. Most metals and objects that are wet or contain water (including the human body) are good conductors. Because electric currents tend to follow paths of least resistance, a person can be injured when a body part is accidentally positioned in line with such a path so that a circuit is completed. Most urban electrical injuries result from faulty electrical equipment, careless use of appliances, or accidental contact with a power line. Handling an electrical appliance while sitting in a bathtub is particularly dangerous.

Lightning is the main electrical hazard in remote areas. If caught in an electrical storm, avoid bodies of water and take shelter away from high points, exposed ridges, and solitary trees. All of these features attract lightning strikes. Return small boats to shore at the first threat of storm. Avoid small caves where body parts are close to cave walls or the ceiling, since ground currents may flow through the body instead of taking a longer course through the cave wall.

If caught in the open, retreat as far down on the side of a ridge or other exposed area as possible and move away from ice axes, ski poles, and other metal objects. Squat on your heels until the danger is over. This position shortens the body and minimizes ground contact, decreasing the tendency for the body to act as a lightning rod and making it less likely that ground currents will pass through the body.

During electrical storms at alpine ski areas, ski lifts and exposed summit structures should be cleared of skiers. Avoid metal structures such as lift towers.

AVALANCHE INJURIES

Even if uncovered within the first half hour after burial, an avalanche victim has less than a 50 percent chance of being alive. If found alive, the patient will be suffering from suffocation, and frequently from hypothermia, frostbite, shock, and trauma.

Fig. 19.9

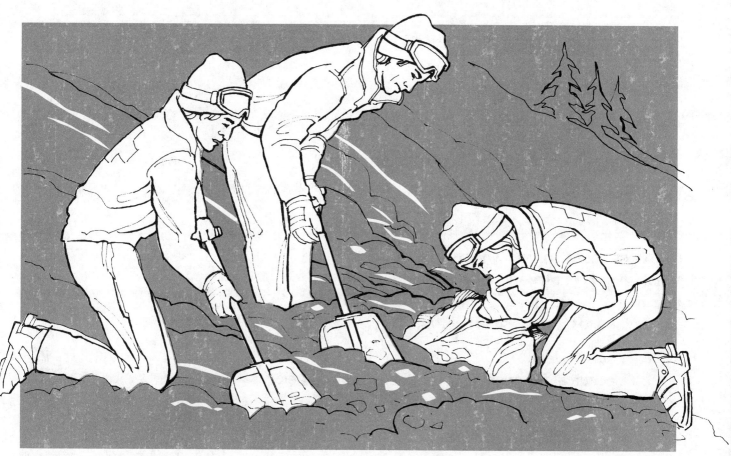

As soon as the patient's head is uncovered, open the airway, and start rescue breathing unless the patient is breathing spontaneously (Fig. 19.9). Water, snow, blood, and/or vomitus usually must be removed before the airway can be cleared. A portable suction unit is useful under these circumstances and is included in most avalanche rescue caches. A patient in cardiac arrest must be fully uncovered before CPR can be given.

Meanwhile, add insulating materials over and around the patient to prevent further heat loss. Although the patient almost always is hypothermic, rewarming usually is impossible under these circumstances and may even be counterproductive for patients requiring CPR. Give oxygen in high concentration, if available.

After breathing and circulation have been restored, examine the patient and treat any fractures or other injuries using the usual techniques.

Fig. 19.9 *Rescue Breathing Performed on an Avalanche Victim*

20

Extrication and Transport

One does not ask of one who suffers:
What is your country and what is your religion?
One merely says: You suffer, this is enough for me:
you belong to me and I shall help you.

> *—Louis Pasteur*
> Speech at the opening of the Philanthropic Society's
> Refuge for Mothers, June 8, 1886

Preceding chapters present the assessment and emergency care of patients, regardless of location. This chapter describes rescue techniques for obtaining access to, extricating, packaging, transferring, and transporting patients who may be found in inconvenient locations (Fig 20.1).

Search and rescue literally begins with a **search** for the patient, often a complicated process. **Rescue** involves obtaining access to and giving emergency care to the patient, extricating, transferring, packaging, and transporting the patient.

After the patient is located and given initial emergency care, the patient must be transferred to a spine board, litter, or toboggan. This process, called **extrication**, may require removing the patient from a tangled thicket or from a tight or awkward place. In the next step, **packaging**, the patient is properly positioned, strapped in securely, and protected from the elements and hazards such as rockfall. After being packaged, the patient can be **transported** to definitive medical care.

When the patient is first sighted, note his or her location and position compared to your own and determine the fastest and most efficient way to reach the patient with all necessary equipment. Also note hazardous aspects of the rescue scene that may endanger the patient and/or rescuers. The patient may be in a precarious position that poses imminent danger of falling, drowning, or suffocating. Rescuers may run the same risks in attempting to reach the patient. Rescuers may endanger the patient by accidentally knocking down loose rock or dislodging the patient from an unstable position. As a general rule, rescuers should not approach a patient from directly above or directly below unless there is no alternative. The safest route of access may be difficult to determine.

Hazards can include potential rockfalls, steep slopes, heavily traveled ski slopes, technical terrain, snow avalanches, whitewater, flash floods, approaching storms, and forest fires.

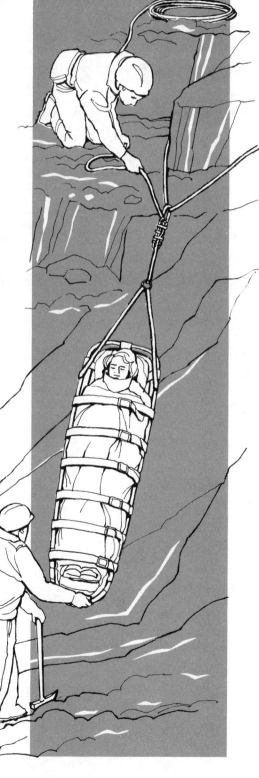

Fig. 20.1 *A patient being lowered down a steep snow field.*

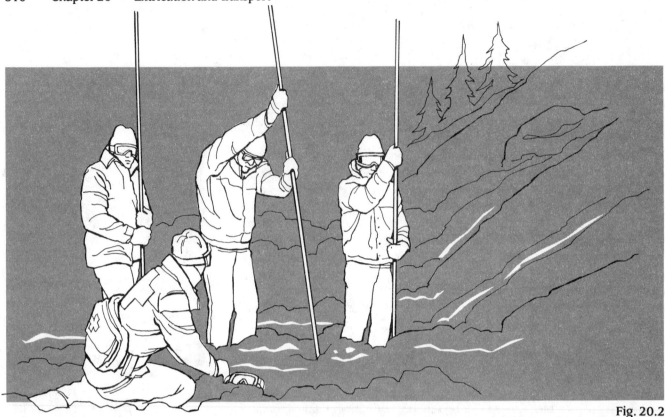

Fig. 20.2

Fig. 20.2 *Avalanche Hasty Search*

Remember that, despite altruism, your first responsibility should be to yourself, second to your companions, and third to the patient. In extreme cases, rescue may be impossible.

If the terrain is steep or technically challenging, search and rescue should be conducted only by rescuers comfortable with the terrain; otherwise, technical rescue teams should be called in. Hard hats should be worn routinely in steep terrain where falls or rockfall could occur. It may be necessary to work quickly to reach shelter in advance of an approaching storm. Dangerous slopes may have to be crossed to reach a person buried in an avalanche; rescuers may be endangered if unstable slopes feed into the avalanche track above the site (Fig. 20.2). Gaining access to the patient may require cutting away trees and brush, moving rocks and other obstacles, and using special techniques such as rappeling.

After the patient has been reached, urgent care is given at the scene using the standard techniques of assessment and emergency care discussed in previous chapters.

Impedances may have to be cleared by sawing, cutting, prying, or digging before equipment for transportation can be brought in and the patient can be extricated. The general principle is to remove the impedance from the patient, *not* the patient from the impedance. Special short backboards and litters, such as the Kendrick extrication device (KED) and the SKED stretcher (see Chapter 9), have been designed for difficult extrications (Fig. 20.3).

In general, a patient should not be moved until all necessary emergency care has been given, all injured parts have been immobilized, and it is clear that the patient will not be further injured if moved. The various techniques for moving a patient to a location where packaging can take place are divided into **emergency** and **nonemergency moves**, depending on whether the patient must be moved before emergency care and stabilization are completed.

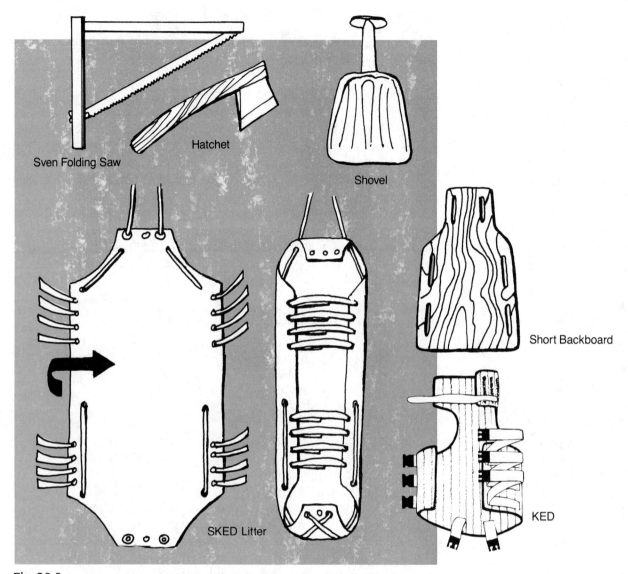

Sven Folding Saw

Hatchet

Shovel

SKED Litter

Short Backboard

KED

Fig. 20.3

Fig. 20.3 *Extrication Tools and Litters*

EMERGENCY MOVES

Emergency moves are used when there is immediate danger to the patient or to rescuers, a need to gain access to other patients with life-threatening injuries, or a need to move a patient to a flat, level surface for CPR. The main danger of an emergency move is *aggravating a spine injury*.

If there is no time to immobilize injuries before moving a patient, the spine and other injured areas should be protected as much as possible by using a multi-rescuer lift and transfer (described below), or by pulling the patient in the direction of the long axis of the body, so that the back, neck, or an injured extremity undergo minimal twisting or rotation.

NONEMERGENCY MOVES

Rescuer protection is an important requirement in nonemergency moves. Rescuers should know how to lift and carry heavy loads without injuring their backs or other parts of their bodies. It is unwise to lift or carry too heavy

Fig. 20.4 *Proper Lifting Procedure*
Fig. 20.5 *Fireman's Drag*

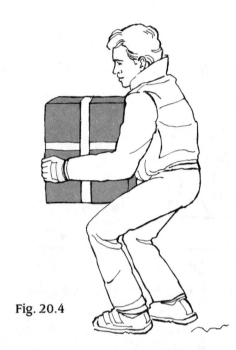

Fig. 20.4

a load without adequate assistance. The back is vulnerable to injury during common mishaps such as lifting and twisting to the side with the feet mired in mud or snow, and lifting while bending forward with the knees straight, hips bent, and arms extended forward (as when removing a cooler from the trunk of a car).

Lift with the *hips* and *legs* rather than the back. Keep the back *straight*; do not twist or bend forward or to the side (Fig. 20.4). Hold the load as close to the body as possible, and avoid sudden jerky movements.

It is important to pay attention to footing and balance, especially on slippery rocks, icy stairs, and wet or snowy inclines. Movements must be made *smoothly* and in unison with fellow rescuers. During multi-rescuer lifts and carries, one rescuer should be designated as the *leader*–usually the rescuer maintaining manual stabilization of traction on the head and neck – and all movements should be made on agreed-upon signals from the leader.

LIFTS AND CARRIES

Lifts and carries can be divided into the following categories: emergency and nonemergency, spine injury and no spine injury, and single rescuer and multiple rescuers.

Examples of Lifts and Carries

1. **Emergency, One-rescuer Techniques–Spine Injury Unlikely**
   (These techniques are used only when there is a bona fide emergency and no time to obtain assistance.)
   a. **Fireman's Drag** (Fig. 20.5). As the name implies, this carry was invented for removing a patient from a burning building. Roll the patient onto the back and tie the wrists together with a cravat or belt. Face the patient, kneel straddling the patient, raise the patient's arms and place them around your neck and shoulders so the patient's hands are behind your neck. As you raise your shoul-

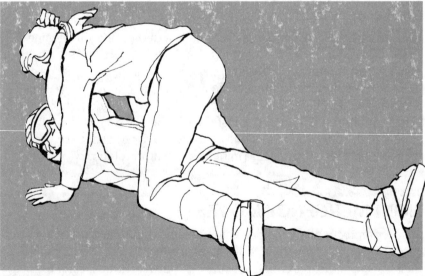

Fig. 20.5

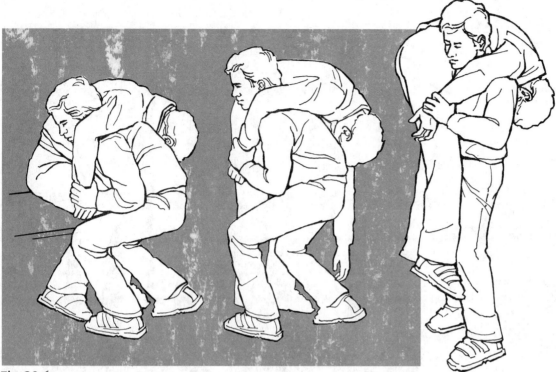

Fig. 20.6

Fig. 20.6 *Fireman's Carry*

ders and begin to crawl, the patient's trunk is lifted clear of the ground and the patient's legs are dragged along the ground between your knees.

Even though this carry is one of the least desirable from the standpoint of patient comfort and safety, it is useful for removing a patient from a low, confined space where there is room for only one rescuer and for removing a patient from a smoke-filled room, since the freshest air is near the floor.

b. **Fireman's Carry**. Stand facing the patient, who must be either sitting or standing, and grasp both the patient's wrists; bend your knees into a partial squat and pull the patient toward you so that he or she is slung across your shoulder with hips and legs anterior and chest and head posterior (Fig. 20.6). Keep holding on to the patient's wrists, and walk with your legs spread for increased stability.

c. **Human Crutch**. A person who is conscious and not seriously ill can be assisted in walking to safety. Have the patient put one arm around your shoulders while you put an arm around the patient's waist (Fig. 20.7a). If two rescuers are available, they should flank the patient and each put an arm around the patient's waist; the patient puts his or her arms around the rescuers' shoulders (Fig. 20.7b).

d. **Front Cradle**. A strong rescuer can carry a small, light patient in his or her arms. Place one arm around the patient's chest below the armpit and the other arm under the patient's knees. The patient's near arm goes around your neck (Fig. 20.8).

e. **Back Carries**. In difficult terrain, a one-person carry is easier if the patient can be placed on a strong rescuer's back. The patient must be conscious and without serious injuries. A seat can be fashioned

Fig. 20.7 *Human Crutch*

Fig. 20.8 *Front Cradle*

Fig. 20.9 *Nylon Webbing Carry*

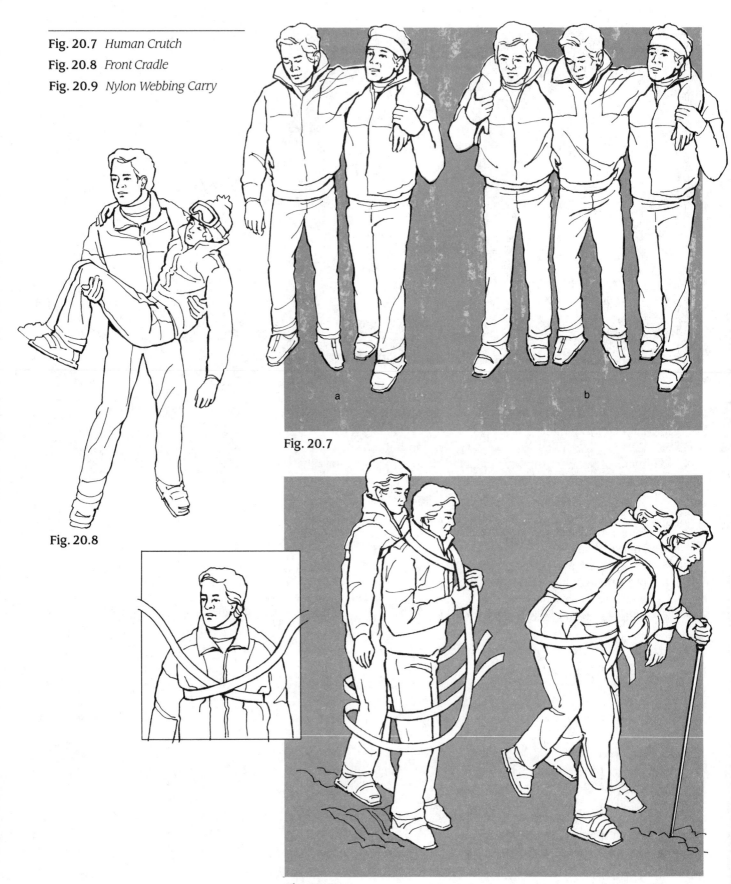

Fig. 20.7

Fig. 20.8

Fig. 20.9

from a long nylon sling (Fig. 20.9) or from a climbing rope (Fig. 20.10), as recommended by the National Outdoor Leadership School (NOLS).

To fashion a seat, double a climbing rope and wind it into two large coils by passing the doubled rope under your feet and over a hand held at waist level, leaving about 16 feet of rope at the two ends. The coils are secured by a large coil or knot in the middle. The coils are then separated and laid side by side on the ground.

The patient sits and inserts one foot in each coil; the coils are pulled up so that the patient is sitting on the knot. The rescuer squats, inserts an arm through each coil as if putting on a back-pack, and stands up, assisted by helpers if necessary. The loose ends are crossed over the patient's back and held by the rescuer to stabilize the patient. The patient is carried piggyback on the rescuer's back. An assistant walks on either side to steady the rescuer.

One-person back carries are tiring for the rescuer and uncomfortable for the patient and should not be used for long-distance carries. They are best suited for moving patients short distances over very rough terrain or for short vertical stretches when the patient and rescuer are both belayed.

2. **Emergency One-rescuer Moves—Possible Spine Injury**
   a. **Long Axis Drag**. Roll the patient into the supine position. This is difficult for a single rescuer because the patient must be rolled without twisting the neck or back. The patient can be pulled by the feet and dragged feet first (Fig. 20.11), or pulled by the clothing or by grabbing the patient under the armpits and dragged head first.

Fig. 20.10 *Rope Coil Seat*
Fig. 20.11 *Drag Without a Tarp*

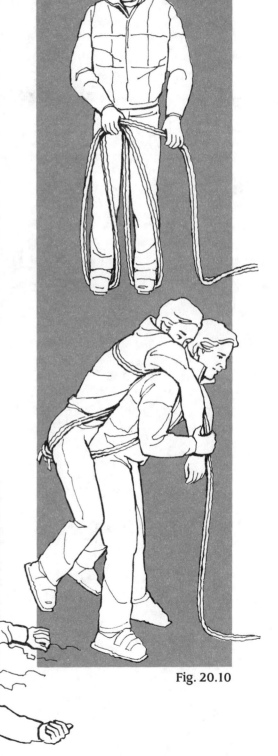

Fig. 20.10

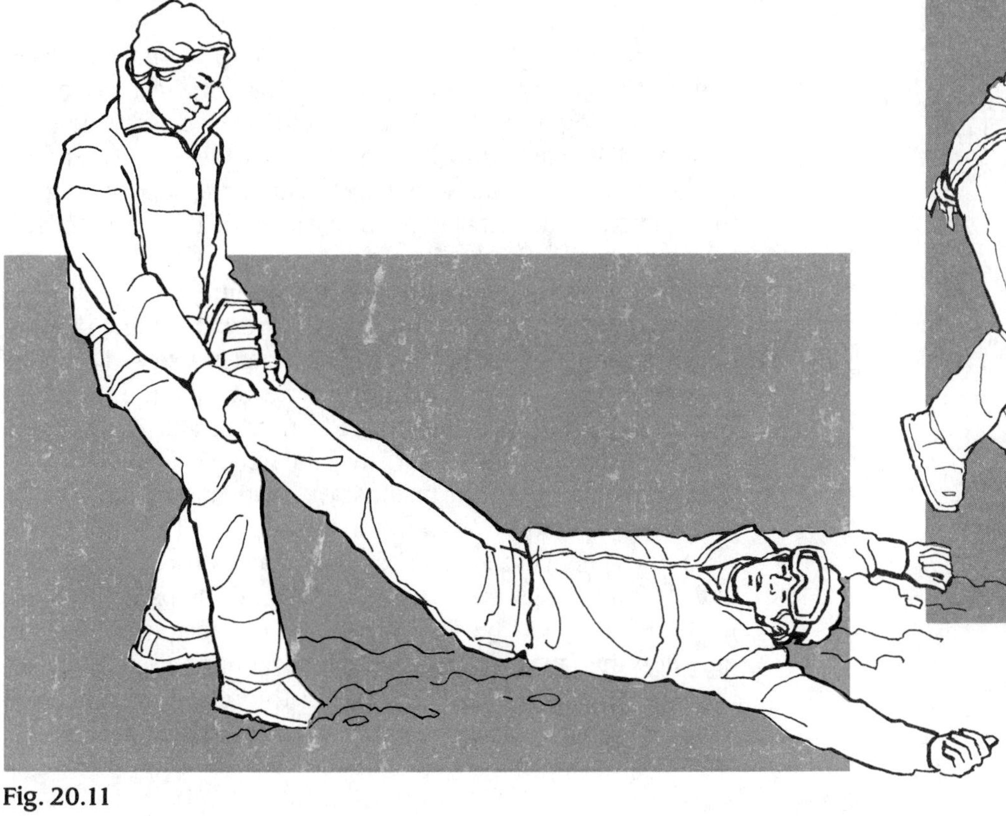

Fig. 20.11

Fig. 20.12 *Placement Procedure and Drag on a Tarp*

Fig. 20.13 *Seated Carry*

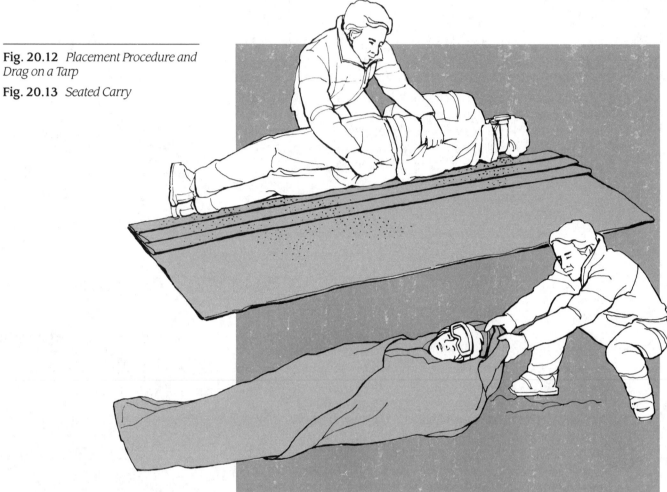

Fig. 20.12

It is preferable to pull the patient on a tarp or space blanket (Fig. 20.12). If a tarp is available, it can be placed under the patient by first pleating or tightly rolling it lengthwise, leaving one-third flat. Place the rolled side of the tarp alongside the patient and push it under the patient's body; pull the tarp from the opposite side so that it unrolls under the patient. If done properly, the tarp unrolls so that the patient ends up at its center.

3. **Emergency Two-rescuer Moves—No Spine Injury**
    a. **Seated Carries**. A patient who has no serious injuries and is conscious but unable to walk can be carried in a seated position by two rescuers with the patient's arms around the rescuers' shoulders (Fig. 20.13). Either a two-handed or four-handed seat (Fig. 20.14) can be used to carry the patient.
    b. **Fore-and-Aft Carry**. An unconscious patient with no serious injuries can be moved as shown in Figure 20.15. The first rescuer raises the patient to a sitting position, squats or kneels behind the patient, and wraps his or her arms around the patient's chest under the armpits. The second rescuer faces the patient, kneels between the patient's legs, and places a hand under each of the patient's knees. On command, the rescuers both rise. Before walking, the second rescuer should turn around facing the other way.

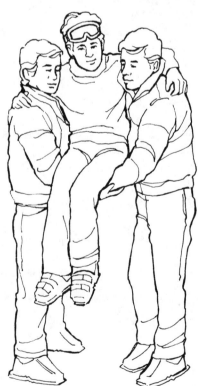

Fig. 20.13

4. **Nonemergency Moves--One or Two Rescuers**
   a. In nonemergency situations, patients with minor injuries may be carried as described above for emergency moves. In general, nonemergency moves are best deferred until more help arrives, especially if the patient has injuries that are more than trivial.

5. **Nonemergency Moves—Multiple Rescuers**
   a. **Direct Ground Lift and Carry – No Spine Injury**. This method requires at least three rescuers. The rescuers kneel at the patient's least-injured side. One rescuer is positioned at the patient's shoulder, one at the hip, and one at the knee (Fig. 20.16). A fourth rescuer, if available, kneels at the patient's opposite hip (Fig. 20.17). The rescuers kneel on the knee closer to the patient's feet. The first rescuer puts one arm under the patient's head, neck, and shoulders and the other arm under the patient's upper back; the second and fourth rescuers, kneeling at opposite sides, each put one arm under the patient's lower back and the other arm under the patient's thighs; the third rescuer puts one arm under the patient's knees and the other arm under the patient's ankles.

   On command, the rescuers simultaneously lift the patient to knee level (Fig. 20.18). At this point, one of the rescuers or an assistant can slide a litter or toboggan under the patient and, on command, the patient can be lowered into it (Fig. 20.19). If the rescuers must first carry the patient some distance, they simultaneously stand on command, roll the patient's body toward their chests, and walk in unison. The procedure is reversed to lower the patient to the ground or into a litter.

Fig. 20.14 *Hand Positions for Two-handed and Four-handed Seats*

Fig. 20.15 *Fore-and-aft Carry*

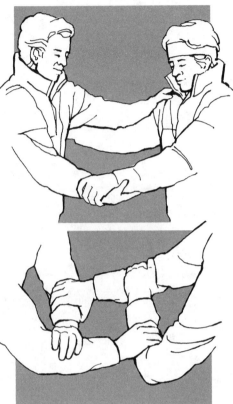

Fig. 20.14

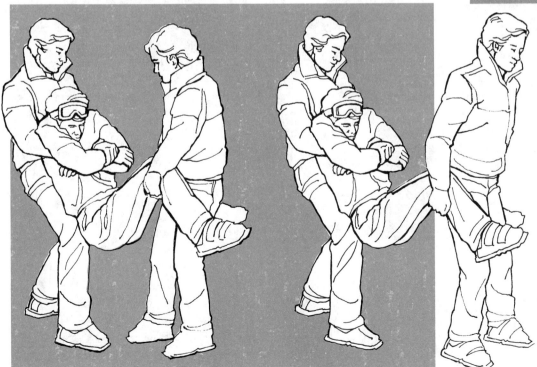

Fig. 20.15

Fig. 20.16 *Direct Ground Lift for a Patient with no Spine Injury*

Fig. 20.17 *Direct Ground Lift Using a Fourth Rescuer*

Fig. 20.18 *The first rescuer coordinates a simultaneous lift.*

Fig. 20.16

Fig. 20.17

Fig. 20.18

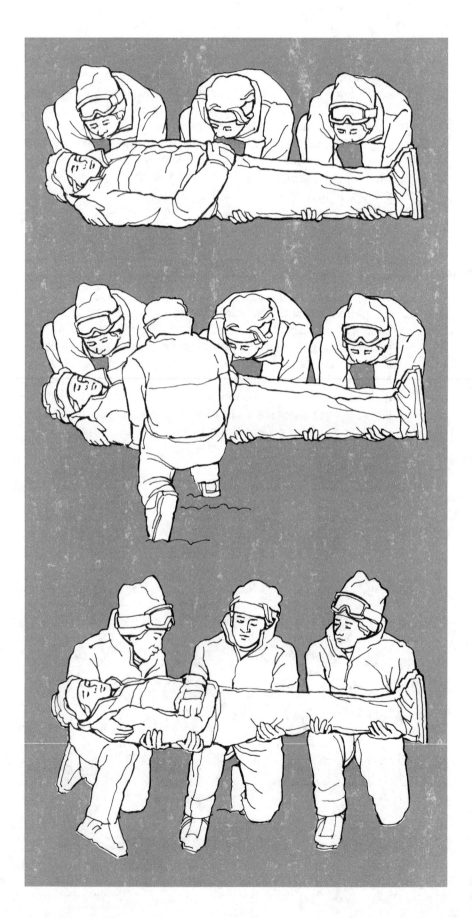

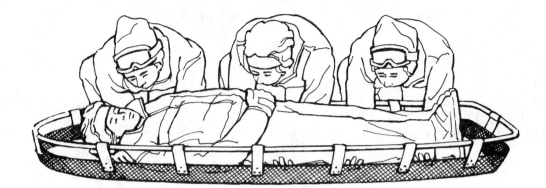

b. **Direct Ground Lift and Carry – Possible Spine Injury**. This method is similar to a. except that four rescuers are required. The additional rescuer is the leader, who maintains manual stabilization of the head and neck during the procedure and calls out the commands. The lift and carry are performed without bending or rotating the patient's neck or back (Fig. 20.20).

c. **Extremity Lift, Fractures Splinted—Two or More Rescuers**. This lift is frequently used by ski patrollers to move a patient with a splinted lower extremity from the first aid room to a nearby vehicle. It is more suitable for minor lower-extremity sprains and fractures than for major, painful injuries.

The patrollers help the patient stand and provide support from either side. The patient balances on the uninjured foot and puts one arm around each of the patrollers' necks. The patroller on the side of the injury supports the splinted extremity.

The patient, supported and partially carried by the patrollers, then hops to the waiting vehicle (Fig. 20.21). The patient should be oriented so that the splinted leg will be along the back of the seat. To load a patient into the back seat of a four-door vehicle, open both rear doors so a third patroller can enter the far door to help pull the patient onto the seat (Fig. 20.22). If a station wagon is available, the patient can be loaded into the rear compartment in a similar manner.

Fig. 20.19 *Technique of Lowering a Patient into a Litter*

Fig. 20.20 *Direct Ground Lift for a Patient with a Suspected Spine Injury*

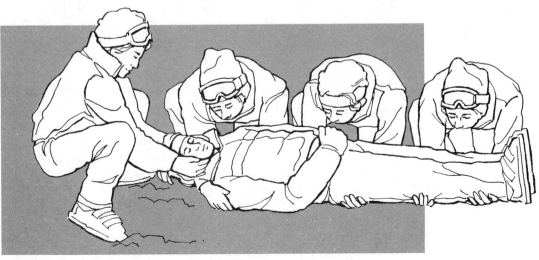

Fig. 20.20

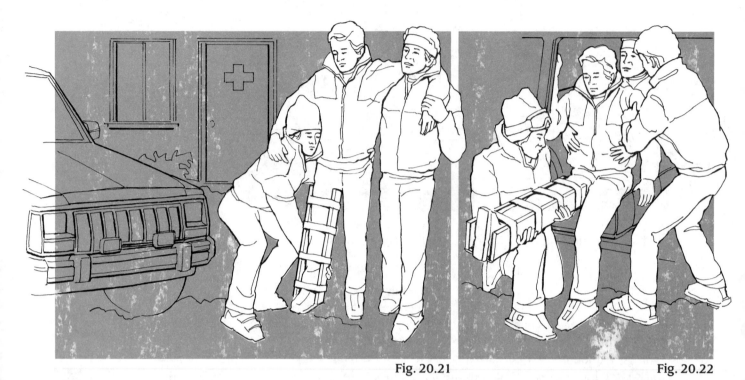

Fig. 20.21   Fig. 20.22

Fig. 20.21 *Technique of Assisting a Patient from the Patrol Room*

Fig. 20.22 *Technique of Positioning a Patient in a Vehicle*

d. **Stretcher to Bed Transfer or Vice Versa — No Spine Injury**. If the patient is lying on a sheet or blanket, it can be used to lift the patient from a stretcher on the floor to a bed. At least four rescuers are required.

The stretcher is laid next to the bed and two rescuers are positioned on either side (Fig. 20.23a). The sides of the sheet are rolled to provide a better grip. On a signal, the rescuers lean back slightly, lift the patient to the level of the bed (Fig. 20.23b), and transfer the patient to its edge. The two rescuers closest to the bed then move to the opposite side of the bed and pull the sheet toward them, moving the patient to the center of the bed (Fig. 20.23c).

This procedure is easier if an adjustable-height stretcher such as a gurney is used (Fig. 20.24). A three- or four-person direct ground lift technique also can be used.

e. **Canvas Stretcher or Blanket Lift and Carry — No Spine Injury**. Many ski patrols use a heavy canvas stretcher with eight handles to transfer a patient from a toboggan to a first aid room cot (Fig. 20.25). The stretcher is laid flat inside the sleeping bag or blanket roll in the toboggan pack, and the patient is placed directly on it when loaded into the toboggan. On arrival at the first aid room, the sleeping bag is opened and the stretcher and patient are lifted and carried to the cot by four patrollers.

A strong sheet or blanket can be used as a substitute for the stretcher. The sides of the sheet or blanket should be rolled tightly lengthwise to fit the contours of the patient's body. Two patrollers are stationed at each side. They should space their hands evenly along the sides of the blanket and grasp it tightly. On command, the patrollers lean back slightly, lift the patient to waist level (Fig. 20.26) and place the patient on the cot as described in d. above.

Fig. 20.23 *Using a Blanket Lift to Transfer a Patient from a Stretcher to a First Aid Cot*

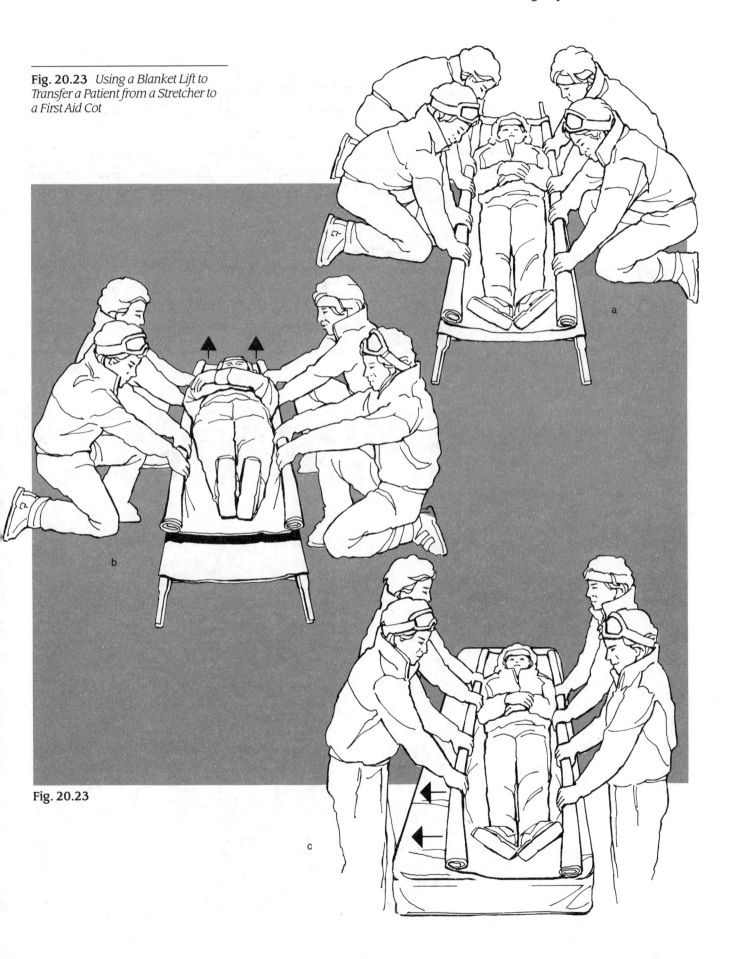

Fig. 20.23

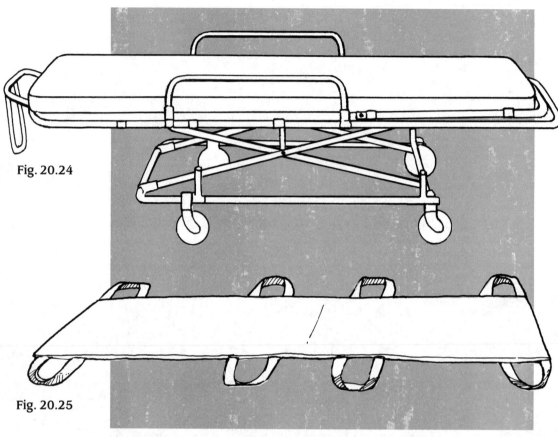

Fig. 20.24

Fig. 20.25

Fig. 20.26

Fig. 20.24 *Gurney Adjustable-height Wheeled Stretcher*

Fig. 20.25 *Canvas Stretcher*

Fig. 20.26 *Blanket Litter Carry*

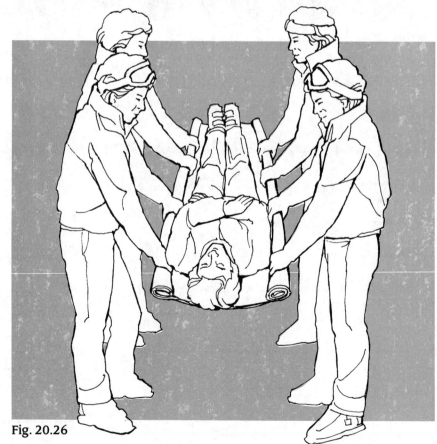

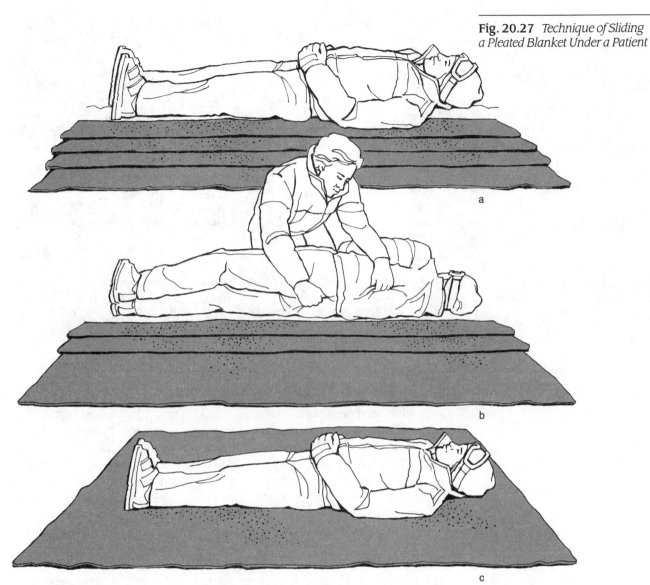

Fig. 20.27 *Technique of Sliding a Pleated Blanket Under a Patient*

a

b

c

To slide a blanket under a patient from the side, pleat it lengthwise for two-thirds of its width and place the pleated side alongside the patient (Fig. 20.27a). Logroll the patient about 45 degrees away from the blanket (for logrolling technique, see Chapter 14), push the pleated side of the blanket as far under the patient as possible (Fig. 20.27b), and roll the patient back onto the pleats and then 45 degrees to the opposite side. Next, pull the blanket under the patient (Fig. 20.27c) so that it is smooth. This should position the patient in the center of the blanket.

Fig. 20.27

LITTERS AND STRETCHERS

Litters and stretchers include toboggans, rigid and semirigid litters such as the Stokes, plastic basket litters, short and long spine boards, scoop stretchers, gurneys, soft stretchers, and improvised litters. Soft stretchers, except for the canvas type described above, are rarely used now because they do not

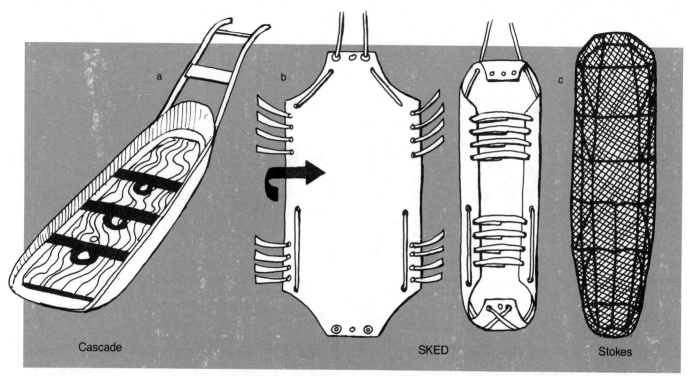

Fig. 20.28

Fig. 20.28 *Rigid and Semirigid Litters*
   a. Cascade
   b. SKED
   c. Stokes

Fig. 20.29 *Technique of Carrying a Litter with a Nylon Sling*

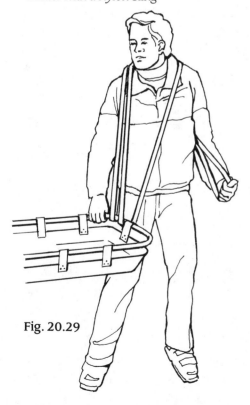

Fig. 20.29

protect an injured spine. Spine boards and scoop stretchers are discussed in Chapter 14, and toboggans in Chapter 21.

Rigid and semirigid litters (Fig. 20.28) are used by wilderness rescue groups for lowering, raising, and transporting patients. These include the familiar wire basket Stokes litter and heavy-duty plastic modifications such as the Thompson, Jakes, Cascade, and SKED litters. Some newer versions can be broken down for easier transport to the accident site. Rigid and semirigid litters can be used with a short backboard such as the Kendrick extrication device or Oregon spine splint for patients with neck and back injuries.

Most litters have handholds or nylon loops for lifting and carrying. Carrying a litter over a boulder field or along a rough trail is a tiring endeavor that requires many trained rescuers. At least two teams of six rescuers each should be available. The teams should be frequently rotated, and the rescuers should frequently switch from one side of the litter to the other.

The most comfortable way for rescuers to carry a litter is to shift the strain from their hands and arms to their shoulders using long nylon slings. One technique is to form a sling for each rescuer from 15-foot pieces of 1-inch tubular nylon tied into a loop with a water knot (double overhand knot). The rescuer brings the loop over the head so that it rests on the shoulder farthest from the litter. The loop is pulled across the rescuer's chest, inserted through a litter handhold, brought in front of and over the inside shoulder, then down across the back to the waist, where it is held by the outside hand (Fig. 20.29). This method distributes the weight of the litter fairly evenly across both shoulders.

Three rescuers are needed for each side of the litter; additional rescuers can precede the litter to clear away obstacles, warn the party of hazards, and set up belays, if necessary. The litter should be belayed down steep or very rough slopes. As a convenience, a detachable wheel can be mounted on the litter when traversing easier trails (Fig. 20.30).

Gurneys (Fig. 20.24) and similar adjustable, wheeled stretchers were developed for ambulance use. The height of these stretchers can be easily changed to the best position for patient transfer, transport, and ambulance loading–a useful feature for ski patrol first aid rooms. Adjustable stretchers can be elevated to bed level, making it easier to carry out assessment and provide emergency care. The patient's trunk and legs can be independently raised or lowered as needed.

Improvised stretchers and litters are uncomfortable and insufficiently rigid to be used for patients with spine and neck injuries. They should be used for short-distance moves only.

Fig. 20.30 *Stokes Litter with Detachable Wheel*

Fig. 20.31 *Technique of Using a Folded Blanket as a Stretcher*

Fig. 20.32 *Stretcher Made from Two Parkas*

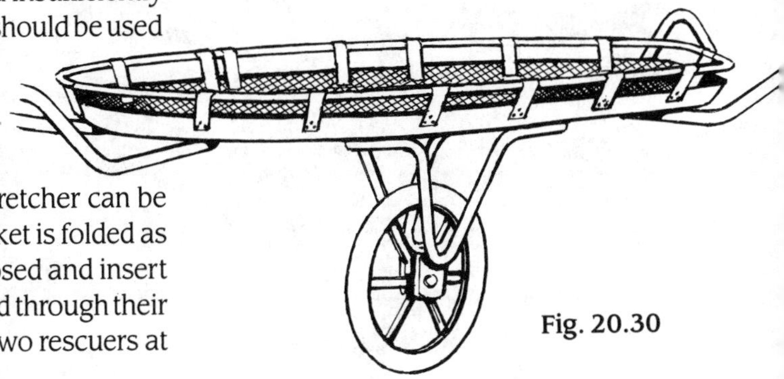

Improvised Stretchers and Litters

1. **Blanket and parka stretchers**. An emergency soft stretcher can be improvised from a blanket or several parkas. The blanket is folded as shown in Figure 20.31. If parkas are used, zip them closed and insert two long poles, one on either side, inside the parkas and through their arms (Fig. 20.32). The poles can be carried by one or two rescuers at each end and other rescuers at the sides.

   An easier method is to tie the ends of the poles to backpacks, preferably packs with external rather than internal frames. The packs are then worn by rescuers. The poles should be long enough so that the rear rescuer can see his or her feet while walking.

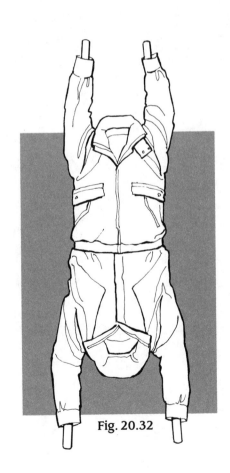

Fig. 20.30

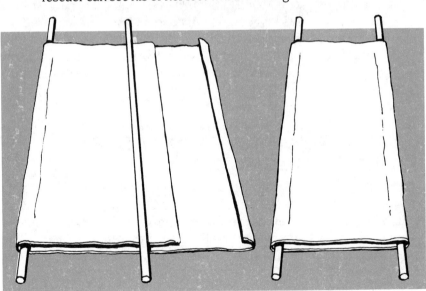

Fig. 20.31

2. Stretchers also can be made from **climbing ropes** or **pack frames**. The National Outdoor Leadership School makes a semirigid litter using three or four external pack frames, tied end to end in pairs, with the pairs tied together one on top of the other, overlapping by at least a foot (Fig. 20.33).

   A rope stretcher can be improvised from a 150-foot climbing rope. Uncoil the rope and locate the center. Then, lay 16 180-degree bends on the ground, eight on each side of the center of the rope (Fig. 20.34). The total distance between the first and last bend should be slightly

Fig. 20.32

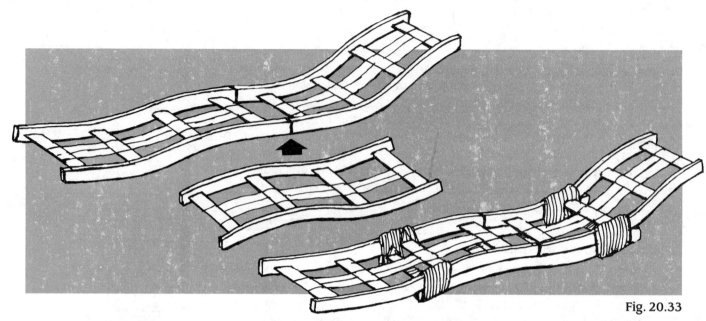

Fig. 20.33

Fig. 20.33 *Stretcher Made from Pack Frames*

longer than the patient's height, and the distance between bends slightly longer than the patient's width. Bring the two free rope ends around, one on each side of the stretcher. Tie a clove hitch in these ends at each bend, and insert the end of the bend about 2 inches into the hitch to form a loop.

After all bends have been inserted into a hitch, the remaining rope ends are threaded around through the loops until no rope is left. The clove hitches are snugged up, the ends are tied off, and an Ensolite pad or sleeping bag is laid on the stretcher. A rescuer should try out the stretcher to locate uncomfortable areas that should be padded before the patient is placed in the stretcher. Four to six rescuers can carry the stretcher, or it can be tied to poles as described above.

EXTRICATING A PATIENT FROM A DIFFICULT POSITION OR LOCATION

After locating the patient, the first rescuer assesses the scene for possible hazards to the patient and rescuers. When the patient is reached, the rescuer forms a first impression and performs the primary survey, identifying and giving care for life-threatening conditions such as respiratory or cardiac arrest, serious bleeding, or a sucking chest wound, as described in previous chapters of this textbook. These conditions are treated immediately. Less critical injuries then are identified, and any wounds or fractures are treated. If the patient is unconscious because of trauma, or if injuries to the neck or back are suspected, stabilize the patient's head and neck during these initial procedures and position a short backboard under the patient as soon as possible.

During examination and treatment, the patient must be protected against wind, cold, rain, snow, strong sun, excessive heat, rockfall, and other dangers. A hard hat, dark glasses, extra clothing, sleeping bag, and rescuers' backpacks may be needed.

These emergency procedures are carried out before the patient is moved, unless there is significant hazard to the patient or rescuers. While waiting to extricate and transport the patient, perform as much of the secondary survey as possible.

Meanwhile, other rescuers should prepare the extrication route. In the case of a skiing accident, the patient may be entangled in trees, dense brush, snowmaking equipment, a snow fence, or a crowd of other skiers. A skier may have slid into a gully or tree well. In other situations, patients may be found jammed between boulders, in a crevice, in a crevasse, on a ledge, in a narrow cave passage, or on rocks in midstream. It may be necessary to cut trees, move rocks, shovel snow, chip away ice, or set up lowering, raising, or traversing rope systems. Axes, saws, shovels, and special technical rescue equipment may be required.

The patient should be moved only after the route is ready and the patient is stabilized. The patient must be transported so that no further injury is caused and existing injuries are not aggravated. It usually is possible to safely transport the patient using a short backboard such as the KED or a narrow, semirigid litter such as the SKED, plus small fixation splints, compact traction splints such as the Sager, cravats, and swathes.

Occasionally, a litter or backboard cannot be brought to the patient. If the patient must be carried a short distance, it is preferable to use at least a three-person direct ground lift and carry. An alternative is to drag the patient in the direction of the long axis of the body as described above. Maintain the best possible stabilization of the head, neck, and back during these maneuvers.

When the patient is on stable ground, conduct the secondary survey to detect additional injuries and other problems. Perform the secondary survey so that the patient's body receives minimal exposure to inclement weather. Alpine ski patrollers usually delay undressing the patient until reaching the first aid room.

As soon as possible, and certainly after reaching stable ground, place the patient in a toboggan or litter. If evacuation will be prolonged, allow the patient to urinate or defecate, if necessary, before being packaged (see Appendix B).

Transport requires sufficient manpower and must be done with deliberate speed yet in a gentle and safe manner so that the patient is not jarred or jostled unnecessarily and injuries are not aggravated. It may be necessary to control onlookers and crowds.

During a wilderness evacuation, send runners ahead to alert the responsible authorities and the EMS system, or to maintain radio contact with the authorities. Arrangements should be made as far in advance as possible if a rendezvous with a helicopter or ambulance will be required.

Fig. 20.34 *Rope Stretcher*

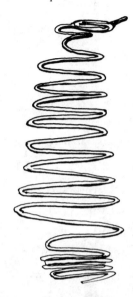

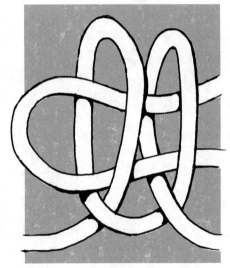

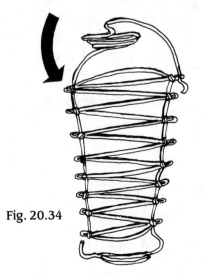

Fig. 20.34

21

Ski Injuries

There was blood upon his bindings,
There were brains upon his skis.
Intestines were a-hanging from the highest
of the trees.
We scraped him up from off the snow
And poured him from his boots.
Well, he ain't a-gonna race no more.

— *Traditional ski song*

A comparison between recent data and data collected 15 to 20 years ago reveals changes in the ski injury rate and the relative frequency of certain types of ski injuries. The overall alpine injury rate, which had been falling for 20 years, has remained static at about three accidents per 1,000 skier visits for the past several years. While ankle sprains and fractures are now less frequent, lower leg fractures are relatively more frequent, probably because ski boots are higher and stiffer. Leg fractures at the top of the boot (boot-top fractures) continue to be common, but the incidence of spiral fractures of the tibia and fibula has decreased. The decrease in these fractures apparently results from the reduction of friction between the ski and boot and from advances in lateral toe release technology.

Lacerations and contusions continue to occur at high rates, while the rate of upper body and head injuries shows a relative increase. Upper body injuries include rib fractures, shoulder sprains and separations of the acromioclavicular joint, shoulder dislocations, sprains of the hand and fingers, and fractures of the humerus, clavicle, and forearm. Skier's thumb is the most frequent upper body injury and probably the second most frequent ski injury.

Knee sprains remain the most common ski injury. Knee injuries present a challenge to equipment manufacturers to design a binding that will provide better knee protection, and a challenge to ski instructors to perfect techniques that prevent the types of falls that injure the knee.

An ominous development has been the increase in serious injuries to multiple body areas, including various combinations of injuries to the head, spine, chest, and abdomen that resemble the injuries seen in motor-vehicle accidents. This worrisome trend, noted both in Europe and North America, is probably a by-product of improvements in equipment, technique, and slope grooming, which have lead to higher speeds, harder falls, and more frequent collisions. As a consequence, ski areas now emphasize control of fast skiing and better hill design.

The equipment used in skiing and the characteristics of the motions involved in skiing produce injury patterns not seen in other sports. The ski boot is designed to hug the foot and is fixed tightly to the ski by the binding. This allows the boot to accurately reflect movements of the lower extremity and transmit them to the ski.

Modern alpine skiing technique is possible because the heel is held down rather than being free to lift. However, if the skier suddenly changes momentum or direction, the lever action of the ski magnifies the resulting forces that act on the extremity. Release bindings are designed to both free the boot from the ski before these forces exceed the body's threshold of injury and to withstand the smaller forces produced during normal skiing without releasing.

An ideal binding would allow both the heel and toe to release to either side and upward and the foot to release in a roll-out fashion to either side. No currently available binding is capable of releasing under all test conditions without injury to the lower extremity. The difficulty seems to be in designing a binding that will provide release in multiple directions without releasing prematurely. Intermediate and expert skiers tend to choose the convenience of step-in bindings that release laterally at the toe and upward at the heel, and

Fig. 21.1 *Two Basic Types of Ski Accidents*

prevent premature releases. Beginning skiers are advised to select a multi-directional release binding.

There probably always will be an irreducible rate of skiing accidents despite the most sophisticated advances in ski boot and binding technology, skiing technique, and ski hill design. Nonetheless, skiing is relatively safe when compared with other sports. Injury rates of three per 1,000 skier visits in downhill skiing and less than one per 1,000 in nordic skiing contrast favorably with injury rates of 810 per 1,000 in high school football, 30 per 1,000 in tennis, and 10 per 1,000 in swimming (figures courtesy of Dr. James Garrick). Also, only about one in 500 skiing falls produces a significant injury.

TYPES OF SKI ACCIDENTS

There are two basic types of ski accidents: **collisions** and **falls** (Fig. 21.1). Collisions occur in many different ways and can injure almost any part of the body. Falls can be divided into two general types: **rotational** (twisting) and **nonrotational** (nontwisting). The specific type and degree of injury produced by a fall depend on the type, magnitude, and direction of the resulting forces and whether these forces are concentrated on a body part in a manner that exceeds the threshold of injury. The type of equipment (i.e., high, low, stiff or soft boots, ski poles with straps) may be important, as well as the skier's physical condition, flexibility, weight, and bone structure. Another factor is whether the bindings release normally, prematurely, or not at all.

A **rotational fall** (Fig. 21.2) most commonly rotates the foot *outward* and forces the leg outward at the knee, e.g., when a skier catches an inside edge while falling forward or to the side. This fall can sprain the medial ligaments of the knee joint, sprain or fracture the ankle (usually the lateral malleolus), or fracture one or both bones of the leg. If the leg is fractured, the fracture line usually spirals around the shaft of the bone in contrast to the more horizontal fracture line produced by a nonrotational fall. A less common type of

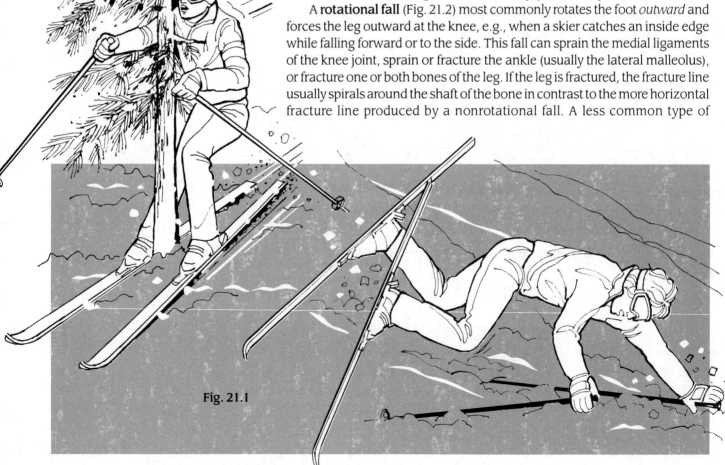

Fig. 21.1

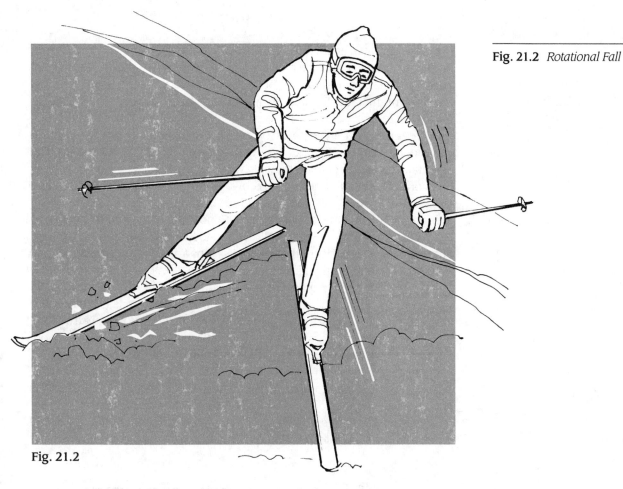

Fig. 21.2 *Rotational Fall*

Fig. 21.2

rotational fall rotates the foot *inward*, e.g., when beginning skiers cross the tips of their skis. This fall can cause fractures and sprains of the ankle, particularly of the medial structures; fractures (usually spiral) of the leg bones; and knee sprains.

A **nonrotational fall** typically occurs when a skier falls forward over the ski tips, which tends to bend the leg over the front edge of the boot. This can sprain the ankle or knee, rupture the Achilles tendon, or fracture the ankle or lower leg (boot-top fracture).

Landing on an outstretched hand may sprain the hand, wrist, or shoulder; dislocate the shoulder; or fracture the clavicle, arm, forearm, or hand.

A skier who wears high, stiff boots or who "sits back" may suffer a boot-top fracture during a backward fall. The lack of an upward toe release in most modern bindings contributes to this injury. The repeated impact of a stiff, poorly padded boot top against the outer leg can cause isolated fibular fractures. The anterior cruciate ligament may be injured more readily when high boots are worn.

Lacerations and contusions are caused by collisions or by blows from a ski or pole during a fall. A sharp pole tip can cause puncture wounds, and blows from the butt of a pole grip can cause serious eye injuries.

The shoulder, forearm, hand, or fingers can be fractured or dislocated if a pole basket is caught on a tree when the pole straps are around the skier's wrists (Fig. 21.3). Skiers who use breakaway pole grips or who do not use wrist straps can avoid this injury, but these precautions will not prevent a common ski injury, skier's thumb (also called gamekeeper's thumb), which

Fig. 21.3 *A skier can be injured if a pole basket catches on a tree.*

Fig. 21.4 *Skier's Thumb*

occurs when a skier tries to break a fall with an outstretched hand while holding onto a ski pole. The pole grip holds the thumb so that it is easily bent backward on impact, spraining or fracturing the medial structures of the first thumb joint (metacarpophalangeal joint, Fig. 21.4). The only way to prevent this injury entirely seems to be for skiers to discard their poles during a fall.

The late ski safety expert Gordon Lipe called attention to a common cause of medial knee ligament injury unrelated to binding malfunction. The skier falls forward between the skis while skiing in the stem or snowplow position. The ski and boot press sideways into the hill, preventing binding release, the knee hits the snow, and the skier's body rotates over the knee, tearing the ligament (Fig. 21.5). It may be possible to prevent this injury by teaching beginning skiers to fall to the side rather than falling forward between their skis. Devices that prevent ski tips from crossing also are useful.

The tibia and fibula, like other bones, are viscoelastic structures that behave like a viscous liquid under some stresses and like an elastic solid under others. A slow twisting force of 60 to 70 foot pounds is sufficient to cause a spiral fracture of a man's tibia. However, if the force is applied quickly, it must be considerably greater before the tibia will break. This phenomenon, combined with the lesser likelihood that bindings will release in a slow fall, explains the relatively high rate of fractures incurred by beginning skiers during slow twisting falls compared to the lower rate of fractures from hard falls suffered by experts who "load" the tibia at a much more rapid rate.

Other studies have shown that the amount of comminution produced when a bone is fractured is related to the magnitude of the forces involved.

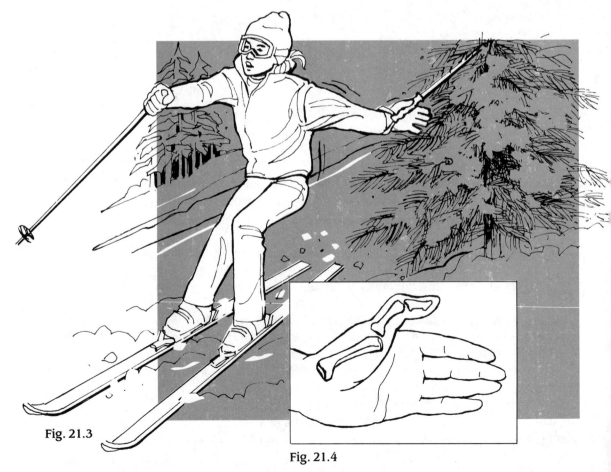

Fig. 21.3

Fig. 21.4

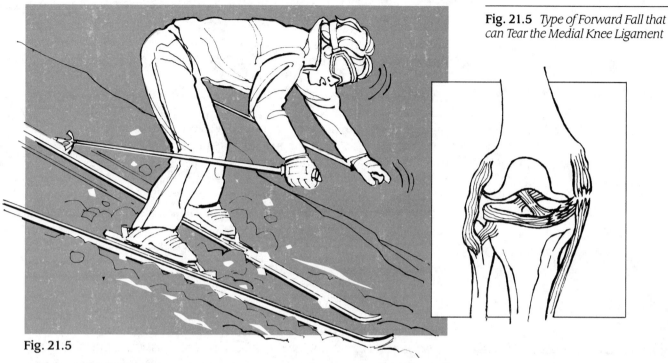

Fig. 21.5 *Type of Forward Fall that can Tear the Medial Knee Ligament*

Fig. 21.5

A high-speed fall that generates heavy forces that have to be dissipated by the lower leg will cause more comminution of the fractured bone and more injury to the soft tissues than a fall involving lesser forces.

LIKELIHOOD OF INJURY

Currently, more than 55 million skier visits are recorded in the U.S. each year. There are approximately 160,000 ski injuries in the U.S. each year, many of which are trivial. Deaths and serious injuries are rare; combined, they occur at an annual rate of one for each million skier visits.

For data on ski injuries to be meaningful, their sources must be specified. It is necessary to know whether the injuries occurred at a single ski area or at several areas, during a single year or over several years, and if snow conditions were typical or unusual. Injury rates at a small, weekend ski area with a single T-bar lift may differ from injury rates at a large, destination ski resort or at a resort that serves a large, metropolitan area.

In addition, because only 25 to 50 percent of injuries are reported to the ski patrol, it is important to state the distance from the ski area to the nearest large town or medical center and indicate whether data come from the ski patrol, a local medical clinic, or both. It also is important to indicate whether the services of the patrol are free – as in the U.S., Canada, Japan, New Zealand, and Australia–or whether a fee is charged, as in most of Europe.

Any comparison of injury rates in different classes of skiers must take certain variables into account. For example, fractures and other serious injuries are more likely to be reported than trivial injuries. Also, beginning skiers, children, ski school students, women, and older people are more likely to report their injuries than are younger people, expert skiers, and men.

Nevertheless, certain general statements can be made. *Ability* and *experience* are probably the most important factors in determining a skier's

Fig. 21.6 *Binding Release Check*

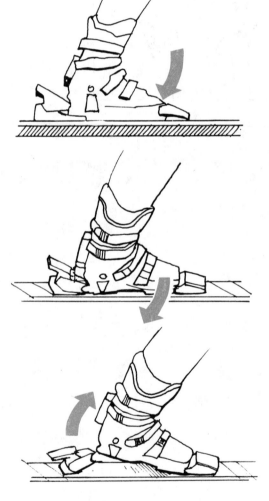

Fig. 21.6

likelihood of injury. The decline in the overall injury rate over the last 20 years probably has resulted because of increased numbers of older and experienced skiers on the hill, better teaching methods, better slope grooming, shorter skis, better bindings, better rental equipment, and the use of ski brakes and antifriction devices.

Beginning skiers, women, and children have proportionally more injuries than experienced skiers, men, and adults. The higher incidence of injuries during the late afternoon is largely because more skiers are on the hill at that time, although fatigue, poor lighting, and deteriorating snow conditions undoubtedly play a role. Skiing in large groups or when the slopes are crowded also seems to increase the injury rate, which is lowest on weekdays. In alpine ski racing, almost half of the injuries occur on the last third of the course, a statistic that reflects the importance of fatigue as a contributor to ski injuries.

The various types of nordic skiing continue to be much safer than alpine skiing. Although the informal nature of nordic skiing makes data collection difficult, injury rates are estimated to be less than one per 1,000 skier visits.

In nordic skiers, upper-extremity injuries occur more often than lower-extremity injuries; most injuries result from falls while going downhill. Although thumb, knee, and ankle sprains are the most common injuries, lower leg and femur fractures, shoulder dislocations, and serious head and trunk injuries may occur. In track skiing, devices that restrain lateral motion of the heel on the ski (e.g., heel wedges and heel locators), increase the lower-extremity injury rate.

In backcountry and telemark skiing, the use of higher boots and more rigid bindings results in a higher proportion of lower-extremity injuries than the use of three-pin bindings and low nordic boots. Skiing in convertible mountaineering bindings with the heels locked down would be expected to produce lower-extremity injury rates approaching those of alpine skiing. If a releasable three-pin binding were developed, it would be expected to further reduce the low nordic injury rates. Nordic skiers with previous experience in alpine skiing have a lower injury rate than those without it.

BINDING CARE

Modern alpine bindings are safer than the old cable bindings, but the perfect binding has yet to be developed. Such a binding would have to be inexpensive, simple to install, and easy to adjust and maintain. It would have to release during a fall but not during a hard turn, release equally well during all types of falls, and be unaffected by dirt, snow, ice, or corrosion.

To improve skiing and increase safety, skiers should take good care of their bindings.

Techniques of Binding Care

1. Skiers should understand the mechanics of their bindings and keep them properly maintained, lubricated, and adjusted. Keep bindings clean and free of snow and ice, and regularly spray them with a silicone lubricant.

2. Regularly test toe releases for proper setting using the following method (Fig. 21.6):
   a. Buckle the boots tightly.
   b. Put a ski on a flat surface (snow, a rug, etc.) and place one boot in its binding.
   c. Bend the knee, put the ski on its inside edge or against a wooden block, and twist the binding inward at the toe. Release should occur without excessive pressure. Repeat the test with the ski on its outside edge, twisting outward at the toe.
   d. Take off the ski, place the other boot in its binding, and repeat step c.
3. Test the heel release as follows:
   a. Buckle the boots tightly.
   b. Put a ski on a flat surface (snow, a rug, etc.) and place one boot in its binding.
   c. Push the knee toward the tip of the ski. Do not have anyone stand on the rear of the ski because a hard lunge may injure the Achilles tendon if the heel does not release. It is useful to hold onto a set of railings during this maneuver. The heel piece should release without undue pressure.
4. Use an antifriction device.
5. If necessary, obtain cants, which improve skiing ability because the skier will edge better and catch fewer edges. Many modern boots have built-in canting adjustments.
6. Cover bindings to protect them from dirt and corrosion, especially when carrying skis on top of a car.
7. Use ski brakes instead of safety straps to decrease the likelihood of being hit by a windmilling ski during a fall. Powder skiers should use powder cords to avoid lost skis, and all skiers who use ski brakes should be careful not to accidentally release a binding while riding on lifts.

OTHER SKI EQUIPMENT

Goggles should be unbreakable, ventilated to avoid fogging, and equipped with light-sensitive or interchangeable yellow and dark lenses. The dark lenses should filter all but 2 to 15 percent of the sun's ultraviolet rays.

Ski pole length should be determined by the height and experience of the skier. To avoid eye injuries, the top of the pole grip should be at least 25 square centimeters in surface area (12 square centimeters for children). If pole straps are used, they should be a breakaway design; the pole tip should be hollow and round to provide a good grip on ice. Wear hard hats during giant slalom and downhill races, and when "timber-bashing."

APPROACH TO THE INJURED SKIER

Unless there are specific local instructions to the contrary, the first patroller on the scene of injury is considered to be in charge. The patroller places his or her crossed skis upright in the snow several yards above the accident to cau-

Fig. 21.7 *Approaching an Injured Skier*

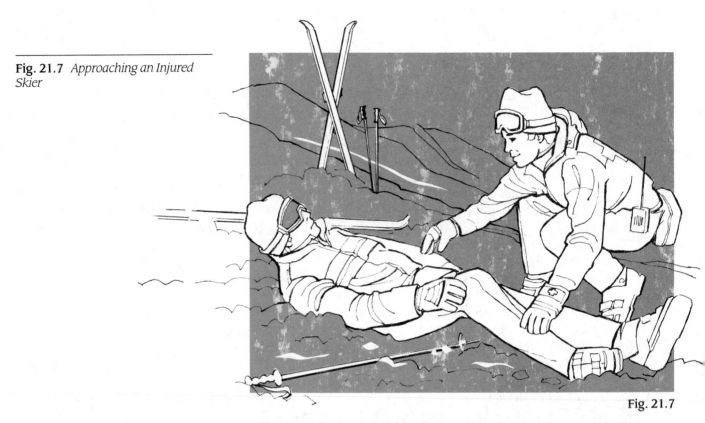

Fig. 21.7

tion other skiers and to help toboggan handlers find the accident (Fig. 21.7). Examine the patient as described in Chapter 4, and place warm clothing over and under the patient.

If it will be necessary to call for a toboggan, first determine the need for special equipment such as a backboard or traction splint. If a radio is unavailable, send a responsible skier to the nearest phone or lift shack to notify the ski patrol. Make sure that the messenger can accurately describe the patient's location. In confusing areas, use map coordinates. If the patient is critically injured, radio ahead so that an ambulance or helicopter can be summoned.

The toboggan generally is brought to the patient from the side and is parked securely in a safe location below the patient. It should be close enough to aid loading yet not so close that it interferes with emergency care. Anchor the toboggan with skis or a rope belay. On very steep hills, it may be easier to load the patient onto a toboggan parked above rather than below. Before parking the toboggan, turn it so that its head end is nearer the part of the patient's body that will be downhill during transport.

Positioning the Patient in the Toboggan

The general rule is to position the *injury uphill* to keep the patient's weight from jamming the injured extremity against the end of the toboggan. However, no rule is absolute, and the patient's comfort should be the final determinant.

Positioning Guidelines

1. *Head downhill* for patients with shock, hypothermia, lower-extremity injuries, and abdominal injuries (unless they are short of breath).

2. *Head uphill* for patients with injuries to the head, face, neck, chest and upper extremity, as well as for patients who are short of breath, unconscious, or are suspected of having a heart attack, and perhaps when the terrain is very steep.
3. *On the injured side*, for a one-sided chest injury.
4. *Semiprone* or NATO position for patients with any condition that produces nausea and vomiting and for unconscious patients who have not suffered trauma.

Some cases may present conflicting requirements (see Chapter 14).

After splinting and providing other emergency care, lift the patient into the toboggan (Fig. 21.8) being careful not to aggravate injuries (see Chapter 20). Wrap the patient in a blanket or sleeping bag covered with a tarp or other snowproof and windproof cover, and strap the patient in securely. Toboggan straps should not put pressure on the site of injury. A jacket or fanny pack can be used as a pillow, if indicated. Take the toboggan down the hill to the first aid room by the safest, smoothest, and shortest route. Avoid jostling and bumping. Strap the patient's skis and poles to the side of the toboggan opposite the injury with their tips pointing toward the patient's feet. Or, have a patroller carry the equipment. Never leave a loaded toboggan unattended.

Fig. 21.8 *Preparing a Patient for Downhill Transportation from a Ski Slope*

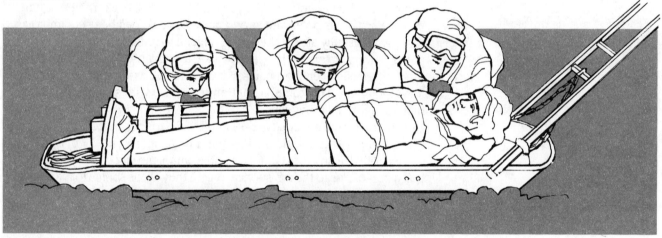

Fig. 21.8

OVERSNOW RESCUE TECHNIQUES FOR NORDIC PATROLLERS AND SKI MOUNTAINEERS

Cross-country skiers and ski mountaineers can become sick or injured in difficult terrain or terrain that is far from roads and trails. Members of nordic patrols and other winter rescue groups should be familiar with the techniques of backcountry oversnow rescue and toboggan handling taught by appropriate units of the National Ski Patrol.

If the site is accessible by snowmobile or helicopter, the best practice often is to stabilize the patient and send for such help. Otherwise, the patient will have to be moved by a toboggan, which can be brought to the site or built from available materials.

A toboggan loaded with a heavy patient can be very difficult to pull uphill or handle in deep snow with insufficient manpower. Toboggans should be belayed on steep terrain and dangerous sidehills.

Ready-made Backcountry Toboggans

Ready-made toboggans are available from many different manufacturers and come in various sizes. Backcountry toboggans, which are lighter than those used by alpine ski patrols, usually have two long front handles and are pulled by a single skier by means of a waist belt; some models have rear handles as well.

Some toboggans have detachable shoulder straps and are light enough to be carried on one's back. Otherwise, the toboggan will have to be pulled to the scene. When transporting a patient, one or more ropes should be attached to the front of the toboggan when going uphill or through difficult snow so that additional skiers can help pull; another skier should guide the toboggan from the rear, using the rear handles or a tail rope. A disadvantage of most practical backcountry toboggans is that they are too small to satisfactorily transport a patient with a back or neck injury.

Improvised Backcountry Toboggans

Improvised toboggans are made from one or more pairs of skis held together by a frame that forms a platform to which the patient can be strapped. Skis can be attached to commercially available frames; pack frames or natural materials such as poles and strong branches also can be used. Improvised toboggans usually are weaker, more difficult to handle, and more difficult to pull over long distances than ready-made toboggans. However, they do save time, especially over short hauls, if it would otherwise be necessary to send for a toboggan. The commercial frames for use with skis are much lighter than ready-made toboggans.

There are two general types of improvised toboggans. One type is made of a long, narrow, flat piece of aluminum flashing or heavy plastic that is carried rolled up in the pack. To assemble, unroll the piece so that it is flat, and bolt a pair of skis to the top surface, where they act as splints to maintain the shape of the toboggan (Fig. 21.9a). A second type is made of one or two pairs of skis held side by side with a frame that fastens to the top surface of the skis (Fig. 21.9b).

Improvised toboggans are handled like ready-made toboggans. Front and back handles can be improvised from ski poles; ropes should be attached so that extra rescuers can help pull the toboggan uphill or help slow it on downhill stretches.

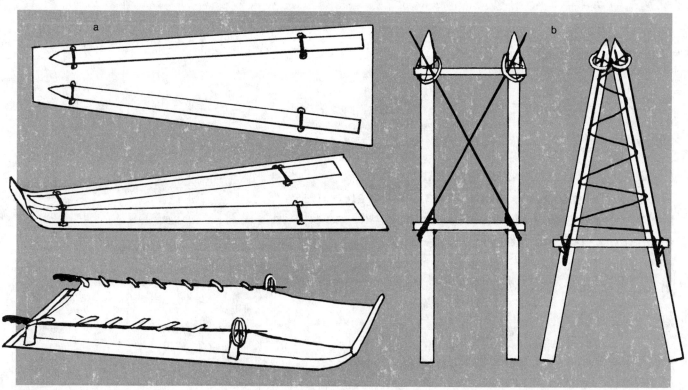

Fig. 21.9

Fig. 21.9 *Improvised Backcountry Toboggans*

22

Triage

Good fortune will elevate even petty minds,
and give them the appearance of a certain greatness
and stateliness, as from their high place they look down
upon the world; but the truly noble and resolved spirit
raises itself, and becomes more conspicuous
in times of disaster and ill fortune.

> −*Plutarch*
> *Eumenes*

The French word **triage** means to choose or sort out. In emergency care, triage refers to the technique of handling a disaster with so many patients that the capabilities of the rescuers are initially overwhelmed and the resources of the community are stretched to the limit or exceeded. This type of disaster is called a **mass-casualty incident** (MCI). When limited resources do not allow everything possible to be done for *every* patient, rescuers must be guided by the principle of *doing the greatest good for the greatest number*. In a patient with multiple injuries, triage also can refer to the proper order in which to treat each injury.

Triage in the outdoors follows the same principles as triage under urban conditions, except that terrain, weather, equipment, manpower, communication, and distance from definitive medical care often make decisions more difficult and may require modifications of standard triage protocols.

In any mass-casualty incident, there are three general categories of patients:

1. Those who will live no matter what is done.
2. Those who will die no matter what is done.
3. Those for whom what is done will make a difference.

In triage, the rescuer identifies and concentrates time and effort on patients in the third category, remembering always that *life takes precedence over limb*.

The most experienced and best-trained rescuer should be in charge of triage. Priorities for both care and transportation to a hospital must be set for each patient, remembering that, in isolated areas, emergency care can be given, but early transportation may be impossible.

By international convention, four color-coded categories of priority have been established.

Triage Categories

1. **Red**, the category for immediate or highest priority, includes patients with the following signs and symptoms:
   a. Hypoxia or shock is either present or imminent.
   b. Survival is highly probable with immediate care and rapid transportation to a hospital.
   c. The patient can be stabilized without constant attention.
   Note that patients with severe injuries of the head and chest do *not* meet these criteria.
   Red priority patients include those with an obstructed upper airway, a sucking chest wound, a flail chest, tension pneumothorax, major external or internal hemorrhage, burns covering more than 20 percent of the body surface, and pericardial tamponade.
2. **Yellow** is the category for second or delayed priority. These patients are considered urgent but not as urgent as red priority patients based on injury type or less rapid progression of the injury. They are able to wait longer than red priority patients before being transported. This priority includes:
   a. Those who are seriously injured but not yet hypoxic or in shock and who appear able to wait without serious risk for 45 minutes or longer before being transported to a hospital.

b. Those who have a poorer chance of survival.

Stabilize yellow priority patients, give necessary care, and transport them after the red priority patients have been transported. Examples of yellow priority patients include those with burns covering less than 20 percent of the body area, back injuries, multiple fractures, pelvic or femur fractures, stable abdominal injuries, eye injuries, and severe head or chest injuries.

3. **Green** is the category for patients whose injuries have third priority. These patients have minor injuries that do not present a risk to life or that can be stabilized after a minimum of emergency care; they may be ambulatory and are regarded as able to wait several hours before being transported to a hospital. Examples of green priority patients include those with localized soft tissue injuries or minor fractures.

4. **Black** is the category for patients who are dead, who die during emergency care, or who have lethal injuries and no chance of survival even in a hospital. Examples of black priority patients are those who have suffered cardiac arrest, decapitation, or a severing injury of the trunk.

Table 22.1

TRIAGE CATEGORIES

Priority	Handling	Color Code	Description	Examples
1	Immediate	Red	1. Hypoxia or shock present or pending. 2. Survival likely with rapid care and transport. 3. Care is not time-consuming.	Upper airway obstruction. Major hemorrhage. Sucking chest wound, flail chest. Tension pneumothorax. Open abdominal wound. Shock. Heart attack. Cardiac tamponade. Severe burn (more than 20 percent).
2	Delayed	Yellow	1. Serious injuries without hypoxia or shock. 2. Able to wait more than 45 minutes before transport.	Burns less than 20 percent. Back or spinal cord injuries. Multiple or major fractures. Stable abdominal injuries. Eye injuries. Severe head or chest injuries.
3	Hold	Green	1. Injuries not a risk to life. 2. May be ambulatory. 3. Minimum of emergency care needed. 4. Able to wait several hours before transport.	Minor fractures and wounds. Burns less than 10 percent. Psychological problems.
4	Dead	Black	1. Vital signs absent or soon to be absent.	Cardiac arrest. Decapitation or other lethal injuries. Obvious death.

TRIAGE TECHNIQUE

In triage, the task is to sort a large number of patients as rapidly and accurately as possible, concentrating first on identifying and caring for patients with critical *yet correctable* conditions, and then on setting priorities for transportation. Priorities may change both as the condition of patients changes and as more help arrives, so that more attention can be given to those with less chance of survival.

Standard techniques of first impression, primary survey, and secondary survey are too time-consuming for triage and must be replaced by techniques that are rapid, effective, easily taught, and easily remembered. An excellent technique is the START (Simple Triage and Rapid Treatment) plan, developed at Hoag Memorial Hospital Presbyterian, Newport Beach, California. This simple plan, designed to be used by the first rescuer or rescuers responding to a mass-casualty incident, allows the rescuers to rapidly identify salvageable, high risk patients and to provide basic salvaging maneuvers. It includes four steps:

1. Identification of the "walking wounded."
2. Assessment and basic care of ventilation.
3. Assessment and basic care of circulation.
4. Assessment of mental status.

Immediately upon reaching the MCI site and determining the presence of any danger to rescuers, the first rescuer indicates a large tree or other easily identifiable site and shouts: "All of you who can walk, move over there."

This step immediately sorts out most of the green priority patients – the walking wounded – and allows concentration on the remainder.

Beginning with the *nearest* patient, the rescuer carries out a rapid survival scan of each patient, spending only a minute or two with each. After being examined and given any necessary salvaging maneuvers (described below), each patient should be tagged with the appropriate triage identification tag (Fig. 22.1). If triage tags are unavailable, write the initial of the appropriate color (R, Y, G, or B) on a piece of tape and attach it to the patient's forehead.

The survival scan begins with a rapid observation of the patient's breathing. The patient is then classified as not breathing, breathing normally, or breathing more than 30 times per minute.

While evaluating breathing, the rescuer should check the airway. If necessary, clear the airway of foreign bodies and open the airway with the head-tilt/chin-lift or jaw-thrust maneuver. In these circumstances, the usual cautions about guarding the cervical spine may have to be ignored. Patients who are not breathing are immediately classified as dead or nonsalvageable (black). Patients who are breathing normally are not classified at this step. Patients who are breathing more than 30 times per minute are classified as red priority.

Because there is insufficient time to count respirations, rescuers should learn to detect a respiratory rate over 30 per minute by observing others simulate this rate until they can detect tachypnea at a glance. If there is doubt, the patient is assigned red priority.

Patients with slow respirations also may be at risk, but they usually can be classified more precisely after their mental function is assessed. The rescuer cannot remain with the patient to maintain the airway; time may permit

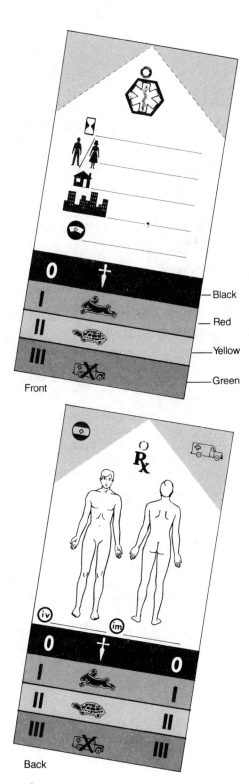

Fig. 22.1 *Triage Identification Tag (front and back)*

— Black
— Red
— Yellow
— Green

Front

Back

Fig. 22.1

only simple techniques such as positioning the patient or inserting an oral airway before moving on to the next step or the next patient. If necessary, recruit one of the walking wounded (green priority patients) to maintain the airway. Patients with airway problems are always classified as red priority.

The next step for patients who are breathing normally is to assess their circulation by performing the capillary refill test on the nailbed of an uninjured extremity. The lip also can be used. If the capillary refill time is more than two seconds (say "capillary refill," or "one thousand one, one thousand two"), the patient's circulation is inadequate, and the patient should be tagged red priority. If lighting is poor, checking the radial pulse can be used as a substitute for the capillary refill test. If the pulse is palpable, it is considered normal; if it is not palpable, the patient is classified as red priority. When capillary refill or pulses indicate inadequate circulation, rapidly check the patient for bleeding, and elevate the patient's legs 12 inches. If external bleeding is found, have the patient or one of the walking wounded apply direct pressure (Fig. 22.2).

Table 22.2

ALGORITHM

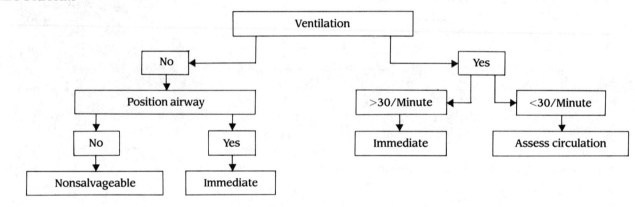

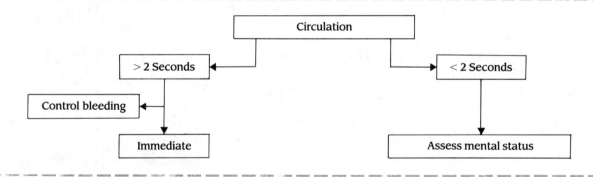

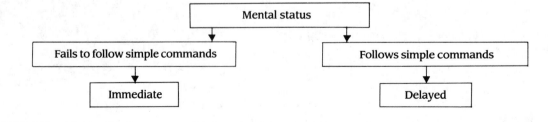

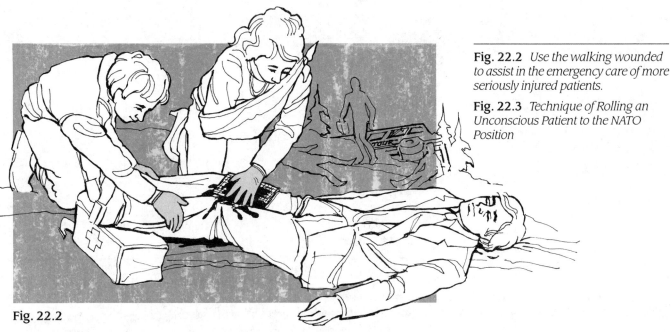

Fig. 22.2 *Use the walking wounded to assist in the emergency care of more seriously injured patients.*

Fig. 22.3 *Technique of Rolling an Unconscious Patient to the NATO Position*

Fig. 22.2

For patients with normal breathing and circulation, the next step is to assess their mental function. By this time, the rescuer has had a chance to see whether these patients can follow simple commands. If in doubt, ask the patient to open or close his or her eyes or to squeeze your hand. Patients who are *unable* to follow the command are classified as red priority; those who are *able*, are triaged as yellow priority. Unconscious patients are rolled into the semiprone (NATO) position to keep the airway open (Fig. 22.3).

After an initial evaluation of all patients is completed, and as additional rescuers arrive, patients assigned to the red group can be transported. Patients designated yellow and those in the red group who are awaiting transportation can be monitored and given more extensive assessment and care. Patients whose condition has deteriorated are moved to a higher priority category.

Another triage device, the CRAMS scale (Table 22.3), is useful in assigning patients to one of two clearly divided groups, one with a score of 6 or less and a high mortality rate (62 percent), and the other with a score of 7 or more with a low mortality rate (0.15 percent).

In some cases, factors other than the type of injury may influence the category to which a patient is assigned. An injured rescuer or relative of a rescuer is automatically assigned to the red category regardless of the severity of injuries. This is done to minimize distraction and maintain rescuer morale. An injured child, hysterical patient, or patient with a hysterical relative also should be assigned a higher priority than the injury might otherwise warrant.

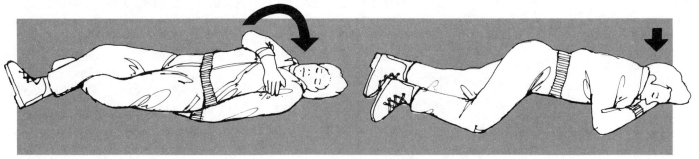

Fig. 22.3

Table 22.3

CRAMS SCALE

(**C**irculation, **R**espiratory, **A**bdomen, **M**otor, **S**peech)

Category	Score
Circulation:	
Normal capillary refill, blood pressure above 100 systolic.	2
Delayed capillary refill, blood pressure 85-99 systolic.	1
No capillary refill, blood pressure below 85 systolic.	0
Respiration:	
Normal.	2
Abnormal (labored, shallow, or rate above 35/minute).	1
Absent.	0
Abdomen:	
Abdomen and thorax not tender.	2
Abdomen and thorax tender.	1
Abdomen rigid, thorax flail, or deep, penetrating injury to either the chest or abdomen.	0
Motor:	
Normal (obeys commands).	2
Responds only to pain, no posturing (extension or flexion).	1
Postures or gives no response.	0
Speech:	
Normal (oriented).	2
Confused or inappropriate.	1
No speech or makes unintelligible sounds.	0

Significance of CRAMS Scale: A score of 6 or less indicates a critically ill person (62 percent overall mortality rate even in a hospital, and an expected mortality rate close to 100 percent if the patient does not reach a hospital within two hours). A score of 0 means the patient is essentially dead or will be dead within a few minutes. A score of 7 or above is favorable, with an overall hospital mortality rate of 0.15 percent.*

*Clemmer, et. al., *Journal of Trauma*, 25:188, 1985.

One of a rescuer's more difficult jobs is dealing with the emotions of seriously injured patients and of their friends and relatives, who may not understand why a certain patient is being "neglected" by being placed in a lower category.

EXAMPLE OF TRIAGE IN ACTION (Fig. 22.4)

Imagine that you are a professional ski patroller at XYZ, a large ski area served by a gondola as well as multiple chairlifts. Your station is at the top of the gondola. You hear over the radio that there has been a derailment; eight gondola cars have fallen to the ground. You arrive at the first gondola car, point to a spot, and say, "All of you who can walk, move over here." Three of the eight patients are able to do so. Your survival scan reveals the following:

    1. A middle-aged woman who is screaming hysterically. She has a large lump on her forehead and a fractured wrist. Her respirations and cap-

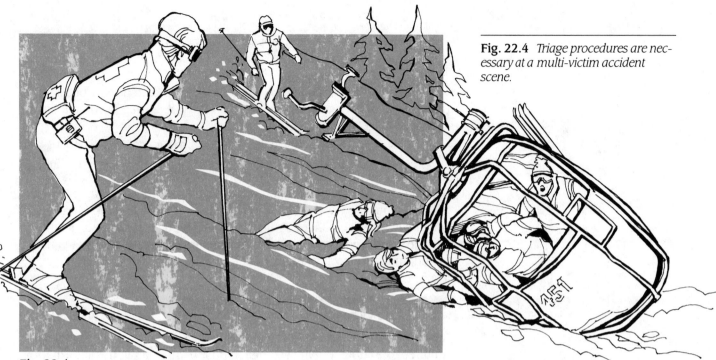

Fig. 22.4 *Triage procedures are necessary at a multi-victim accident scene.*

Fig. 22.4

illary refill are normal; she tells you that she hurt her head and wrist when the gondola fell.

2. A middle-aged man who is lying in the gondola wreckage, unconscious, breathing normally, groaning, and spontaneously moving all four extremities. His capillary refill time is one second.

3. An elderly man with an obvious crushed chest. He has no detectable pulse and is not breathing.

4. A young woman who is lying quietly. Her skin is pale, cold and clammy, her pulse is fast, her respirations are rapid and shallow, and her capillary refill time is delayed. She complains weakly of abdominal pain.

5. An obnoxious, middle-aged man who is yelling, cursing, and threatening to sue the ski area. He does not appear to be hurt.

6. A young man who is lying quietly on his side, complaining of pain in the back between the shoulder blades. He says that he cannot move his legs. His breathing and capillary refill time appear to be normal.

7. An elderly woman who appears basically healthy and vigorous for her age. She is in respiratory distress and is complaining of chest pain. A brief inspection of the site of pain discloses a flail segment of chest wall.

8. A middle-aged woman who seems calm and does not appear to be injured.

How should these patients be classified, and what do you do?

Analysis

Patients number 4 and 7 are assigned red priority because of impending shock and hypoxia, respectively. Patients 2 and 6 are assigned yellow priority because, although seriously injured, they appear to be stable. Patient 3 is classified black priority and patients 1 and 8 are assigned green priority.

If patient 8, who is calm, appears to be sensible, she may be drafted to talk to and try to quiet patient 1; if this is unsuccessful, patient 1 should be moved to yellow priority.

Patient 5, who would otherwise be assigned green priority because he appears uninjured, should be bumped up to the red category for immediate transport to get him out of everyone's hair.

As the rescuer, you perform basic salvage maneuvers on patients 4 and 7. These actions include a rapid search for external bleeding and elevating the legs 12 inches for patient 4, and stabilizing the flail chest for patient 7. If no other patrollers have arrived yet, you will need to move on to the next patient; if necessary, one of the green priority patients can be recruited to manually stabilize patient 7's flail chest. If adequate help has arrived, you should spend your time caring for and preparing transportation for patients 4 and 7 and monitoring patients 2 and 6.

TRIAGE OF A PATIENT WITH MULTIPLE INJURIES

By now, the student has learned about basic life support and managing injuries to various organ systems, and is ready to draw this information together to provide the proper sequencing of emergency care for a patient with multiple injuries.

It goes without saying that all such patients should be taken to a hospital as soon as possible. If transportation is available, the rescuer should not spend unnecessary time stabilizing the patient in the field.

It is important to remember the concept of the "golden hour," which refers to the average amount of time that elapses before a patient with multiple injuries starts to deteriorate rapidly. For every half hour following this first hour, the patient's chances of survival are cut in half. To increase the patient's chances of survival, the rescuer must be knowledgeable, experienced, and able to establish priorities and work quickly and efficiently. There will be no time to go back and reread the emergency care manuals; important things must be done right the first time. The rescuer should be aware of the dramatic appearance of a seriously injured person and of the normal tendency to feel panic and inadequacy when faced with several simultaneous, life-threatening problems in one or several individuals.

Rescuers also should remember that their job is to buy time for the patient until a hospital is reached or an ambulance or helicopter arrives. Advanced life support attendants have extensive training and sophisticated life-support equipment, and deal with serious injuries every day. They should be summoned as soon as it is apparent that a serious injury has occurred.

Emergency personnel have recognized the need for developing a method of taking fast action and making rapid decisions based on limited data in an emergency situation. This type of response is stereotyped but is applicable to any emergency situation and should be practiced and thought about *beforehand* so that, in an emergency, it can be called forth automatically.

Many of the procedures listed below should be done simultaneously if enough rescuers are present. As in caring for any patient, the steps represented by the acronym ABCDE (Table 22.4) apply, with ABC being the most

Table 22.4

ABCDE

Airway and cervical spine.
Breathing.
Circulation, bleeding, shock.
Disability.
Expose.

important. Remember that extremity fractures are dramatic injuries that may overshadow more serious and important injuries such as major head, chest and abdominal injuries. Musculoskeletal injuries generally are not life-threatening, so their management is *not* part of ABC.

The first consideration is the **airway**, which is opened by the jaw-thrust maneuver, since every seriously injured patient is considered to have a cervical spine injury. Remove obstructing material such as snow, vomitus, and blood using the finger sweep method or suction. Stabilize the head and neck while other procedures are carried out and, if there is time at this point, apply a rigid extrication collar. Perform the Heimlich maneuver if the jaw-thrust maneuver does not open the airway after obvious foreign matter has been removed. If the patient is unconscious, put an oral airway in place.

If the airway cannot be maintained with the above techniques, particularly if there is an injury to the neck or face, advanced airway maintenance such as an endotracheal tube will probably be required. If no one at the scene is trained in this technique, the patient probably will die unless taken immediately to a doctor or hospital.

After the airway has been established, check the patient's **breathing**. If there is respiratory distress, examine the chest to detect major causes such as a sucking chest wound or flail segment, which can be treated in the field, or tension pneumothorax, which can only be treated by someone adequately trained in the proper procedures. Give oxygen in high concentration, if available.

If the patient is not breathing, give artificial ventilation. If oxygen is available, use a pocket mask or bag-mask so that oxygen can be added.

The next consideration is **circulation**, which also includes controlling **bleeding**, and treating **shock**. Stop bleeding by applying direct pressure. Although cardiac arrest secondary to trauma is almost always fatal, even in a well-equipped hospital, give CPR to a patient without a pulse or heartbeat. A physician or paramedic treats shock with intravenous fluids or a PASG; a rescuer without these special skills and equipment has very little to offer in the field other than controlling external bleeding and elevating the legs.

By following the ABCs, the rescuer will have dealt with the conditions that pose an immediate threat to life.

The next consideration is **disability**, which refers to the search for injury to the central nervous system by determining the patient's level of consciousness and assessing the patient for paralysis, weakness, or loss of sensation in the extremities. The AVPU and Glasgow Coma scales (see Chapter 4) are useful in this part of the assessment.

Finally, the patient should be **exposed**, which refers to removing enough clothing from the chest, abdomen, and extremities so that all injuries to these areas are discovered. Except for exposure needed to detect and treat external bleeding, this part of the ABCDEs usually should be delayed until the patient reaches shelter so that his or her body temperature will remain stabilized. At an alpine ski area, exposure usually takes place in the first aid room.

It is almost always preferable to immobilize the multiple-trauma patient on a long spine board rather than treat fractures and other extremity injuries separately. This is the best care for spine and spinal cord injuries and is effective for any fractures or other injuries that may be present; it also cuts the time needed to stabilize patients before transport.

23

Poisoning

Poison is in everything, and no thing is without poison.
The dosage makes it either a poison or a remedy.
   —*Paracelsus*

Poisons (Fig. 23.1) are substances that damage the functioning of the body through chemical action that interferes with normal metabolic processes. Poisons can be substances not normally taken internally or legitimate drugs taken in excessive doses. They also can be compounds that are produced naturally by the body but for some reason are not detoxified or excreted, e.g., in patients with chronic kidney failure, the normal byproducts of metabolism accumulate in toxic amounts.

Many poisonous materials are present in nature, such as the elements arsenic and selenium in soil, poisonous mushrooms, and poisonous higher plants such as water hemlock and baneberry. Certain types of seafood, such as California mussels, are safe to eat at some times of the year and poisonous at others, usually because they eat toxin-containing microorganisms and concentrate these toxins in their tissues. Other poisonous creatures introduce toxic materials into the body through stings, bites, and poisonous appendages such as spines.

Poisonous substances can enter the body through ingestion, inhalation, injection, or absorption through the skin or mucous membranes.

This chapter discusses poisoning in general and urban poisoning in particular. Chapter 24 discusses hazardous animals and plants.

Each year in the United States, more than a million poisonings occur, causing 3,000 deaths. Few specific antidotes for poisons exist and those few are available only in a hospital. Therefore, emergency care for poisoning consists of removing or diluting the poison, treating its signs and symptoms (such as convulsions, vomiting, and unconsciousness), and taking the patient to a hospital as soon as possible. In the hospital, poisoning is treated by preventing the absorption of the poison, curtailing its conversion to an active form, enhancing its excretion or conversion to an inactive form, and/ or counteracting its clinical effects.

In urban areas, most poisonings occur in the home from the ingestion of drugs or household chemicals, either accidentally by children or with suicidal intent by older persons.

It is important to keep all drugs, household cleansers, weed killers, pesticides, and other chemicals safely out of the reach of toddlers. All prescription medicines should be in child-proof containers. Empty soft drink bottles and food containers should not be used to store household cleansers and other chemicals because someone who thinks the original contents are still in the container may accidentally ingest the harmful substance.

If a victim of poisoning is to receive proper emergency care, the rescuer must first suspect poisoning and then identify the poison.

Fig. 23.1 *Be careful with poisonous substances.*

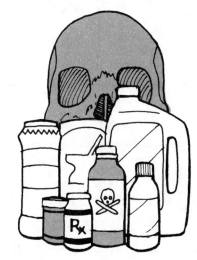

Fig. 23.1

Common Signs and Symptoms of Poisoning

1. Inappropriate behavior or disturbances of consciousness.
2. Suspicious materials, such as bottles, vials, pills, spilled liquids, chemicals, syringes, needles, and the remains of food and drink.
3. Unusual odors associated with the patient.
4. Convulsions.
5. Gastrointestinal symptoms such as abdominal pain, nausea, vomiting, and diarrhea.
6. Excessive salivation or sweating.

Fig. 23.2 *Vomiting can be induced with a spoon handle.*

7. Abnormal respirations.
8. Dilation or constriction of pupils.
9. Redness, blistering, or burns on the skin, especially around the mouth.

It is important to identify the poison once poisoning is suspected or confirmed, even though there are general measures that are useful for any type of poison. Conscious patients can be questioned. The contents of most prescription drugs are labeled, and the contents of many chemicals are listed on their labels. Any spilled tablets, liquids, suspicious plants, partially consumed food or drink, or vomitus should be collected and sent to the hospital along with the patient. Immediately summon an ambulance and contact the nearest poison control center by dialing the local emergency number (often 911) or calling the nearest hospital emergency department. Poison control centers are staffed 24 hours a day. The staff can recommend immediate emergency care measures that can be carried out while awaiting the ambulance. They will need to know the age, size and weight of the patient, and a description of the drug or poison. Containers of prescription medicines list the name, strength, and number of dose units (tablets, ounces of liquid) on the label. The labels of many chemical containers list ingredients as well as recommendations for immediate emergency care.

Unless a poison control center issues specific instructions to the contrary, initial emergency care in general consists of efforts to *remove* or *dilute* the poison by such measures as washing it from the skin, inducing vomiting, or having the patient drink bland liquids such as water or milk.

Emergency Care for Specific Poisons

(If possible, a poison control center should be called for specific directions.)
A. Ingested poisons include drugs, alcoholic beverages, household chemicals, contaminated food and drink, and parts of plants. The general principles are to remove the poison by inducing vomiting or to dilute the poison with milk or water. Vomiting should *not* be induced in the case of:
   • Strong acids or alkalis, since they are corrosive and vomiting may increase damage.
   • Petroleum products, since vomiting may cause serious chemical pneumonia if some of the material is accidentally inhaled into the lungs.
   • A patient who is unconscious or having convulsions, since vomiting is likely to produce inhalation of vomitus into the lungs.
1. If the patient is awake and alert, the first step is to have him or her drink milk or water to dilute the poison. The amount ranges from one glass up to several glasses, depending on the patient's size. Next, induce vomiting by gagging the patient with a tongue blade or spoon handle (Fig. 23.2) or by having the patient drink a cupful of soapy water or a glass of water with a teaspoonful of dried mustard stirred into it. When the patient vomits, guard the upper airway by turning the patient to the side and using suction as necessary.
2. Activated charcoal can be used to absorb any remaining poison *after* the patient has vomited. It usually is given only at the direction of a poison control center. Stir one or two tablespoons of activated charcoal into a glass of water for the patient to drink.

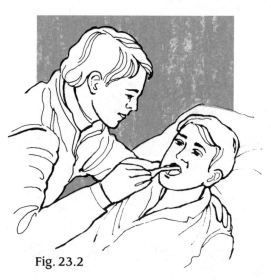

Fig. 23.2

3. Because a poisoned patient's consciousness frequently is impaired, give general care for unconsciousness as needed (see Chapter 13).

B. Inhaled poisons include smoke, industrial gases such as chlorine and hydrogen sulfide, and natural gases such as carbon dioxide and methane, which may accumulate in harmful amounts in wells and caves. One of the most common inhaled poisons is carbon monoxide (see Chapter 18). Inhaled poisons cause damage by directly irritating the lung, by replacing oxygen in the air, or by acting as general body poisons. Emergency care consists of the following:

1. Remove the patient from the contaminated atmosphere (Fig. 23.3). Frequently, there is considerable danger to the rescuer, and all necessary precautions must be taken, including the use of lifelines and gas masks.

Fig. 23.3 *The fireman's drag can be used to move a patient.*

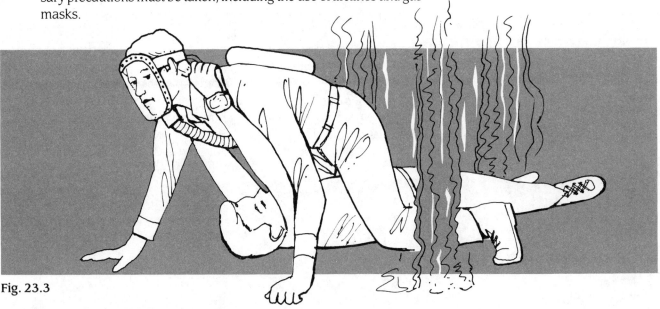

Fig. 23.3

2. Give oxygen in high concentration.
3. Give basic life support, as needed (see Chapter 5).
4. Provide care for unconsciousness, as indicated (see Chapter 13).

C. Injected poisons include a variety of drugs that are deliberately injected, as well as stings and bites of flying insects (bees, wasps, and hornets) and arachnids (spiders, scorpions, mites, ticks), snakebites, and puncture wounds from the spines of marine animals. General principles of emergency care include the following:

1. Remove all watches, rings, and bracelets from an involved extremity before swelling occurs.
2. Wrap an involved extremity with a rubberized bandage, starting as high proximally as possible and extending distally to the tips of the digits. The bandage should be firm but not so tight that it restricts arterial or venous circulation. (Bandaging does not help in cases of snakebite.)
3. Place a cold pack on the injection site to slow absorption, except in cases of snakebite.
4. Injected poisons are rapidly absorbed, which makes them difficult to remove by suction. However, the poison may be removed by using the recently developed Sawyer extractor within 15 minutes after the poison is injected (three minutes for snakebites). The extractor, a

small, powerful suction pump, is currently available from Recreational Equipment, Inc., P.O. Box C-88125, Seattle, WA 98188-0125.

5. Give general care for unconsciousness and convulsions (see Chapter 13), and shock (see Chapter 7), as required.

6. Give basic life support, as necessary (see Chapter 5).

D. Contact poisons include chemical substances such as acids and alkalis, and natural substances such as the sap of poison ivy, poison oak, and poison sumac. General principles of emergency care include:

1. Remove the substance from the skin. If the material is dry, first dust it off, then flush the area with water. Other materials are rinsed off with water; the area then is washed with soap and water.

2. Do *not* rinse off lye, dry lime, elemental sodium, and other materials that react with water; instead dust off the material or remove it with kerosene or mineral oil.

3. Elemental phosphorus catches fire when exposed to air. It should be washed off while the affected body part is immersed in water. An alternative is to coat the affected part with a 1-percent copper sulfate solution and remove the particles with forceps.

4. Remove contaminated clothing as soon as possible.

5. If the eyes are involved, follow the guidelines in Chapter 13.

6. Cover open wounds with sterile, dry dressings.

24

Poisonous Plants and Animals

Beware the Jabberwock, my son!
The jaws that bite, the claws that catch!
Beware the Jubjub bird, and shun
The frumious Bandersnatch.

—*Lewis Carroll (Charles Lutwidge Dodgson)*
"Jabberwocky"

Fig. 24.1 *Dieffenbachia*

POISONING BY PLANTS

Several thousand cases of plant poisoning occur every year in the United States. Because many domestic and wild plants are poisonous, outdoor travelers should be thoroughly familiar with the poisonous plants native to the area and should not taste or eat unfamiliar plant materials. If plant poisoning is suspected, bring the plant or its leaves to the hospital with the patient.

Unless the patient is unconscious or having convulsions, the initial emergency care for all cases of toxic plant ingestion consists of diluting the poison and inducing vomiting as described in the section on ingested poisons in Chapter 23.

Common Reactions and Their Emergency Care

1. **Circulatory collapse**. If typical signs and symptoms of shock are seen, treat them as described in Chapter 7.
2. **Gastrointestinal disturbances**. Little can be done to treat symptoms such as nausea, vomiting, diarrhea, and cramps. If evacuation will be delayed, prevent dehydration by having the patient drink plenty of water and electrolyte-containing fluids. Save any vomitus and take it to the hospital with the patient.
3. **Central nervous system symptoms**. Emergency care depends on the major manifestations, which range from convulsions, excitement and hyperactivity at one extreme to depression, mental confusion, stupor, and coma at the other. As needed, give basic life support (see Chapter 5), give general care for unconscious (see Chapter 13), and manage convulsions (see Chapter 18).
4. **Skin irritation**. Symptoms can include itching, redness, burning, swelling, blister formation, and rash. As soon as possible, wash the area with soap and water to remove the offending substance. A soothing nonprescription lotion such as Calamine may be applied later, if desired.
5. **Swollen mucous membranes**. The common houseplant *dieffen-bachia*, or dumb cane (Fig. 24.1), can cause a unique problem. If the plant is placed in the mouth, it causes the mucous membranes to swell, which makes swallowing and talking difficult and obstructs the upper airway. Emergency care includes keeping the upper airway open and administering oxygen, if available.

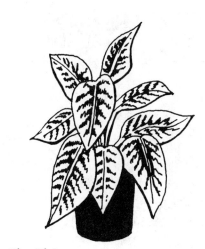

Fig. 24.1

STINGS AND BITES OF ARTHROPODS

The phylum Arthropoda contains many members that are annoying or dangerous to man. Such arthropods include members of the following classes:

1. Class Insecta
   a. Order Hymenoptera (bees, wasps, hornets, yellow jackets, ants)
   b. Order Diptera (mosquitoes, biting flies)
   c. Order Lepidoptera (caterpillars)
   d. Order Homoptera (blister beetles)
   e. Order Hemiptera (true bugs)
2. Class Arachnida (spiders, scorpions, ticks, mites)
3. Class Chilopoda (centipedes)

Fig. 24.2 *Examples of Stinging Insects*

Fig. 24.3 *Technique of Removing A Honeybee Stinger*

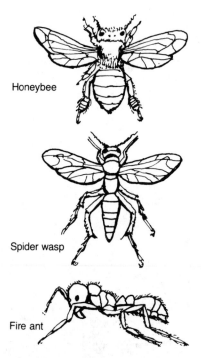

Honeybee

Spider wasp

Fire ant

Fig. 24.2

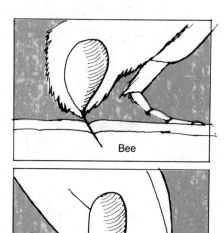

Bee

Knife

Fig. 24.3

Dangerous Insects

Insects are the most numerous of the higher orders of creatures. The stinging apparatus of most stinging insects (Fig. 24.2) is a small, hollow spine that resembles a hypodermic needle. The stinger projects from the end of the abdomen and is attached to a venom sack. The honeybee's stinger is barbed and cannot be withdrawn after it is embedded. The honeybee can sting only once because it is disemboweled when it flies away after stinging. Wasps and other hymenoptera can sting repeatedly. Some hymenoptera, such as the fire ant, both sting and bite.

Local symptoms of an insect sting or bite include sudden pain at the site followed by swelling and redness. A white, itchy swelling resembling a hive may occur. The stinger of a honeybee frequently remains embedded in the wound; it should be removed by gentle scraping with a knife blade so that the venom sac does not squeeze more venom into the wound (Fig. 24.3). Additional emergency care is listed in the section on injected poisons in Chapter 23. If available, apply a small amount of unseasoned meat tenderizer (Adolph's, etc.) to the wound. Some people are allergic to the venom and may develop anaphylactic shock (see Chapter 7).

Contact with stinging insects in the outdoors can be minimized by storing garbage away from living areas, by eating food inside tents and other shelters, and by not wearing brightly colored clothing and perfumed cosmetics. Give a wide berth to hives and nests. When confronted by insects, remain calm and avoid activities that anger insects such as making loud noises and "shooing" motions. If pursued by swarms of stinging insects, seek refuge in tents or vehicles or jump into a body of water.

Although mosquitos, black flies and other biting flies (Fig. 24.4) can carry serious diseases such as malaria, yellow fever, and sleeping sickness, these insects generally are more of a nuisance than a menace. Their bites, unless multiple, usually do not require treatment. Soothing, nonprescription lotions (Calamine, etc.) can be used for local symptomatic relief. Bites can be prevented by using chemical insect repellents and by wearing protective tightly woven clothing with long sleeves, long trouser legs, and tight cuffs. Tents or other sleeping quarters should be protected by suitable netting.

Certain caterpillars, such as the gypsy moth caterpillar and the puss caterpillar, have irritating hairs that can cause an uncomfortable rash (Fig. 24.5). Emergency care consists of removing the hairs with adhesive tape and applying a soothing lotion.

Blister beetles (Fig. 24.6) contain cantharidin, a substance that is very irritating to human skin. Emergency care consists of washing the area with soap and water and applying a soothing lotion.

Some members of the order Hemiptera (Fig. 24.7) can inflict a painful bite that is treated like a bee sting (see above).

Dangerous Arachnids

There are only two dangerous spiders in North America: the black widow and the brown recluse.

Only the female black widow spider is poisonous. This shiny black spider spans about an inch with its legs extended and has a characteristic, red hourglass marking on the underside of the abdomen (Fig. 24.8a). It spins a nondescript scraggly web and prefers to live in garages, basements, out-buildings, and woodpiles. One or more brown egg cases often are visible in the web. The spider is shy and bites only if disturbed. Black widow spiders occasionally spin webs under the seats of outhouses and may bite the nether parts of unsuspecting users if webs are disturbed by falling excrement.

A black widow bite is seldom painful and may be overlooked at first. The toxin produces severe muscle spasms, chest tightness, respiratory distress, dizziness, nausea, vomiting, and burning of the soles of the feet. The abdominal muscles may develop boardlike rigidity that can mimic an acute abdomen. Most patients recover with symptomatic care, but the toxin can be quite dangerous to small children. Emergency care is described under the section on injected poisons in Chapter 23. Suctioning to remove the poison is effective only when done immediately following the bite.

The brown recluse spider is found mostly in the Southern United States, although it occasionally is carried to other areas in the personal belongings of travelers. This dull brown spider has a smaller body than the black widow, with a characteristic violin-shaped marking on its cephalothorax (Fig. 24.8b). It inhabits dark, sheltered areas such as basements, vacant buildings, and woodpiles. The bite causes a large, slowly developing ulcer that enlarges over several weeks and heals very slowly. There is no effective emergency treatment for a brown recluse spider bite. One frequently used medical treatment is to excise the site of the bite as soon as possible. Heat should *not* be applied.

Scorpions (Fig. 24.9) are found primarily in the Southwest. They have a long, jointed, tail-like abdominal projection with a stinger on the tip. The stings of most scorpions are no worse than a bee or wasp sting, causing only localized pain, redness, and swelling. However, one scorpion found in the Southwest, the Arizona scorpion (*Centruroides exilicauda*), has a venom that causes a severe systemic reaction with shock, muscle spasms, convulsions, and heart failure. It is a slender, nocturnal, yellowish brown scorpion with a small swelling at the base of the stinger.

The emergency care for a scorpion sting is the same as for any injected poison. If a sting by the Arizona scorpion is suspected, the patient should be taken to a hospital as soon as possible. It may be necessary to provide basic life support and general care for unconsciousness and convulsions (see Chapters 5 and 13).

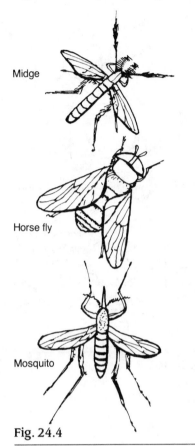

Fig. 24.4 *Examples of Biting Insects*

Midge

Horse fly

Mosquito

Fig. 24.4

Fig. 24.5 *Saddleback Caterpillar*
Fig. 24.6 *Blister Beetle*
Fig. 24.7 *Blood-sucking Bug*
Fig. 24.8 *Poisonous Spiders*
Fig. 24.9 *Scorpion*

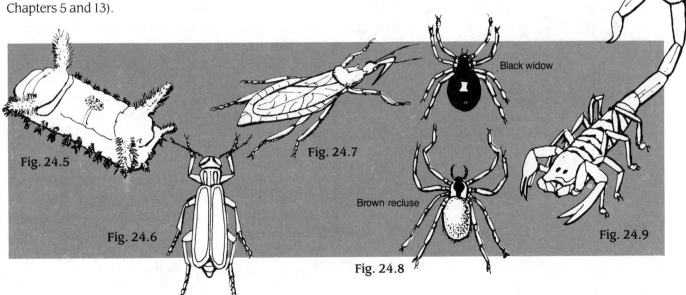

Fig. 24.5

Fig. 24.6

Fig. 24.7

Black widow

Brown recluse

Fig. 24.8

Fig. 24.9

Fig. 24.10 *Tick Removal with Forceps*

Fig. 24.11 *Venomous Snakes*

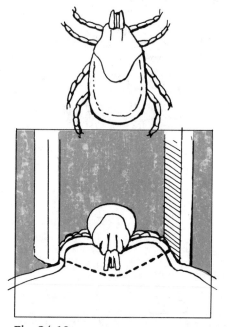

Fig. 24.10

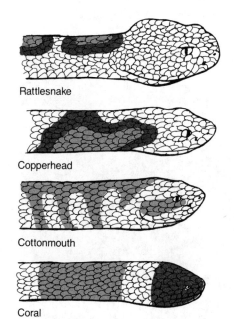

Rattlesnake

Copperhead

Cottonmouth

Coral

Fig. 24.11

Prevention of spider bites and scorpion stings consists mainly of avoiding contact with these creatures. It is unwise to place hands, feet, and other body parts in uninspected places. When camping in the desert or tropics, shake out clothing, footgear and bedding before use to remove unwanted tenants.

Although ticks (Fig. 24.10a) can carry serious diseases, they usually are more of a nuisance than a hazard. The incubation period of such tick-born diseases as Colorado tick fever, Lyme disease, and Rocky Mountain spotted fever is long enough that the outdoor traveler usually is back home before the disease develops.

One exception is tick paralysis, an interesting disease characterized by extreme fatigue and weakness of the arms and legs. If a member of a party traveling in tick country complains of these symptoms, conduct a thorough search for ticks. Removing the tick usually cures the disease within 24 to 48 hours.

Ticks should be removed with forceps rather than with the fingers. To avoid leaving the mouthparts of the tick in the wound, remove a small area of surrounding skin along with the front end of the tick using a sturdy pair of splinter forceps (Fig. 24.10b). If forceps are not available, touching the tick with a hot match or covering it with a substance that clogs its breathing pores (sunscreen lotion, camp stove fuel, etc.) may induce it to back out.

During the tick season, outdoor recreationists should inspect each other for ticks nightly. It is important to inspect all hidden and hairy areas carefully, particularly the scalp, armpits, perianal and genital areas.

SNAKEBITES

Venomous snakes are the animals most dangerous to man. Worldwide, there are 50,000 deaths from snakebite each year. In the United States, about 7,000 poisonous snakebites occur each year, causing about 15 deaths. Most of these bites occur in the South and Southwest, mainly between the months of April and October. A third of snakebites occur when snakes are purposefully handled. The relative frequency of snakebites caused by exotic poisonous snakes kept as pets is increasing.

There are two general types of poisonous snakes in the United States: pit vipers and coral snakes (Fig. 24.11). Pit vipers account for almost all bites by native snakes. Pit vipers have long, slender, hollow fangs that resemble hypodermic needles; they inject their venom deeply into the tissues (Fig. 24.12a). Coral snakes have solid fangs (Fig. 24.12b); they chew rather than stab.

It is important to distinguish poisonous snakes from harmless ones. All pit vipers, which include rattlesnakes, copperheads and water moccasins, have triangular heads and vertical elliptical pupils, while harmless snakes they may resemble have tubular heads and round pupils (Fig. 24.13a). Pit vipers have a characteristic depression, or pit, midway between the eye and nostril on each side of the head. They tend to be thicker and heavier for their length than harmless snakes. Rattlesnakes are distinguished by their rattles, which they do not always use. Pit viper bites characteristically show two fang marks (occasionally three or four marks if older fangs have not been shed), while harmless snakebites leave a horseshoe pattern of small puncture wounds (Fig. 24.13b).

A pit viper does not jump but can strike up to two-thirds of its length. In striking, the snake opens its mouth widely, erects its fangs so they point forward, and lunges. The snake buries its fangs in the victim's flesh with a thrusting motion and injects a dose of venom. Pit viper venom contains many different enzymes and toxic proteins that damage local tissue, blood vessels, blood components, the heart, and the muscles.

Coral snakes are small, shy snakes related to the cobras. They have brilliant red, black, and yellow bands, which make them resemble the similarly colored but harmless scarlet king snake. The mnemonic "red on yellow, kill a fellow; red on black, venom lack" helps in remembering the different markings of the two snakes (Fig. 24.14). Their venom acts principally on the nervous system.

The signs and symptoms of snakebite depend on the type, age and size of the snake, and the amount of venom injected. Twenty percent of snakebites do not involve envenomation. Most snakebites occur on the extremities.

Signs and Symptoms of Pit Viper Bites

Immediately following a pit viper bite, the patient experiences burning at the site. Inspection reveals bite marks ³⁄₁₆ to 1½ inches (½ centimeter to 4 centimeters) apart. Local swelling occurs within five minutes and slowly progresses proximally to involve the entire extremity. The swelling frequently is accompanied by ecchymosis and blood-filled blisters and blebs. In severe cases, systemic signs and symptoms develop, including nausea, vomiting, sweating, weakness, generalized bleeding, and tingling of the scalp, face, and lips. Damage to blood vessels may cause hypovolemic shock and pulmonary edema.

Emergency Care of Pit Viper Bites

Most patients who are bitten by pit vipers are within a few hours of an urban center where definitive treatment with antivenin is available. The major aim of emergency care is to *do no harm*. Bites unaccompanied by envenomation require no emergency care other than arranging for tetanus prophylaxis. If burning pain or swelling do not develop at the bite site within a few minutes of the bite, envenomation has not occurred.

Fig. 24.12 *Fangs of Venomous Snakes—Pit Viper and Coral*

Fig. 24.13 *Head and Bite Patterns of a Pit Viper and a Harmless Snake*

Fig. 24.14 *Comparison of the Color Patterns of Coral and Scarlet King Snakes*

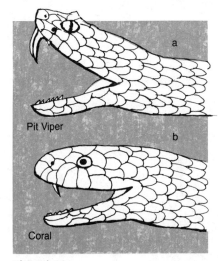
Fig. 24.12

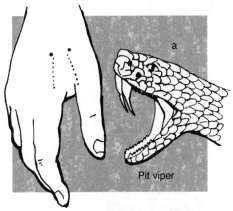
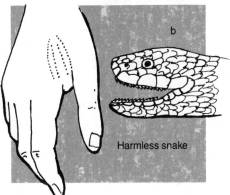
Fig. 24.13

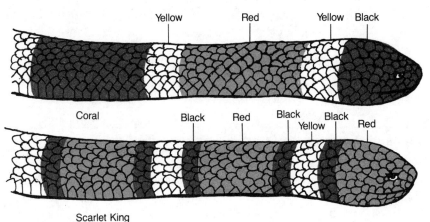
Fig. 24.14

Emergency Care of Bites with Envenomation

1. Do not allow the patient to walk or run, because muscular activity may increase venom absorption. Carry the patient from the site to the nearest transportation. A person who is bitten while alone should walk slowly to help.
2. The patient and bystanders should get out of the snake's way. If possible, kill the snake and bring it to the hospital in a bag. Because reflex biting may occur, a snake's head remains dangerous even after death.
3. Because any motion or muscular activity will speed absorption of the venom, splinting is indicated for snakebites on an extremity.
4. Mark the boundary of swelling with a pen and write the time the mark was made on the patient's skin. Repeat this procedure every 15 minutes until the patient reaches a hospital. It is important for the emergency department physician to know how rapidly swelling has progressed.
5. Take the patient to a hospital as soon as possible.
6. Additional suggestions for emergency care when definitive medical care cannot be reached for many hours:
   a. Applying suction after incising the wound through the fang marks has not been shown to be helpful and cannot be recommended. Incisions performed by excited, inexperienced rescuers may cut important structures or lead to infection.
   b. Laboratory studies in animals and field studies in humans have shown that the Sawyer extractor can remove significant amounts of venom if used *within three minutes* of a bite (see the section on injected poisons in Chapter 23). This inexpensive device is recommended first aid equipment for everyone traveling in areas where pit vipers are found.
   c. Send a party member for help.
   d. Wash the bite with soap and water and cover it with a sterile compress.
   e. Tourniquets, constricting bands and elastic wraps are probably of no value and may be dangerous. Because the swelling associated with snakebite is caused by plasma spreading through the subcutaneous tissues, restricting the swelling in an extremity provides no benefit and may be harmful.
   f. Splint the extremity.
   g. Give the patient electrolyte-containing fluids to replace fluid lost from the blood into the bitten area.
   h. Set up camp and keep the patient at rest until help arrives. If the party is large enough and a litter can be improvised, the patient may be carried out.

Signs and Symptoms of Coral Snake Bites

Coral snake bites usually involve much less local burning than pit viper bites. Local swelling, blistering, and ecchymosis usually are minimal. Within an hour or so, the effects of the venom on the nervous system begin to develop. First, the bitten extremity becomes numb and weak. Later, central nervous system symptoms such as dizziness, impaired consciousness, nervousness, involuntary movements, drooling, and increased salivation occur. These symptoms are followed within several hours by difficulty in talking and swallowing, double vision, and, in untreated cases, death because of cardiac arrest and respiratory failure.

Emergency Care of Coral Snake Bites

1. Have the patient lie down and remain as calm as possible.
2. Flush the bite area with several quarts of clean water.
3. If the bite is on an extremity, splint the extremity.
4. Provide basic life support and treat shock as necessary (see Chapters 5 and 7).
5. Incision and suction or use of the Sawyer extractor are ineffective and contraindicated in coral snake bites, even if there will be a delay in reaching medical care.
6. Transport the patient to medical care.

To avoid snakebites in snake country, outdoor travelers should never put a hand, foot, or other body part in a place that is not in full view. Use caution when reaching overhead to grasp a rocky ledge or when stepping over a log. Wear sturdy boots that extend to mid-calf. Special snakeproof boots are available. Avoid hiking at night without a light and always avoid hiking alone.

WARM-BLOODED ANIMAL BITES

Most warm-blooded animals will not attack man unless cornered, teased, or otherwise provoked. In addition to soft-tissue damage, the bites of animals commonly cause infection because their mouths harbor large numbers of bacteria. The greatest danger is contracting **rabies**, a universally fatal disease of the central nervous system. The rabies virus, present in the saliva of infected animals, can be transmitted by biting or licking. Because vaccination of pets for the prevention of rabies is required by law, *wild* animal bites present the greatest danger to humans. Prevention of bacterial infection and prevention of rabies are discussed separately.

Prevention of Bacterial Infection

1. Irrigate the wound thoroughly with clean water and wash it with soap and water, or, preferably, an antiseptic solution such as povidone-iodine (Betadine) or benzalkonium (Zepharin).
2. Do not close the wound with tape or sutures; leave it open and cover it with a sterile dressing.
3. Splint large-extremity wounds.
4. Have the patient see a physician as soon as possible. Tetanus prophylaxis is desirable.

Prevention of Rabies

1. When the bite is caused by a domestic pet with a current rabies vaccination tag, there is very little danger of rabies. Notify the county health department about the incident.

Fig. 24.15 *Marine Animals that Bite*

If the animal has no rabies vaccination tag, attempt to capture or identify the animal. If at all possible, avoid killing or hurting a pet animal. Turn over the animal to the health department for confinement and observation. If the animal is healthy at the end of 10 days, there is little danger of rabies.

If the animal must be killed, cut off its head, preserve the head on ice, and take it to the health department.

If the animal cannot be captured or identified, the patient should receive the rabies vaccine.

2. Bites from a wild animal (fox, skunk, bat, wolf, squirrel, raccoon, wildcat) should be given the same emergency care as recommended above for bites from uncaptured or unidentified domestic animals.

Human Bites

The mouth is so bacteriologically ''filthy'' that a human bite can cause virulent infection. One common method of injury occurs during a fistfight when an assailant strikes an adversary's jaw, and the adversary's tooth cuts the assailant's hand. Emergency care is the same as for any warm-blooded animal bite except that measures to prevent rabies are unnecessary.

INJURIES FROM MARINE ANIMALS

People who live in coastal areas or who practice scuba diving and other salt-water sports should be thoroughly familiar with hazardous marine animals they are likely to encounter. An excellent reference book is *Medicine for the Outdoors*, by Paul S. Auerbach, M.D., published by Little, Brown & Co., Boston, 1986.

Emergency Care of Injuries from Marine Animals

1. Bites by sharks and barracuda or other large fish (Fig. 24.15) can cause terrible wounds with serious tissue damage and massive blood loss. The emergency care of such bites includes the following:
   a. Remove the patient from the water as soon as possible to avoid exposure to further danger and to expedite emergency care.
   b. Control hemorrhage by direct pressure. A tourniquet may be needed to control bleeding from large wounds involving major arteries.
   c. Give basic life support as necessary (see Chapter 5).

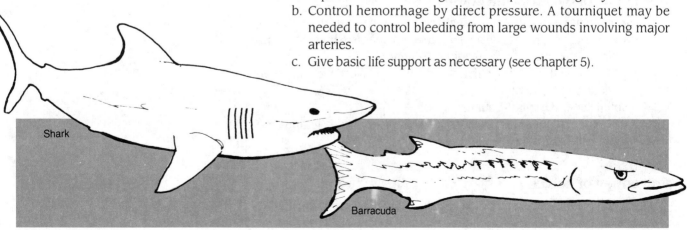

Shark

Barracuda

Fig. 24.15

   d. Anticipate and treat shock as described in Chapter 7.

   e. Irrigate and clean the wound as described above for warm-blooded animal bites. Bandage the wound but do not close it. If an extremity is involved, apply a splint.

   f. Transport the patient rapidly to a hospital. Tetanus prophylaxis is advisable.

2. Jellyfish, sea anemones, corals, hydras, and the Portuguese man-of-war (Fig. 24.16) can inflict painful stings. The purpose of emergency care is to *inactivate the toxin* as follows:

   a. Remove the patient from the water.

   b. Wash the affected area thoroughly with sea water (*not* fresh water).

   c. Remove any remaining large tentacle fragments with forceps.

   d. Next, wash the affected area with one of the following solutions (listed in order of preference): rubbing alcohol, vinegar (or 5-percent acetic acid solution), or household ammonia diluted to one-quarter strength.

   e. Apply shaving cream and gently shave the affected area.

   f. Reapply rubbing alcohol or soak the area in vinegar for 15 minutes.

   g. On rare occasions, anaphylactic shock may occur. Treat it as described in Chapter 7

   h. Tetanus prophylaxis is advisable after the patient reaches definitive medical care.

3. The spines of sea urchins, stingrays, catfish, scorpion fish, and stonefish (Fig. 24.17) can cause puncture wounds. The main purpose of emergency care is to control pain by *inactivating the toxin with hot water*, as follows:

   a. Soak the affected area in the hottest water the patient can tolerate (up to 115°F or 46°C) for 30 minutes.

   b. Remove any visible spines with forceps.

   c. Take the patient to a physician for tetanus prophylaxis and removal of deeply imbedded spines.

   d. In rare instances, anaphylactic shock may occur. Treat it as described in Chapter 7.

4. Sea snake (Fig. 24.18) bites are treated as described under the preceding section on coral snake bites.

5. Food poisoning from ingesting fish is treated as described in the section on ingested poisons in Chapter 22.

Eating improperly preserved scombroid fish (tuna, mackerel, etc.) can produce an allergic reaction with itching, hives, nausea, diarrhea, and asthma. The reaction responds to an antihistamine such as nonprescription diphenhydramine (Benadryl).

Fig. 24.16 *Marine Animals that Sting*

Fig. 24.17 *Marine Animals with Dangerous Spines*

Fig. 24.18 *Sea Snake*

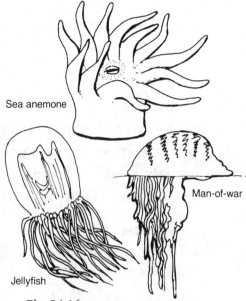

Sea anemone
Man-of-war
Jellyfish

Fig. 24.16

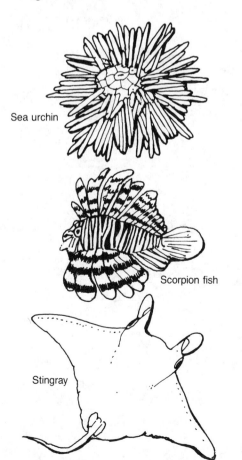

Sea urchin
Scorpion fish
Stingray

Fig. 24.17

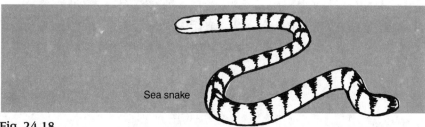

Sea snake

Fig. 24.18

25

Water Emergencies

A man who is not afraid of the sea will soon
be drowned, he said, for he will be going out on a day
he shouldn't. But we do be afraid of the sea,
and we do only be drowned now and again.

—Ernest Rutherford
The Aran Islands

Many outdoor injuries are associated with water sports such as swimming, boating, windsurfing, and scuba diving. These injuries are related to the inherent characteristics of bodies of water, water in motion, and the equipment used in water sports. Even cavers can be subject to hazard from underground bodies of water. Because the number of Americans participating in water sports is growing, more water-related injuries are likely to occur.

In the United States, between 7,000 and 8,000 deaths from drowning occur each year. Use of alcohol or other drugs is a factor in at least half these deaths, and one-third or more involve hypothermia caused by cold water. About half of drowning deaths occur outside the warm months of June, July, and August. Many who drown had not learned how to swim.

Swimmers who dive into shallow water can suffer head injuries, cervical spine fractures and facial injuries. Participants in whitewater and swiftwater sports who capsize their craft or perform poorly executed rollovers can suffer blunt head trauma, contusions, lacerations, broken teeth, chest and abdominal injuries, and fractures. Dislocated shoulders occasionally are caused by paddle maneuvers that force the arm upwards in abduction. Injuries related to overuse of the thumb, wrist and shoulders, such as sprains and tendonitis, are common. People who swallow contaminated water can develop gastrointestinal infections.

Skin diving and scuba diving introduce problems related to anoxia (lack of oxygen), water pressure, and breathing pressurized gas. These include pressure ("squeeze") injuries of the ears and sinuses, nitrogen narcosis, oxygen toxicity, air embolism, and decompression sickness.

Some techniques must be modified when applied to water-related injuries and illnesses, but the principles of emergency care remain unchanged.

Rescuers should have a strong respect for water, especially cold, deep, or fast-moving water. Only a strong, competent swimmer who is well-trained in lifesaving should attempt a direct swimming rescue of a struggling victim. Unless a victim is unable to grasp a floating object, it usually is better to throw or push a lifesaving device to the victim or to use a boat. The maxim to remember is "throw, tow, row, and only then go." Rescuers untrained in lifesaving are likely to become victims themselves.

Those who live in areas where water sports are popular and water accidents are common should take additional training in water safety and water rescue from the American Red Cross, the YMCA, or a similar organization.

SUBMERSION INJURY

Submersion injuries are divided into drowning and near drowning. A drowning victim is dead; a victim of near drowning survives at least temporarily after submersion. Drowning deaths are caused by anoxia, which can irreversibly damage vital organs, particularly the brain, if it lasts more than four to six minutes.

However, at least in theory, there are two mechanisms that can delay the development of serious anoxia in some submersion victims: the **mammalian diving reflex**, which is discussed in the Chapter 19, and **hypothermia**. People who have been submerged in cold water for up to an hour can occasionally be resuscitated with very little residual injury to the brain. The

Fig. 25.1 *Technique of Turning a Submersion Patient from the Prone to the Supine Position*

most successful of these resuscitations have involved infants and people rescued from very cold water, but there have been occasional successes when water temperatures were near 70°F (21°C). These extraordinary survivals appear to be possible because hypothermia slows the body's metabolism and decreases its oxygen requirements.

Wet and Dry Drowning

When people are submerged, they first hold their breath and struggle intensely before losing consciousness because of anoxia. Once unconscious, they lose their breath-holding ability and their gag reflex and aspirate water into the upper airway. The lungs of 85 percent of drowning victims are filled with water at autopsy (wet drowning). The other 15 percent have dry lungs (dry drowning), apparently because the larynx goes into spasm when water is initially aspirated, keeping additional water out of the lungs.

Rescue, Assessment, and Emergency Care of a Submersed Patient

When a person is found floating face down on the water surface or is brought to the surface by a rescuer, there usually is little question about the cause of unconsciousness. When near drowning is unwitnessed or occurs after a dive or a surfing accident, a head injury and a broken neck also should be assumed. Any near-drowning victim–especially a young one–submerged in water 70°F (21°C) or below for less than an hour is potentially salvageable.

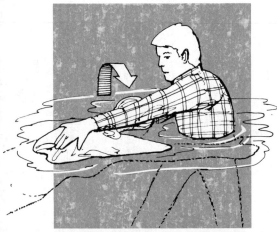

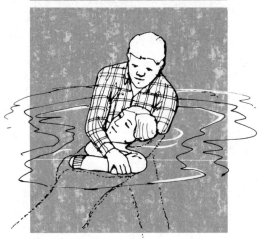

Fig. 25.1

Emergency Care of A Submersion Patient

1. An unconscious submersion patient found floating prone should be turned to the supine position. Turn the patient's entire upper body as a unit, using the following method (Fig. 25.1):
   a. Approach the patient from the patient's head end.
   b. Place one arm over the side of the patient's back and the other arm under the patient's opposite armpit, so that the patient's head is sandwiched between your arms.
   c. Rotate the patient's trunk, bringing the patient to a supine position, with the back still supported by one of your arms.
2. Open the airway immediately using the head-tilt/chin-lift maneuver (or the jaw-thrust method, if a neck injury is suspected) and start rescue breathing as soon as possible, usually as soon as the patient has been towed into shallow water where the rescuer can stand (Fig. 25.2). In some cases, rescue breathing can be started in deep water or under water if the rescuer is experienced and is a powerful swimmer. If two rescuers are available, one can support the patient while the other gives rescue breathing. It is especially important to maintain a watertight seal over the patient's mouth and nose, preferably with a tight-sealing pocket mask. CPR is almost impossible to perform in deep water; there is no point in wasting time attempting it. If CPR is needed, move the patient to dry land or a firm surface as soon as possible.
3. If possible, use a spine board to remove the patient from the water

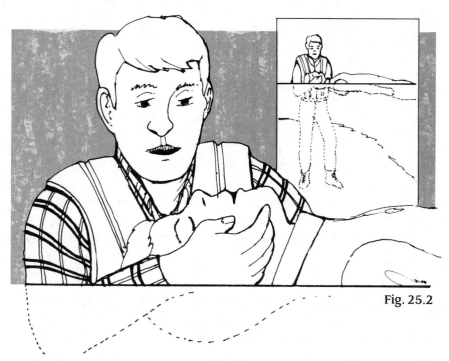

Fig. 25.2 *Start rescue breathing as soon as possible.*

Fig. 25.3 *If possible, use a spine board to remove a patient from the water.*

Fig. 25.2

(Fig. 25.3). Slide the board underneath, allow it to float up underneath the patient, secure the patient to it, and tow the patient to dry land on the board. If a spine board is unavailable, use the four-person direct ground lift (see Chapter 20) when shallow water is reached.

4. After reaching dry land, determine the presence or absence of heart action and start CPR if indicated. Give oxygen in high concentration using a bag-mask or pocket mask. Search for lacerations, fractures, and other injuries as time and personnel allow.

5. Following near drowning, the patient's stomach usually is filled with water and the patient will vomit. Anticipate vomiting and turn the patient to one side to avoid aspiration. Suction is useful, if available. The Heimlich maneuver (see Chapter 5) should *not* be used to remove water from the stomach.

6. Take the patient's rectal temperature, preferably with a low-reading thermometer. Hypothermia is protective in near drowning and should not be corrected in the field if spontaneous breathing and heart action are absent. Prevent further cooling by insulating the patient's trunk while leaving the extremities uncovered (see Chapter 19).

7. Take *all* submersion patients to a hospital as soon as possible, even if they appear normal after they have been revived, since serious delayed complications may occur. On the way, give rescue breathing or CPR if indicated. Frequently monitor and record vital signs. The emergency room physician will need to know the patient's initial rectal temperature and any subsequent readings, the water temperature, the patient's age, the probable length of submersion, and any other important factors such as injuries.

8. A hypothermic victim of near drowning who has spontaneous respirations and heart action can be rewarmed according to the guidelines found in Chapter 19. The techniques appropriate for rewarming depend on the patient's core temperature.

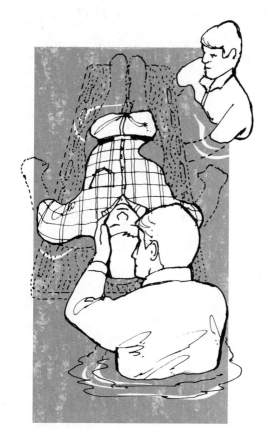

Fig. 25.3

Fig. 25.4 *Flotation Devices*

Prevention of Near Drowning

1. Teach all children to swim.
2. If possible, fence all swimming pools and other bodies of water in inhabited areas. Keep the water level of swimming pools close to the pool rim to enable swimmers to climb out easily.
3. Wear U.S. Coast Guard-approved flotation devices such as life jackets or partial exposure suits while aboard small water craft, particularly rafts, sailboats, rowboats, canoes, and kayaks (Fig. 25.4).
4. Use helmets when kayaking.
5. When swimming, skin diving or scuba diving, use the buddy system. Partners should keep track of each other at all times.
6. Do not leave infants and small children unsupervised near open water.
7. Do not use alcohol and/or "recreational" drugs while participating in water sports.
8. People engaged in cold-water sports should wear suitable clothing (wet or dry suits, partial or full exposure suits) to prevent or delay hypothermia if unexpected immersion occurs.

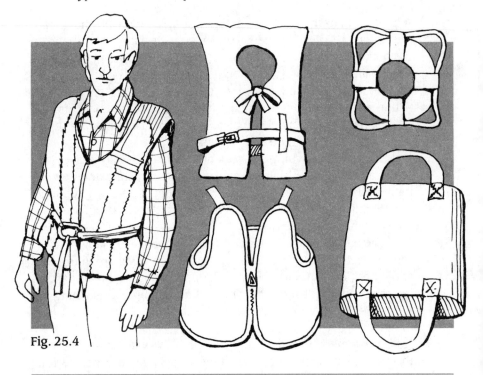

Fig. 25.4

Ice Rescue

The popularity of ice fishing, ice skating, and snowmobiling on frozen lakes increases the likelihood that rescuers may have to aid a person who has broken through the ice.

To allow the victim to reach shore or a rescuer to reach the victim, an ice rescue must be performed so that weight is widely distributed over the ice surface. An excellent rescue device is a lightweight ladder with a lifeline tied to the lowest rung. The ladder is shoved out on the ice to the victim, who crawls onto the ladder and edges along it to safety. If the victim is unable to

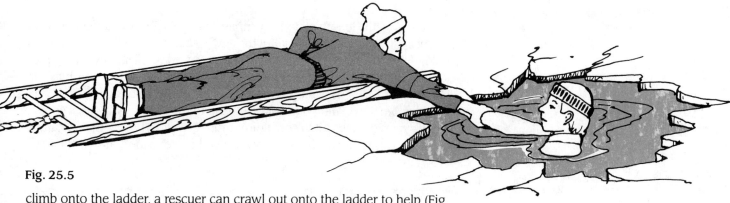

Fig. 25.5

climb onto the ladder, a rescuer can crawl out onto the ladder to help (Fig. 25.5). If the ice breaks under the ladder, the far end will dip and the near end will rise, making it easier to pull the ladder back to safety by the lifeline. If a ladder is unavailable, wide boards or a stout tree branch can be used instead. Alternatives, especially if the ice is too fragile to support these devices, are to shove canoes or rowboats out onto the ice, or to throw a spare tire or ring buoy to the victim. Helicopters have been used successfully, especially in multiple-victim disasters. If no equipment is available, a human chain can sometimes be formed by having several rescuers lie on the ice in a line, each grasping the ankles of the person in front.

A person who falls through the ice should attempt self-rescue by extending the arms forward over the ice, kicking the legs up so that the body is in a level position, and working forward onto the ice by kicking and carefully pulling with the arms. A pocketknife can be used to increase traction (Fig. 25.6). This maneuver can be successful even if the ice continues to break ahead of the victim; it should be continued until firm ice is reached. After pulling the entire body onto firm ice, the victim should carefully roll or edge toward shore, distributing body weight as widely as possible.

All victims of ice breakthroughs are assumed to be hypothermic and are cared for according to the guidelines in Chapter 19.

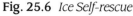
Fig. 25.5 *Ice Rescue Using a Ladder*

Fig. 25.6 *Ice Self-rescue*

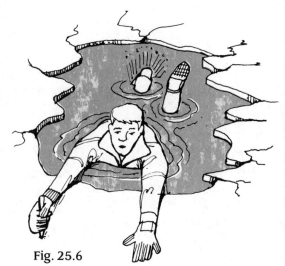

Fig. 25.6

OTHER AQUATIC PROBLEMS

Swimmer's Ear

Swimmer's ear is an infection of the outer ear canal, seen in swimmers and divers whose ears are continually wet. Symptoms include pain in the ear, a white or yellow discharge, and partial deafness. Patients should see a physician for specific treatment. Swimmer's ear can be prevented by putting several drops of a solution of vinegar diluted to half strength with tap water in each ear after emerging from water. Do not use alcohol-based nonprescription preparations for preventing swimmer's ear.

Breath-holding Blackout

The loss of consciousness that occasionally results when a swimmer hyperventilates before swimming under water is called **breath-holding blackout**. Hyperventilation lowers blood levels of carbon dioxide (PCO_2) and increases levels of oxygen (PO_2) (see Chapters 1 and 17). Because the breathing control center in the brain uses blood PCO_2 as a guide to regulate the rate and depth of breathing, the length of time swimmers can hold their breath underwater is proportional to the PCO_2 level. If the PCO_2 is below normal, swimmers can hold their breath longer. The danger is that PO_2 may fall so low during prolonged breath-holding that swimmers lose consciousness from hypoxia before their PCO_2 rises sufficiently to compel them to surface for a breath. Because breath-holding blackout can lead to drowning, swimmers should avoid hyperventilating before swimming underwater. The emergency care of breath-holding blackout is the same as that described above for near drowning.

Associated Injuries

Kayaking, canoeing, sailing, windsurfing, motorboating, water skiing and surfing can all cause injuries. The additional danger of submersion is always a possible complication. The patient must be removed from the water before emergency care can be given effectively. Give basic life support and care for soft-tissue, bone, and joint injuries as outlined in previous chapters. The emergency care of injuries caused by hazardous marine life is discussed in Chapter 24.

SCUBA DIVING INJURIES

The increasing popularity of diving with self-contained underwater breathing apparatus (**scuba**) has led to increasing numbers of accidents and injuries related to diving techniques, equipment, and the nature of the underwater environment. Many sport dives take place in exotic tropical environments where sophisticated medical care may be unobtainable. The medical problems of diving result from the human body's lack of gills and consequent dependence on technology to survive underwater, the effects of water pressure and of breathing compressed gas, and the hazards of the underwater environment.

Anyone who wants to scuba dive should learn the proper technique by taking an approved course taught by the YMCA or a similar organization.

Diving problems can be divided into those of **descent**, those of the **bottom**, and those of **ascent**.

Descent Problems

Ear and sinus injuries occur frequently, making them a major problem for the diver. These injuries can involve the ear canal, middle ear, inner ear, or sinuses. The basic cause is the difference between the air pressure within the ears and sinuses and the water pressure. Accessory factors include wax buildup within the ear, failure of the Eustachian tube to open properly, and swelling of the lining of the nose, all of which can prevent the gradual pressure adjustments that normally occur during a properly conducted dive. Divers should be thoroughly familiar with methods of equalizing pressure by blowing with the nostrils closed or swallowing and should not dive if they have an upper respiratory infection.

Depending on the area involved, symptoms of ear or sinus squeeze can include a feeling of fullness, pain or ringing in the ear, headache, deafness, and loss of balance. A diver who experiences these symptoms should halt the dive and return to the surface as soon as possible to reduce the pressure differences. Failure to surface may result in an eardrum rupture or serious injury to the inner ear.

The lungs and upper airway rarely give trouble during descent. However, if divers hold their breath or their scuba apparatus malfunctions, they may suffer lung squeeze with bleeding into their lungs. Air in the gastrointestinal tract usually causes trouble only on ascent. Masks can cause face squeeze unless the pressure differences that develop during descent are equalized by blowing air into the mask through the nose.

Bottom Problems

Bottom problems are uncommon, and those that occur usually are related to equipment malfunction. Drowning or near drowning can occur if air is lost from leaking equipment or if the diver runs out of air because of a miscalculation. Malfunctioning air compressors or improper filtering of air when tanks are filled can add small amounts of carbon dioxide or carbon monoxide to scuba tanks; the deleterious effects of these gases are magnified by the increased pressure at depth. Nitrogen narcosis, or "rapture of the deep" is caused by breathing nitrogen at depths below about 90 feet (27 meters) and has an effect similar to alcohol intoxication. Oxygen poisoning with convulsions can occur if pure oxygen is breathed below 33 feet (10 meters) or if compressed air is breathed below 297 feet (91 meters).

Ascent Problems

Aside from drowning and near drowning, the most serious underwater problems occur on ascent. Ascent problems, including **air embolism** and **decompression sickness**, are related to the effects of decreasing water pressure on the air in the lungs and on the nitrogen dissolved in the body fluids.

Air Embolism

During ascent, the air in the lungs expands as the water pressure decreases. If air expands too quickly or too much, the pressure may rupture the alveoli and force air bubbles into the small blood vessels of the lungs. **Air embolism**, a danger during rapid ascent, can be prevented if divers *continually exhale* during ascent to reduce the volume of air in their lungs. Scuba divers should *never* hold their breath while under water. Ascent should be *controlled* at a rate of about 60 feet/minute (1 foot/second). This rate can be estimated by ascending at the same rate as the smallest visible air bubble.

Air bubbles that enter the blood are carried through the circulatory system until they reach a narrow vessel where they may become lodged, plugging the vessel and preventing blood from reaching the tissues the vessel normally supplies. Because bubbles can lodge in almost any organ, the signs and symptoms of air embolism are variable. Sudden loss of consciousness upon reaching the surface is a characteristic occurrence.

The most common signs and symptoms of air embolism are caused by involvement of the circulatory, respiratory, and nervous systems. They include chest pain, shortness of breath, cough, hemoptysis, and signs and symptoms of pneumothorax (see Chapter 15); signs and symptoms of heart attack (see Chapter 18); dizziness, confusion, stupor, unconsciousness, and seizures (see Chapters 13 and 18); loss of vision, hearing or speech; and paralysis or loss of sensation.

Emergency Care of Air Embolism

1. Remove the patient from the water and place the patient on the left side with the chest *lower* than the feet. This position tends to trap the air bubbles in the heart and prevent them from entering important arteries, particularly those supplying the brain.
2. Give basic life support (see Chapter 5) and care for unconsciousness (see Chapter 13), as required.
3. Give oxygen in high concentration.
4. The best medical treatment for air embolism is *recompression in a pressure chamber* (hyperbaric chamber). Recompression makes the air bubbles smaller and drives them into solution. Some diving centers have hyperbaric chambers as part of their medical facilities. All scuba divers should know the location of the nearest hyperbaric chamber. Usually a chamber is within a few hours by air. The aircraft used to transport the patient should fly low or be pressurized at near-sea-level pressure. The Diving Accident Network (DAN) can be contacted at (919) 684-8111 for assistance in locating hyperbaric chambers and for advice on emergency care. Medical personnel will need to know the following information, which can be obtained from the patient or companions:
   a. Age and sex of the patient.
   b. Signs, symptoms, elapsed time between surfacing and onset of illness, and duration of illness.
   c. Depth and bottom time of dive or dives.
   d. Conditions under which the ascent was made, i.e., breathing or not breathing, whether scheduled decompression stops were made.
   e. The first aid that has been given.

If a hyperbaric chamber cannot be reached, take the patient to the nearest hospital as rapidly as possible.

Decompression Sickness

Atmospheric nitrogen is much less soluble than oxygen and carbon dioxide in body fluids. However, during a dive, the increasing water pressure forces a higher proportion of the nitrogen in the lungs into solution than would occur on land. If ascent is too rapid, this nitrogen will come out of solution, forming bubbles in small blood vessels, instead of being excreted normally through the lungs. Because the nitrogen bubbles can form or lodge in any organ, the signs and symptoms of **decompression sickness**, like those of air embolism, are variable and depend on the organs involved.

Common Signs and Symptoms of Decompression Sickness

1. Mottling and/or itching of the skin.
2. Pain in muscles, joints, or the abdomen (the "bends").
3. Weakness, paralysis, and loss of sensation, particularly of the lower extremities.
4. Difficulty in urinating.
5. Chest pain, cough, and shortness of breath.

Decompression sickness can be prevented by carefully controlling the depth and duration of the dive. Sport divers are advised *not* to dive in a way that requires stops on ascent for decompression. Tables are available that indicate the safe times at given depths for single and repetitive dives, and the depths and times of decompression stops required on ascent if the safe limits are exceeded.

Emergency care for decompression sickness is the same as for air embolism. The signs and symptoms of air embolism and decompression sickness usually are reversible with treatment in a hyperbaric chamber. Permanent injury may result if recompression is delayed or if the vessels that supply vital organs – such as the heart, brain and spinal cord – are plugged. Therefore, treat serious ascent problems as an emergency and arrange for recompression as soon as possible.

26

Childbirth

Every child comes with the message that God
is not yet discouraged of man.

—*Rabindranath Tagore*

Childbirth (Fig. 26.1) is a natural process that usually proceeds in a normal and safe manner. Early labor commonly begins slowly enough to allow ample time to obtain medical help. However, labor often proceeds more rapidly for women who have already had one or more children than for women having their first child. Occasionally, because of distance, lack of ambulance services, or difficulties in transportation, it may be impossible to obtain medical help before the baby is delivered. Rescuers should be familiar with the basic sequence of childbirth and be prepared to assist as needed. Afterwards, take the mother and infant to a hospital as soon as possible.

Before continuing, review the anatomy and physiology of the female genitourinary system in Chapter 2.

Signs a Pregnant Woman Should Be Taken to a Hospital for Delivery

1. A sudden gush of fluid from the vagina (rupture of the membranes or "bag of waters"). This fluid is the amniotic fluid that supports and protects the fetus; it is *not* urine.
2. The onset of uterine contractions, which eventually are spaced at regular intervals of about two minutes.
3. Sudden passage of bloody mucus from the vagina (more than spotting alone).

Fig. 26.1 *Anatomical Drawing of a Baby Inside the Uterus*

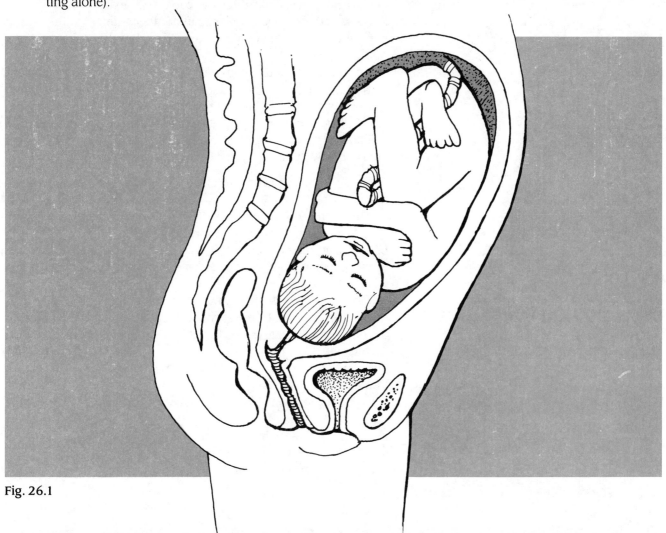

Fig. 26.1

Fig. 26.2 *Vaginal Opening during Contractions with the Baby's Head Visible*

Fig. 26.3 *Delivery of the Head*

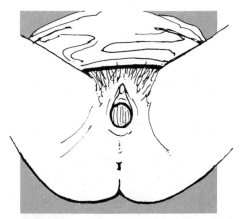

Fig. 26.2

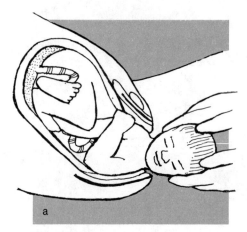

Fig. 26.3

If the mother begins to strain or push down with contractions or cries out that the baby is coming, delivery is imminent and it may be too late to reach a hospital in time. Quickly gather the following supplies:

Two clean sheets	Four clean towels
Sterile material to	Scissors or a razor blade
tie off the umbilical cord	Sanitary napkins
(strong cotton string	Diaper
or a white shoelace	Soft rubber bulb syringe
can be sterilized by	Sterile compresses
boiling for 10 minutes)	Soap and warm water
Rubbing alcohol	Disposable rubber gloves
One or more flannel	Safety pins
blankets for baby	
Newspapers and plastic sheets	
or bags to protect bed,	
rug or car upholstery	

Assessment of a Pregnant Woman

1. Arrange for as much privacy as possible.
2. Remove all clothing below her waist.
3. Have her lie on her back on a flat surface (bed or floor) with both knees bent, feet flat, and thighs spread widely apart.
4. Lay a waterproof piece of plastic under the woman's buttocks and cover it with clean material such as a sheet, towels, or several layers of paper.
5. Wash your hands and put on disposable rubber gloves, if available.
6. Inspect the vaginal opening during a contraction to see if the baby's head is visible (Fig. 26.2). If so, you will see an area of wrinkled skin and dark hair. Important considerations in deciding whether there is still time to take the woman to a hospital are the size of the visible area and how many children the woman has had previously.

There probably still is time to reach a hospital less than 20 minutes away if:

a. The head is not visible or barely visible during a contraction and the woman has had one or more previous children.
b. The head can be seen during a contraction and the visible area is *smaller* than a fifty-cent piece, and the woman is having her first child.

Tell the woman not to bear down with contractions, but to take fast, shallow breaths (pant) with each contraction. Immediately gather the supplies listed above as well as the following items for the automobile ride:

Flashlight	Blanket
Container for placenta	Pillow
(washbasin or pan of	Warm bathrobe for patient
similar size)	

If the visible area of the baby's head is larger than the size of a fifty-cent piece, especially if the woman has had previous children, delivery probably will occur within the next few contractions (10 minutes or less). When a hospital cannot be reached in time, home delivery is preferable to delivering the baby in an automobile.

7. However, if the umbilical cord or any part of the baby's body other than the head is seen at the vaginal opening or if the umbilical cord has fallen out of the vaginal opening, it will be extremely difficult or impossible for a rescuer untrained in obstetrics to deliver the baby safely. Any of these conditions constitutes an *emergency*. Preparations for home delivery should be stopped and the woman should be rushed to the nearest hospital.

Delivery

1. Delivery of the head
   a. The head usually emerges following or during a contraction. Hold the baby's head gently, maintaining it in its normal position with respect to the body. If necessary, allow the head to rotate with the rotation of the baby's body, and guide and support the head as it emerges (Fig. 26.3a).
   b. The head may be covered with the bag of waters. If the bag does not rupture spontaneously, tear it with your fingers or nick it with a scissors blade to free the head (Fig. 26.3b).
   c. If the cord is wrapped around the baby's neck, unwrap it quickly by passing the loops over the baby's head (Fig. 26.3c). If this cannot be done, tie and cut the cord as described below in step 4. If the cord must be cut before it can be tied because it is strangling the baby, pinch the ends until they can be tied. Be aware that the cord is slippery and be especially careful not to lose your grip before it is tied. Otherwise, the baby may suffer serious, potentially fatal bleeding.
   d. Usually, there will be a minute or two between the time the baby's head is delivered and the time the shoulders are delivered. During this interval, wipe out the baby's mouth with a clean cloth. If a soft rubber bulb syringe is available, it can be used instead to gently suction the mouth and nose (Fig. 26.3d).
      Squeeze the bulb and gently insert the tip about 1½ inches into the baby's mouth. Squirt out any material before reinserting the tip. Suction the mouth and each nostril two or three times.

2. Delivery of the shoulders
   a. After the head is delivered, the baby's shoulders will start to emerge. One usually will emerge before the other. Guide out one shoulder at a time with one hand while supporting the baby's head with the other hand. Do *not* try to pull a shoulder out by hooking your finger under the baby's armpit, and do *not* tug on the baby's head to get the shoulders out faster.
   b. After the shoulders have been delivered, the rest of the body usually will emerge rapidly. Be prepared so that the baby can be caught and not dropped (newborn babies are slippery!).

3. Care and resuscitation of the baby
   a. Turn the baby prone, and support the chest and head with the palm of one hand while grasping the feet with the other hand. Insert an index finger between the baby's feet while encircling the

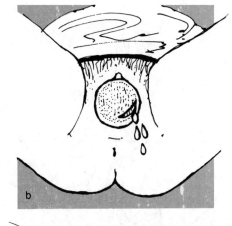

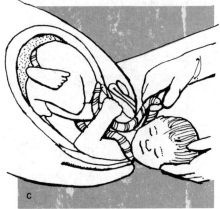

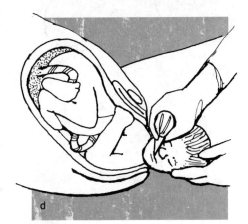

Fig. 26.3

Fig. 26.4 *Care and Resuscitation of the Baby*

Fig. 26.5 *Technique of Tying and Cutting the Umbilical Cord*

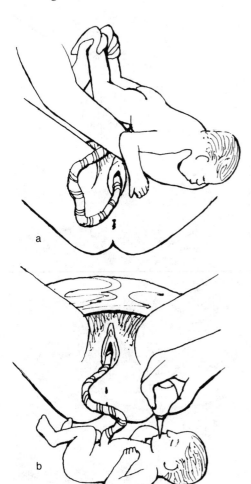

Fig. 26.4

feet with the thumb and other three fingers to provide a more secure grip (Fig. 26.4a).

b. If the baby does not start breathing immediately, suction out the mouth and nose again with the bulb syringe (Fig. 26.4b) and pat the baby's back gently or flick the feet with a finger, several times if needed. If this is ineffective, give rescue breathing (Chapter 5).

c. Wrap the baby in one or more flannel blankets as soon as possible to keep him or her warm. Newborn babies lose heat rapidly because of their large surface-to-volume ratio.

4. The umbilical cord rarely needs to be cut in the field unless it is strangling the baby or there will be a long delay in reaching the hospital. In the hospital, it is customary to delay cutting the cord until it stops pulsating; this allows the maximum amount of blood to flow to the baby from the placenta. If the cord *has* to be cut:

a. Tie off the umbilical cord at intervals 6 inches and 8 inches from the baby using a clean, preferably sterile (boiled for 10 minutes) cotton cord (Fig. 26.5a).

b. Cut the cord between the two ties with scissors or a razor blade sterilized by boiling or by wiping with rubbing alcohol (Fig. 26.5b).

5. Delivery of the placenta ("afterbirth")

a. After the baby is born, the uterus will begin contracting again to expel the placenta. Do *not* push on the abdomen or pull on the cord to speed this process.

b. As soon as the placenta emerges, *gently* massage the uterus through the abdominal wall for a few minutes with one hand to stimulate the uterus to contract firmly and control bleeding. The uterus will feel like a firm, smooth, rounded, grapefruit-sized object in the midline of the lower abdomen just above the pubic symphysis. This massage is uncomfortable, and you should explain to the mother what you are doing and why.

c. Repeatedly massage the uterus every few minutes until the mother arrives at the hospital, or for about an hour total. If the

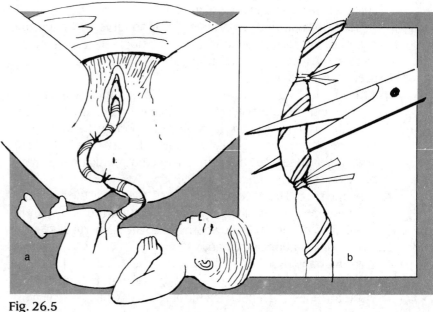

Fig. 26.5

uterus begins to feel soft and there is increased blood flow from the vagina, increase the vigor and frequency of the massage.

6. Care after delivery
    a. Keep the mother and infant warm and check the infant periodically to make sure breathing is normal.
    b. Cleanse the mother's vaginal area by pouring warm, soapy water over it. Rinse with warm water. Do this while the mother is still lying on her back, so that the water flows over the pubis toward the rectum.
    c. Lay a sanitary napkin over the vaginal opening.
    d. If the vagina or perineum are lacerated, control bleeding with a sterile compress and direct pressure.
    e. Dry the baby to avoid evaporative cooling, but do not attempt washing or cleansing.
    f. Take the mother and baby to a hospital.

Legal Aspects of Emergency Care

Jus est ars boni et aequi (Legal justice is the art of the good and the fair).

—Latin saying

In traditional Western society, only physicians have been permitted to diagnose and treat the injured and ill. Preparation for the practice of medicine is long, rigorous, and subject to strict regulation and licensing. Over the years, however, types of medical care that can properly be provided by nonphysicians have been identified through experience and general agreement. These levels have been called by various names: first aid, self-help, and more recently – as sophistication has increased – emergency medical technique, first response, or emergency care. The following discussion will use the term "emergency care" to refer to nonphysician medical care.

Emergency care is appropriate under many circumstances, including but not limited to:

1. Medical emergencies when no physician is present and the patient is in danger of death or serious harm unless something is done immediately.
2. Illnesses or injuries in which certain preliminary care is appropriate during the time before the patient is turned over to a physician.
3. Illnesses or injuries that are not serious enough to normally require a physician's care.

Although written material is available for self study, in most cases people who want to learn about emergency care have enrolled in a specific course taught by a recognized organization such as the American Red Cross. Upon successful completion of the course, students receive a card specifying that they completed the course and fulfilled its requirements. Such people then are regarded as competent to provide the care that they have been taught. To maintain this competency, they attend refresher courses at intervals.

Because of the informal and voluntary way that emergency care has developed in the past, there has been no formal licensing until recently. With the formation of the EMS system, people trained in emergency care who work in ambulances, helicopters, hospital emergency departments, and similar places have been required to obtain a state license. With the exception of licensed members at the higher levels of the EMS system – such as paramedics under physician supervision – emergency care providers are not allowed to start intravenous infusions or perform invasive procedures such as needle thoracotomy (use of a needle to drain air or fluid from the chest) and endotracheal intubation, to administer drugs, or to perform defibrillation and other advanced life support procedures. To do this without EMS authority would be "practicing medicine without a license," which is prohibited by the medical practice statutes of every state.

Under common law, emergency care providers at every level are expected to perform as any other reasonable, prudent person with similar training and experience would perform under similar circumstances, with due regard for the safety and welfare of both the patient and fellow providers. This is called the **standard of care.**

To adhere to this standard, it is necessary to obtain good training, practice skills appropriately and correctly, have basic equipment on hand and know how to use it, keep abreast of advances in the field of emergency care, and have **documentation** of training, refreshing and reevaluation of competency in required skills and knowledge. It is very important that there be *detailed* documentation of the emergency care provided to each patient: this is required by most rescue organizations, which provide report forms to be filled out in each case.

It also is important that the record of signs and symptoms match the record of care given. In general, the law presumes that *emergency care not recorded* in the written report is *emergency care not given*. In addition, an incomplete or untidy report implies that the emergency care given also may be incomplete or careless. The rescuer should remember that, in the case of litigation, he or she may be required to testify in court many months or years after the occurrence in question. It is much better to have a complete and accurate report to refer to than to rely on memory alone.

Generally speaking, in the United States no ordinary citizen has a legal obligation to rescue or go to the aid of another individual who is sick, injured, or endangered unless he or she has caused the sickness, injury, or danger. However, in several states a citizen is obligated either to act personally or to notify competent authorities so that rescue or aid can be given by them.

If the citizen *does* go to another person's aid, the law obliges him or her not only to act reasonably and prudently but to continue to care for the patient until the patient's care is transferred to another qualified person. Failure to do the latter is called **abandonment** and can result in legal constraints or a lawsuit. If a citizen has a role or job that implies an obligation to provide rescue or emergency care, or is a member of a ski patrol or other organized rescue group that has represented itself to the public and to the authorities as an organization of trained, qualified and responsible rescuers, a legal obligation *does* exist to search for, rescue, and care for the injured and ill within the specific area of operation when requested. Even if the rescuer is an unpaid volunteer, he or she is not "ordinary" and does not have the option of arbitrarily refusing such a request.

In the eyes of the law, a person's body is inviolate. Interfering with it or even touching it without permission may constitute **battery**, an illegal act in many states. Because any person usually has a right to refuse emergency care, when first approaching a patient, the rescuer should identify himself or herself as a trained rescuer and provider of emergency care, and ask "Can I be of help?" The patient may either specifically give consent or may cooperate with your assessment and care in a way that can be taken as actual consent.

If the patient is unconscious, irrational, or a minor and urgently needs care for a life-threatening or serious illness or injury, consent may be "**implied**." This means that the law presumes that the patient, if able (or the patient's parents or guardian, if present), would consent to the care.

In some cases, a patient who initially refuses care can be pursuaded to accept help by a calm discussion of the risks of not obtaining care. If the patient persists in refusing, it is wise to have responsible witnesses present and have statements from them for the record specifying that care was offered and refused.

If an irrational or unreasonable patient refuses urgently needed care for a life-threatening or very serious condition, it is probably better to at least try to give the care despite the refusal, since the risk of being accused of abandonment usually is greater than the risk of being accused of battery.

Further, under the legal doctrine of "choice of evils," a rescuer may be protected from liability for battery if he or she preserves the life and health of a seriously ill or injured person who may have refused treatment but who was not in a physical or mental condition to evaluate the situation or to refuse treatment in a rational manner. However, at this point, *proper docu-*

mentation is essential, and law enforcement authorities should be called, if possible, so they can become involved as well. The student also should refer to **The Psychology of Dealing With Injured or Ill Persons** in Chapter 4.

Despite the best emergency care, unexpected results may occur or the patient may allege that the care or transportation was improper. The result, especially in our current legal climate, may be litigation, which is both costly and time-consuming, even if the rescuer is eventually exonerated. For this reason, every rescuer must be certain that he or she is covered by sufficient liability insurance to protect against both *successful claims* and the *expenses of defending against suits*.

Although a disgruntled patient may allege anything, he or she has the burden of proving four things in court to prevail on a claim of negligence:

1. That the rescuer had a *duty* to the patient.
2. That the rescuer *failed to perform*, or "**breached**," that duty because of an error of commission or omission that *violated the standard of care*.
3. That the patient *actually suffered some injury or loss* that is compensable in money.
4. That the rescuer's failure was the *actual cause of the patient's injury or loss*.

These four requirements, which place the burden of proof on the plaintiff, are a strong barrier against frivolous or unjustified lawsuits. Other deterents are the so-called Good Samaritan laws, whose purpose is to encourage people to help out voluntarily in emergencies. These laws have now been passed by every state but differ significantly from state to state. In some states they apply only to physicians and nurses, in others to other recognized emergency care providers as well, and in still others to *anyone* who renders assistance in an emergency. In some states, organized responders are not covered by the Good Samaritan Law because it has been held that they have a duty to respond.

The student should obtain and study a copy of the Good Samaritan Law in his or her state. Although these laws do not prevent suits from being filed, they generally make it more difficult for the plaintiff to win because in theory they absolve from liability anyone covered by the statute who gives care gratuitously, in good faith, and in accordance with his or her training and expertise in a bona fide emergency – except in the case of **gross or willful negligence**. In some states the assistance also must be given "without objection" from the patient.

Negligence can be defined as the breach (failure to perform) of a duty to exercise the degree of care that any reasonable and prudent person would exercise in similar circumstances, resulting in harm to another person.

Gross negligence can be defined as the breach of a duty to exercise the care that even an unreasonable or imprudent person would exercise in similar circumstances, resulting in harm to another person. If bad or malicious intentions are involved, the negligence is referred to as **willful negligence** or willful misconduct

However, the student should realize that the best protection–and also an ethical obligation–is good, up-to-date training, conscientious refreshing of and maintenance of competency in knowledge and skills, and dedicated patient care. Nonetheless, training and refreshing alone are not sufficient unless records are kept that document them, preferably on standardized forms. Detailed notes should be made of dates, names of rescuers attending, and procedures performed. Rescue groups should keep equipment logs that specify the date, type, and duration of equipment use, especially in the case of ropes. Equipment should be retired before it becomes unreliable. Following these guidelines may well prevent liability-incurring incidents in the first place.

GENERAL PROCEDURES FOR HANDLING DEATH

Non-highway-related fatalities in the outdoors are uncommon but not rare. In remote areas, a serious illness or injury is more likely to result in death because of the necessary delay in obtaining expert medical help. Every member of a backcountry rescue group is apt to see at least one fatality during his or her career. Hunters, cavers, kayakers, scuba divers, climbers, and practitioners of similar hazardous sports may see fatalities as well.

The death rate in wilderness backpacking is very low. The rate in alpine skiing is around 0.2 per 100,000 skier visits, which compares favorably with death rates in football of 2 per 100,000 participants, in water sports of 5 per 100,000, and in highway deaths of 27 per 100,000. Death rates in nordic skiing and ski mountaineering are probably lower than in alpine skiing; the informal nature of these activities makes data collection difficult.

Outdoor, off-highway traumatic deaths most often result from head or chest injuries caused by incidents such as falls, snowmobile and all-terrain-vehicle accidents, and collisions while boating or skiing. Deaths also may be caused by hypothermia, drowning, avalanche burial, lightning strikes, and medical illnesses such as heart attack, acute mountain sickness, pneumonia, and stroke. Although actual pronouncement of death can be made only by a physician or other legally constituted authority, a rescuer can tell from a properly performed patient assessment whether death has likely occurred or is obvious.

Factors to consider in assessing the likelihood of death include:
1. The mechanism of injury may have been such that a lethal injury would be anticipated, or the death may have been preceded by a period of obviously severe illness with the symptoms of pneumonia, heart attack, pulmonary or cerebral edema, or serious infection.
2. Signs of death can be divided into **early** and **late**. Remember that the hypothermic or near-drowning patient may look dead and still be salvageable.
   a. Early signs
      (1) Evidence of lethal injury such as decapitation, severe head injury, massive evisceration, consumption of the body by fire, or a severing injury of the trunk.
      (2) Careful assessment shows no respirations, pulse, or detectable heartbeat over a period of several minutes.
      (3) No response to painful stimuli.
      (4) Widely dilated pupils that do not respond to light.
      (5) Pale, cool skin, blue lips and nails.
      (6) Rapidly glazing eyes.
      (7) Relaxed body sphincters, evacuation of body wastes.

b. Late signs
  (1) Rigid limbs and trunk (rigor mortis). Inability to straighten bent body parts (also may occur in cases of severe hypothermia).
  (2) Mottled, bluish or purple skin, especially the dependent parts (parts closest to the surface on which the body is lying).
  (3) Odor of decay (may be difficult to distinguish from odors caused by incontinent bowels in someone who is still alive).

Because of differences in state and local laws, every rescue group should work with the local coroner and law enforcement authorities to establish procedures for handling a death, and every group member should be familiar with these procedures. The laws of many states prohibit moving a body or anything associated with the death until authorized by a coroner. This is especially important in the case of death from trauma or when a criminal act is suspected. Failure to obey these laws may be a criminal offense. Backcountry rescue organizations in particular should consult with the coroner ahead of time regarding guidelines for handling a body when death occurs in the backcountry and terrain or weather will prevent timely examination of the scene by the authorities.

At a ski area, the area management and local authorities should be involved with the development of procedures for handling a death. These procedures should be available in the first aid room. In general, the following people should be notified:

1. A physician associated with the local patrol, if available. He or she can pronounce the patient dead.
2. The area management.
3. The local U.S. Forest Service or National Park Service representative, if the ski area is on Forest Service or National Park Service land.
4. The county sheriff or coroner.

A person who dies in the first aid room should be covered with a blanket and screened from curious onlookers.

If death occurs in a remote area, rescuers should remember that what they see will never be seen again in the same way. Detailed documentation is necessary both to satisfy the law and for insurance and estate settlement purposes. Also, there is always a potential for learning from the episode to prevent similar problems in the future. Painstaking records should be kept of all aspects of the death scene; records should include the preparation of written reports, diagrams, maps, and photographs, with dates and times noted. Photographs should be taken of the general area as well as the death scene to orient authorities to the overall picture. Close-up photos should be taken from no nearer than three feet and, in daylight, should be taken both with and without flash attachments to record details more accurately. If the commission of a criminal act is suspected, the sheriff or other appropriate authority should be notified before the death scene is disturbed, if at all possible.

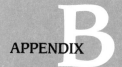

Wilderness Emergency Care Module

On the pitiless slabs of the Nordwand
Where the bivouac sites are few
The Ghosts of the hosts of Old Masters
Are calling this warning to you:
Live it up, fill your cup, drown your sorrow
And sow your wild oats while ye may
For the toothless old tykes of tomorrow
Were the Tigers of Yesterday.

> —Tom Patey, M.D.
> "The Last of the Grand Old Masters"

This module has been prepared as a guide for wilderness travelers, including members of recreational parties, wilderness search and rescue (SAR) teams, mountain rescue groups, and nordic ski patrols. For these purposes, wilderness means any area where modern man is forced to leave behind most of the complex, urban technology that keeps us comfortable and functional. Ancient man lived his life in the wilderness; civilized man, who enters the wilderness only occasionally and for short periods of time, is forced to relearn the knowledge and techniques that enabled his ancestors to survive there.

When most people hear the word "wilderness," they envision thick woods or high, snow-covered mountains. Wilderness also can mean arctic ice, subarctic tundra, desert, seashore, tropical savannah or rain forest, ocean, the underwater world, caverns, and remote, surging rivers.

Exposure to the wilderness may be brief or prolonged. In a sense, an alpine skier caught in a blizzard on a mountaintop is in the wilderness, but only briefly unless he or she strays outside the ski area boundaries. Nordic skiers or hikers out for a day trip are in the wilderness for a time, as are cavers in a deep cavern, rafters on a remote river, scuba divers in the depths, pilots downed in the desert, or mountaineers on the heights. Small-boat sailors, inhabitants of isolated villages, and victims of urban disasters whose electricity is cut off and medical facilities and communications have been destroyed all can be said to be in wilderness.

Successful wilderness existence requires a respect for the forces of nature and at least minimal training and equipment. Rescuers who operate in nonurban areas also need training in wilderness emergency care. The basics of this care are presented in foregoing sections of this text. In most cases, the emergency care of illnesses and injuries in the wilderness is fundamentally similar to outdoor emergency care anywhere. Most differences arise because the rescuer has to care for the patient over a longer period of time, during which the illness or injury may evolve or be modified by the environment.

Rescuers should already have mastered the contents of the preceding sections on basic outdoor emergency care. The information in this module is designed mainly for the reader's personal edification and protection. *Some of this information goes far beyond what rescuers are legally authorized to do at the present time unless they are physicians or physician's assistants. This is particularly true of the sections on the use of prescription drugs and the reduction of dislocations.* Procedures such as inserting Foley catheters, performing cricothyroidotomies, and using a McSwain dart are reserved for those trained to the paramedic level. They are mentioned here because they are basically simple procedures that require minimal equipment and their risk is outweighed by their value in saving lives or relieving distress. *Even though these procedures are medically correct, their inclusion does not imply endorsement by the National Ski Patrol of procedures or practices that go beyond the usual levels of emergency care described in the body of this text.*

Wilderness emergency care differs from the outdoor emergency care described in the preceding sections of this text in the following ways:

1. It is practiced in the wilderness environment, where extreme conditions of heat, cold, altitude, and storm are common and difficulties in

obtaining food, water, and shelter are significant. Dangers such as snow avalanches, rockfalls, flash floods, forest fires, and lightning may be present. Hazardous microorganisms, insects, marine animals, land animals, and plants may endanger the health of wilderness travelers, and preexisting medical conditions may recur or flare up at awkward times.

2. Definitive medical care may be many hours or days away because of distance, adverse environmental conditions, lack of transportation, or difficulties in communication.

3. Illnesses rarely seen elsewhere, such as acute mountain sickness and deep frostbite, may develop.

4. It may be desirable to train intelligent laypeople to carry out advanced procedures for common injuries and illnesses in which a delay in treatment of more than a few hours or days may cause adverse effects.

5. Rescuers should learn basic care of an injured or ill person so they can provide for the patient's ordinary day-to-day requirements until medical assistance can be reached.

Wilderness emergency care can be rendered on several levels of complexity and sophistication. The simplest level is self-help first aid for recreational wilderness groups carrying limited emergency equipment and relying on improvisation. The next level is SAR emergency care, in which rescuers trained to the advanced EMT or paramedic level may be available and rescue kits may include more complex and sophisticated equipment. The highest level is expeditionary emergency care and care given by paramedics in isolated villages. In these situations, personnel are highly trained, medical equipment usually is sophisticated, and there is less emphasis on choosing equipment based on its portability.

To apply Otto von Bismarck's comment on politics to the inherent nature of wilderness travel, wilderness emergency care is "the art of the possible." Rescuers cannot carry the equivalent of a well-equipped hospital emergency room on their backs; instead, they must make do with carefully chosen but limited equipment and rely on thorough training, ingenuity, and their ability to improvise. Patients who are seriously ill or injured may die despite the best care provided in a modern hospital. Thus, rescuers should have a realistic view of their limitations, while at the same time resolving to keep skills sharp and do their best at all times.

Because rescuers who are prepared for potential wilderness hazards can avoid many otherwise inevitable difficulties, prevention is emphasized in previous sections of this text and in this appendix. Enjoyment of the wilderness is enhanced by the knowledge that one has the training to prevent many problems and to deal successfully with those that are unpreventable. Regardless of preparation and training, if a member of a wilderness party is significantly ill or injured, the trip must be aborted and the patient evacuated.

Each member of a wilderness party should start out in good general health, in good physical condition, and free of acute or chronic infectious disease. If health questions arise, the party leader should require a physician's certificate of physical ability sufficient for the level of anticipated physical stress. Many minor physical abnormalities and illnesses can be controlled sufficiently to allow wilderness travel. These conditions include mild hypertension, minor valvular heart disease, hay fever, asthma, diabetes, and similar ailments.

Other conditions are relative or absolute contraindications to wilderness travel because the condition may flare up under the stress of high altitude or long hours on the trail, and/or be difficult to treat in isolated circumstances. These conditions include active peptic ulcers; known kidney, bladder, or gallbladder stones; coronary artery disease; chronic obstructive pulmonary disease; metastatic malignancy; a history of severe, recurrent high altitude illness; and disabilities of the musculoskeletal system such as recurrent, severe back pain and severe knee and hip joint disease. Even in its mild form, sickle cell anemia is a contraindication to high altitude travel and a relative contraindication to severe physical exertion. In borderline or questionable situations, consult a physician familiar with wilderness medical problems.

The party leader should know if any party members have significant health impairments or take any medicines regularly. People who regularly take tranquilizers, antidepressants, beta blockers, and anticholinergics may be more susceptible to wilderness stresses. Beta blockers are mentioned in particular because they are commonly used to treat high blood pressure and can cause chronic fatigue, depression, and deconditioning, with poor exercise tolerance and poor recovery from strenuous exercise.

People who have had anaphylactic reactions to foods, drugs, or arthropod stings should carry emergency kits containing adrenalin and an antihistamine. At least one other party member should know how to use these kits. Those who wear prescription eyeglasses should carry a spare pair, and contact lens wearers should carry a pair of regular glasses as well. Contact lenses can actually freeze to the eyeballs under severe winter conditions.

Routine immunizations, particularly tetanus, should be up-to-date.

PATIENT ASSESSMENT IN THE WILDERNESS

Patient assessment is the same in the wilderness as in the outdoors in general, except that extreme environmental conditions may delay detailed assessment until the patient has reached shelter. Rescuers should be thoroughly familiar with the assessment of both injured and ill patients, as described in Chapters 4 and 17.

CPR IN THE WILDERNESS

Guidelines for starting or stopping CPR are discussed in Chapter 5. These guidelines, while reasonable and proper in an *urban* environment, might not be suitable in a remote, outdoor environment. Eisenberg and associates studied the rate of survival for patients in cardiac arrest from ventricular fibrillation relative to the length of time before basic life support (BLS) and advanced cardiac life support (ACLS) were started. Their findings, reported in the *Journal of the American Medical Association* (241:1905, 1979) indicate that the survival rate is only 10 percent if it takes more than 16 minutes to start advanced life support, even if basic life support is started within four minutes. If BLS is started after more than eight minutes and ACLS after more than 16 minutes, there is no chance of survival.

		Time to Advanced Cardiac Life Support % Survival Rate		
		<8 Min.	8-16 Min.	>16 Min.
Time to Basic Life Support	< 4 Min.	43%	19%	10%
	4-8 Min.	27%	19%	6%
	>8 Min.	7%	0%	

In a remote situation, where advanced life support assistance may be many hours or days away, CPR may have *no* chance of success. In addition, administering CPR under wilderness conditions may put group members in serious danger because of physical hazards and exhaustion.

Based on the above data, several suggestions regarding CPR in remote areas can be made. Even though these suggestions seem reasonable, they should be viewed as tentative and without legal force. At the current time, a rescuer who begins CPR probably is legally obligated to continue unless or until one of the five conditions listed in Chapter 5 are fulfilled.

In a remote environment, giving CPR is useless and probably should not be started if:

1. The patient is in cardiac arrest caused by trauma.
2. The patient is a drowning victim who has been immersed for over an hour.
3. The patient is in cardiac arrest and advanced life support is more than an hour away, especially if the patient must be carried out.
4. The patient experienced unwitnessed cardiac arrest and the time of onset is unknown.
5. The patient appears to be dead, based on rigor mortis (stiffening) or livor mortis (discoloration of the body parts next to the ground), lethal injuries, or a body temperature below 60°F (16°C).
6. Giving CPR would be hazardous to rescuers.

Moreover, after 30 minutes of CPR with no sign of life, further CPR probably is useless and may reasonably be discontinued. Giving CPR to a patient who is being evacuated by litter or toboggan is very difficult, if not impossible. Unless an ambulance or helicopter can be brought in rapidly, chances of survival are small.

Exceptions include patients in cardiac arrest caused by hypothermia per se; patients with another illness or injury complicated by hypothermia (avalanche burial and near drowning in cold water), and patients in cardiac or respiratory arrest caused by lightning injury (see Chapter 19). In these cases, the outlook is probably more favorable and CPR should be given aggressively.

EXTENDED PATIENT CARE IN THE WILDERNESS

In addition to requiring specific care for illnesses and injuries, patients in the wilderness have certain basic requirements for survival, which for the most part rescuers in the wilderness share.

Basic Wilderness Survival Requirements

1. Oxygen.
2. Shelter and maintenance of normal body temperature.
3. Water.
4. Food.
5. Psychological support.
6. Assistance with natural processes such as urination and defecation.
7. Basic faith and the will to live.

Attention to these requirements will ensure the patient is in the best possible physical condition during stabilization and transport to definitive medical care.

The initial care of an ill or injured person is no different in the wilderness than anywhere else. While the primary survey is performed and urgent conditions are treated as described in Chapters 4 and 5, other party members are constructing a shelter and preparing to stabilize the patient's body temperature (Fig. B.1).

In cold weather, insulation is placed beneath and around the patient, the patient's head is covered, and wet clothing is replaced with dry clothing. Rescuers also will lay out a sleeping bag, start a fire or stove, and set up a tent or prepare a snow shelter. In hot weather, a tarp or other shelter is rigged as protection against the sun and a cool surface for the patient to lie on is pre-

Fig. B.1 *Caring for an injured person in the wilderness includes constructing a shelter and stabilizing the patient's body temperature.*

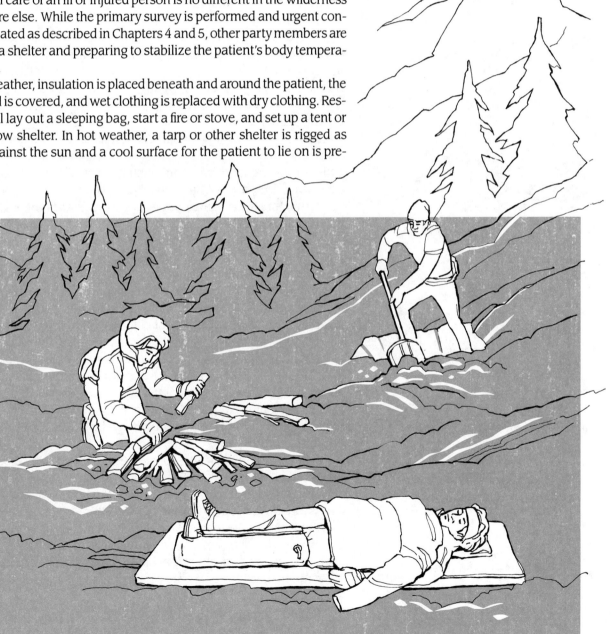

Fig. B.1

pared by either scraping away the upper 6 inches of hot earth or by building a platform with backpacks or natural materials. Clothing is added or subtracted as appropriate to protect the patient against the sun or to lower the body temperature.

The mechanisms for stabilizing body temperature are always impaired by illness or injury, so that both hypothermia and hyperthermia can develop more easily in a patient than in a healthy person. The rescue party must look out for its own safety, since party members are subject to the same environmental stresses as the patient.

After urgent problems are cared for and the patient's body temperature is stabilized, less urgent problems are treated and the secondary survey is performed so that nothing is missed. In cold weather, expose one small body area at a time for examination.

Dietary requirements are discussed in Chapter 1. Normal daily fluid requirements may increase substantially at high altitude, in hot weather, or when the patient has heavy sweating, vomiting, diarrhea, or extensive burns. Give fluids such as plain water, soup, bouillon, or flavored fruit drinks. Because caffeine is a diuretic, caffeine-containing beverages such as tea, cocoa, and coffee may increase fluid loss through the kidneys, thereby contributing to dehydration.

Do not give anything by mouth to patients who are unconscious, have abdominal injuries, or are to have surgery within six to eight hours. When a patient is losing large amounts of fluid because of vomiting, diarrhea, or extensive burns, at least half of the fluid given by mouth should be an electrolyte mixture such as half-strength Gatorade or bouillon. Try to roughly measure the amount of fluid lost because of vomiting or diarrhea and to replace the lost fluid volume-for-volume with electrolyte solutions.

The World Health Organization recommends a standard electrolyte replacement solution for diarrheal illness, designed for use in underdeveloped countries where such illnesses are endemic. This solution, called Oralyte, contains 90 milliequivalents of sodium, 20 milliequivalents of potassium, 80 milliequivalents of chloride, 30 milliequivalents of bicarbonate, and 111 millimoles of glucose per liter. It is prepared by mixing 3.5 grams of table salt, 2.5 grams of bicarbonate of soda, 1.5 grams of potassium chloride (available in many pharmacies), and 20 grams of glucose in a liter of water just before use. The solution can be flavored to taste with small amounts of lemon extract or other flavoring agents. Packets containing the right proportions of these compounds can be made up beforehand and carried in first aid kits.

In patients with diarrhea, fluid losses are sometimes lessened by giving drugs that control diarrhea by slowing the motility of the bowel (see **Stomach and Bowel Problems**, below). Patients who are vomiting because of an illness that does not interfere greatly with stomach or bowel function, such as altitude illness, headache, or mild gastroenteritis, may be able to eat and drink if vomiting can be controlled with an antivomiting suppository such as thiethylperazine (Torecan) or prochlorperazine (Compazine). However, people vomiting because of a head or abdominal injury should not take these drugs or be given anything by mouth.

Some SAR groups include members who are trained and licensed to give intravenous fluids, which are very useful in these circumstances. An average daily IV prescription for a patient unable to eat or drink is 2,500 milliliters of 5-percent glucose in one-half-percent physiological saline solution with 20 milliequivalents potassium chloride added per liter. Estimate additional fluid losses from vomiting or diarrhea and replace the lost fluid volume-for-volume with this solution or with lactated Ringer's solution. In most cases, normal kidneys select what the body needs and excrete the remainder.

Collect and measure the volume of the daily urine output of all patients. If urine output is less than 500 milliliters (17 ounces) per 24 hours, the patient probably is dehydrated and needs more fluid. Urine normally is light yellow when hydration is adequate, but it may be orange-colored in patients with severe illness or injury, cola-colored in patients who have liver disease with jaundice, and bright yellow in people who take vitamin tablets containing riboflavin (Vitamin B2).

Liquids are a more urgent requirement than food, because a previously healthy person can go without eating for many days without permanent damage. Invalids who are able to tolerate solid food should eat a light, bland diet with no spicy or rich foods. Oatmeal, Cream of Wheat, bland soup, broth, gelatin, bread, hard candy and sweet tea usually are well tolerated. The invalid should be allowed to eat as desired and not be forced to eat.

Provisions must be made so that the patient can urinate and defecate. A wide-mouth screw-top polyethylene bottle ("pee bottle") of a 500- to 1,000-milliliter capacity can be used as a urinal. SAR teams can carry lightweight commercially marketed plastic urinals. Patients can defecate in the supine position if they are placed on an Ensolite pad with a hole cut in it, or on carefully arranged clothing, and positioned over a hole dug in the ground or snow. Always ask patients whether they have to urinate or defecate and allow them to do so *before* they are packaged in a litter or on a spine board. Unconscious or severely injured patients may be unable to urinate. Members of SAR groups and expeditions are encouraged to obtain the special training necessary to insert a Foley catheter. Foley catheters should be included in SAR first aid kits. If a catheter is unavailable, nothing can be done except to evacuate the patient with a pee bottle or urinal lying in place to catch urine that may be voided spontaneously.

Adequate pain relief is necessary for humanitarian reasons and to prevent shock. Serious wilderness travelers may wish to have their physician prescribe pain medicines such as acetaminophen with codeine (Tylenol with codeine) meperidine (Demerol), or propoxyphene with acetaminophen (Darvocet-N) so that small amounts of these drugs can be carried for personal use. As with all drugs in first aid kits, the containers should be labeled with the name of the medicine, the rescuer's name, the physician's name, directions for use, and the expiration date. The medication should be first tried at home to ensure that it is effective and does not cause undesirable side effects. Current state and federal regulations do not allow a rescuer to give these drugs to patients unless the rescuer is a licensed EMT or paramedic under physician supervision. However, patients can take such drugs under their *own* responsibility.

For extended wilderness trips and expeditions, injectable pain medication is useful but must be administered by an individual who is trained and authorized to inject it. Wyeth Laboratories markets codeine, meperidine and morphine in prefilled, single-dose Tubex containers. These pain drugs should not be given to persons with head injuries or high altitude cerebral edema (HACE).

Rescuers must not let reliance on pain medication lead them to neglect pain-reducing first aid procedures such as aligning and splinting fractures and dislocations.

Adhere to the usual habits of cleanliness and sanitation as closely as possible in the wilderness. Carry soap, preferably the biodegradable kind, and use it to wash your hands after a bowel movement, after handling vomitus, feces and other secretions of a patient, before dressing open wounds, and before cooking and eating. If soap is unavailable, wash hands in plain water or snow.

All first aid kits should include disposable rubber gloves so that rescuers can avoid direct contact with a patient's secretions.

Defecate *downhill* from and as far as possible *away* from camp, drinking water sources, or snow to be melted for water. Bury feces and burn used toilet paper. Do not camp closer than 100 feet from a water source such as a lake, stream, or spring.

Providing the patient with psychological support (see Chapter 4) is extremely important to reinforce faith and the will to live and to encourage optimism, patience, and cooperation. Discuss plans for emergency care, evacuation, etc., out of the patient's hearing. Attendants should remain calm, unhurried, unharried and deliberate, and should avoid the appearance of indecision, pessimism, fear, or panic. The general situation can be discussed with the patient, adhering to the principle of "emphasizing the doughnut and not the hole." Warn the patient in advance if any unpleasant or painful procedures are to be performed.

Decisions on whether to attempt an evacuation using the party's efforts alone or to send for help will depend on the weather, party size, available equipment, distance involved, the patient's condition, and the availability of local SAR groups, helicopters, and other assistance. Stabilize the patient before he or she is moved. As a general rule, the best course of action is to make a comfortable camp and send for help, unless the weather is excellent, the party is strong and well equipped, the route is short and easy, and the patient is comfortable and stable. Send the two strongest party members for help, and perhaps have them take along any party members who are demoralized or otherwise a liability. If the party is so small that it will be necessary to leave a patient alone so help can be summoned, leave an adequate supply of food, fuel, and water within the patient's reach.

WILDERNESS INJURIES

Wilderness injury management follows the same basic principles as management of any injury, except for certain modifications necessary to avoid infection, restricted circulation, or other complications during the time needed for evacuation. Repeatedly monitor circulation of an injured extremity to detect changes caused by swelling and tight splinting. Reduced circulation introduces the danger of gangrene and frostbite. Maintain the injured patient's normal body temperature.

Lacerations and Other Open Wounds

In the wilderness, improperly treated open wounds can partially immobilize a patient because of pain, stiffness, swelling, and infection, making self-evacuation difficult. All open wounds should be cleaned to prevent infection (see Chapter 8); smaller wounds can be closed with butterfly bandages or sterile tape, while large wounds should be bandaged open. If at all possible, avoid wrapping tape completely around an extremity. If the extremity swells, the tape will cause a tourniquet-like effect. Antibiotics are recommended to prevent infection in patients with very large or contaminated wounds (see **Antibiotics**, below). The patient should consider getting a tetanus booster injection as soon as medical help is reached (see Chapter 8).

Fractures

The proper first aid for any fracture is splinting. Because of weight considerations, few wilderness travelers are able to carry a large variety of premade splints. Splinting material usually must be improvised from natural materials, ski poles, ice axes, ice hammers, and parts of packs such as hip pads and shoulder straps (see Chapter 9 and Fig. 9.10). Wire splints and air splints are lightweight and easy to carry, especially by large parties and SAR groups. Below timberline, tree branches and small trees can be cut and used for improvised splints. Uninjured body parts can act as splints, i.e., a fractured upper arm can be splinted against the chest wall with a sling and swathe, and a fractured hip can be splinted by tying both lower extremities together. A spine board can be made from two skis tied side by side with crosspieces, and an extrication collar can be improvised from a tightly rolled vest or jacket. A patient with an open fracture should take antibiotics (see **Antibiotics**, below) in addition to receiving the care described in Chapter 9.

The most marked modification of traditional splinting in the wilderness involves the emergency care of a fractured femur (Fig. B.2). The standard emergency care for a midshaft femur fracture is traction splinting, but traction applied to a boot for more than a few hours can cause pressure damage to the ankle tissues.

Therefore, unless evacuation time will be short, remove the patient's boot and socks, roll up the pant leg or open it with a seam ripper, and apply a strip of 2-inch-wide adhesive tape from just below the knee down one side of the leg, under the sole of the foot, and then up the other side of the leg so that a stirrup is formed. Next, wrap the leg from toes to knee with an elastic bandage, making sure that the bandage is firm but not too tight. Insert a piece of wood into the stirrup as a spreader to keep pressure off the sides of the ankle. After this, apply a Thomas type of traction splint as described in Chapter 9. Because the stirrup prohibits replacing the sock on the foot, keep the foot warm by wrapping it in a spare jacket. Unwrap the jacket at regular intervals to inspect the toes for warmth and movement.

A Sager splint, Kendrick traction device or Hare splint with a special ankle hitch made of wide nylon webbing is less likely to injure the ankle tissues if the ankle hitch is applied over the sock with the boot off. Nevertheless, the ankle hitches supplied with these devices are probably more likely to injure the ankle tissues than the traction method described above.

Fig. B.2 *Modified Traction Splinting Technique for a Fractured Femur*

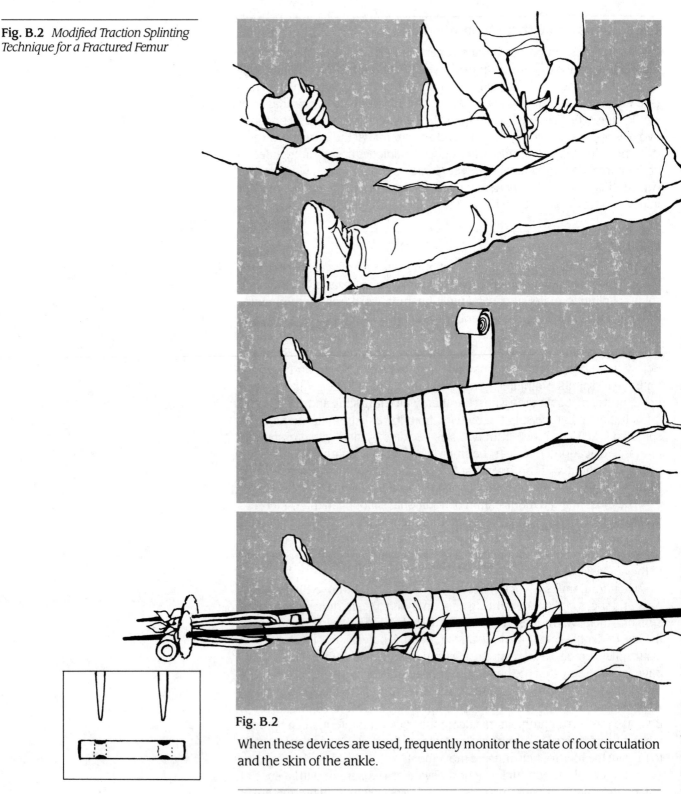

Fig. B.2

When these devices are used, frequently monitor the state of foot circulation and the skin of the ankle.

Dislocations

Standard teaching in this text, as endorsed by the National Ski Patrol, is to treat a dislocation as a fracture, splinting it in the position found without attempting to straighten or align it unless there is interference with circulation or nerve supply. However, a dislocation usually is more painful than a fracture and causes considerable pressure on joint cartilage and other structures, resulting in additional injury and possible permanent disability.

When a dislocation is splinted in the position found, ligaments and tendons are stretched more and circulation is more often impaired than when a fracture is splinted this way. Thus, when medical help is more than a few hours away, there is considerable justification for attempting to align a dislocation so that normal anatomy is restored. Alignment usually provides marked pain relief, makes it much easier to evacuate the patient, and may prevent a great deal of future disability. This type of alignment is called **relocation** of the dislocation. If one attempt at relocation is unsuccessful or causes severe pain, abandon further attempts and splint the dislocation in the most comfortable position.

Relocation works best if it can be done immediately after the dislocation occurs, before the injured part stiffens, and while it is still numb. Otherwise, the patient should take a dose of pain medication, and relocation should be delayed until the medication has had time to work (45 minutes to one hour).

Shoulder Dislocations

In the wilderness, the shoulder is the most commonly dislocated joint; the injury usually is an anterior dislocation (see Chapter 11). Circulation and nerve function should be checked and documented before and after any attempt at alignment. Several methods are available for relocating a simple shoulder dislocation if there is no associated fracture.

The examiner carefully puts several fingers into the patient's armpit. The head of the humerus, which feels like a ball, usually can be palpated. The examiner then moves the extremity slightly. A grating sound or feeling means a fracture also is present. If there is any possibility of a fracture, do *not* attempt to relocate the dislocation; splint it as described in Chapter 11. Fortunately, fracture-dislocations of the shoulder are quite rare in young, healthy persons.

An excellent and safe method for relocating a dislocated shoulder is to have the patient lie prone on an elevated platform such as a large, flat rock or log, high enough to allow the injured extremity to hang free. Tie a 10-pound weight to the patient's wrist (Fig. B.3). The gradual pull usually will relocate the shoulder within one to one-and-one-half hours. If an elevated platform is unavailable, try the following method (Fig. B.4):

The patient sits on the ground with the rescuer kneeling, facing the patient's injured side. An assistant sits behind the patient opposite the rescuer and anchors the patient by wrapping both arms or a sling around the patient's chest. The rescuer ties two cravats together to make a large loop and slips the loop around his or her waist. The loop should be large enough so that it can be pulled out in front of the waist about a foot. The rescuer then grasps the patient's injured upper extremity in both hands and flexes the patient's elbow to a right angle. The loop around the rescuer's waist is slipped over the patient's hand and worked down to where it is just distal to the bend of the elbow. Keeping the patient's forearm bent with both hands, the rescuer slowly leans backward while the assistant applies countertraction in the opposite direction. The shoulder should slip back into place, frequently with an audible pop. The patient often sighs with relief as the pain disappears.

When no help is available, self-relocation of a dislocated shoulder may

Fig. B.3 *Relocating a Dislocated Shoulder by Gravity*

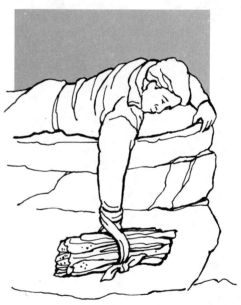

Fig. B.3

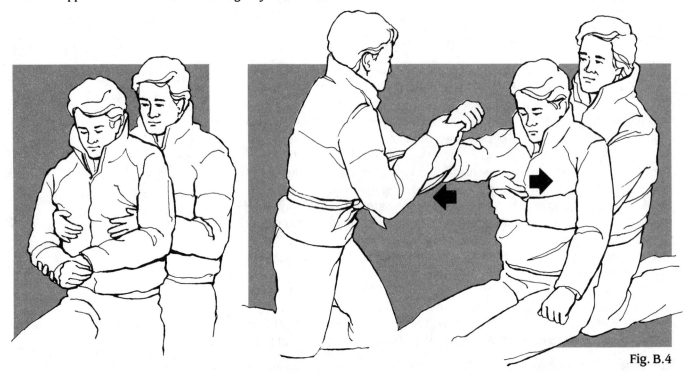

Fig. B.4

Fig. B.4 *Emergency Technique of Relocating a Dislocated Shoulder Using Two Rescuers*

be successful if done immediately. The method is as follows (Fig. B.5):

The injured person sits on the ground with the knees bent, locking both hands together around the knees. The person then slowly leans back and straightens the hips. With luck, the shoulder slips back into place.

After relocation, the injured extremity should be immobilized with a sling and swathe until medical help is obtained, or for a minimum of three days.

Elbow Dislocations

When an elbow is dislocated, the forearm usually is dislocated backward on the upper arm, producing a marked deformity with the point of the elbow much further back than it should be. The circulation and nerve supply of the forearm and hand frequently are damaged. To relocate a dislocated elbow, the rescuer pulls steadily on the forearm with the elbow partially flexed while an assistant holds the upper arm tightly.

Finger Dislocations

To relocate a dislocated finger, the rescuer uses the thumb and forefinger to firmly hold the part of the patient's finger proximal to the dislocation. With the other hand, the rescuer partly flexes the finger distal to the dislocation while pulling on it and pushing the base of the dislocated part back into position (Fig. B.6).

Hip Dislocations

Attempting to relocate a dislocated hip in the field is justifiable since a prolonged hip dislocation frequently leads to death of the head of the femur because its blood supply is interrupted. The most common type of hip dislocation is a posterior dislocation. The lower extremity is characteristically bent at the hip, rotated inward, and adducted. Attempts to move the hip are very painful. The technique is as follows (Fig. B.7):

An assistant straddles the patient, facing the patient's feet, and places one hand on each side of the front of the pelvis to provide countertraction. The rescuer straddles the leg on the patient's injured side, holding it tightly between his or her legs, and gently bends the patient's knee to 90 degrees. The rescuer bends his or her own knees slightly and tightly grasps the back of the patient's leg just below the knee with locked hands. Next, the rescuer exerts steady traction in an upward direction by straightening his or her knees, while the assistant leans hard on the patient's pelvis. After relocation, put padding between the knees and ankles, tie the lower extremities together, and transport the patient on a spine board.

Patella Dislocations

In the case of a patella dislocation, ask the patient to bend the hip to a right angle, which will relax the quadriceps muscle on the front of the thigh. The rescuer then gently straightens the knee while pushing the patella back toward its normal location at the front of the knee joint.

Knee Dislocations

Great force is required to dislocate a knee because of its strong ligamentous and muscular attachments. Most of the major ligaments of the knee must be torn for the joint to dislocate. A dislocated knee usually is unstable, and the circulation and nerve supply usually are impaired. Amputation will likely be necessary if the knee cannot be reduced within six to eight hours. Therefore, there is considerable reason to attempt relocation in a wilderness setting.

Relocation consists of simple axial traction to realign the joint so that the leg and foot are in the most normal position possible. Immobilize the extremity in a long-leg fixation splint, and monitor and document circulation and nerve supply at 15-minute intervals. If either are compromised, remove the splint and realign the injury in the position that gives the strongest pulse.

Ankle Dislocations

A dislocation of the ankle is almost always a fracture-dislocation; impairment of the circulation and nerve supply are the main danger. Relocation consists of simple axial traction (Fig. B.8) and immobilizing the extremity in the most natural position with a fixation splint. Monitor and document circulation and nerve supply at 15-minute intervals after relocation. If either are compromised, remove the splint and realign the injury in the position that gives the strongest pulse.

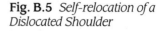

Fig. B.5 *Self-relocation of a Dislocated Shoulder*

Fig. B.6 *Technique of Relocating a Dislocated Finger*

Fig. B.7 *Technique of Relocating a Dislocated Hip*

Fig. B.8 *Technique of Relocating a Dislocated Ankle*

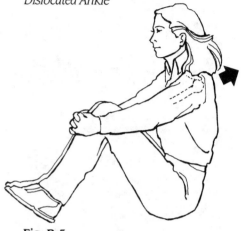

Fig. B.5

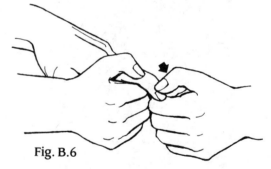

Fig. B.6

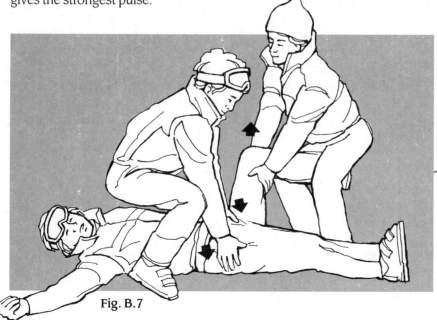

Fig. B.7

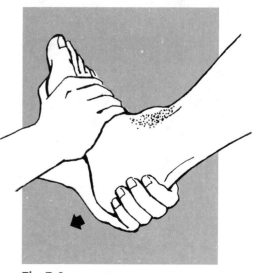

Fig. B.8

Fig. B.9 *An adhesive tape boot can support a sprained ankle.*

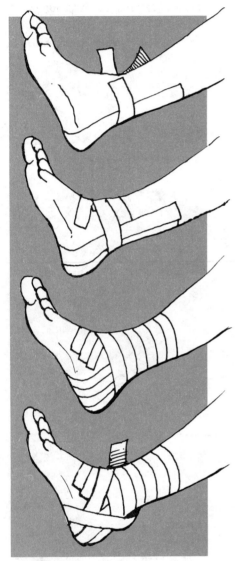

Fig. B.9

Sprains

The standard assessment and emergency care for an ankle sprain is discussed in Chapter 12. Under wilderness conditions, a patient with an ankle sprain may have to self-evacuate. A sturdy hiking, mountaineering, or telemark boot alone may provide the necessary support, but an adhesive-tape boot (Fig. B.9) usually is needed to stabilize the sprain enough to allow walking.

Hold the patient's foot at a right angle and apply overlapping vertical and horizontal strips of tape that are 1-inch wide and 20 to 30 inches long. Run vertical strips from the lower leg on the *uninjured* side across the sole of the foot and up the opposite side of the ankle; run horizontal strips from the top of the foot around the back of the heel to the other side of the top of the foot. Alternate application of the vertical and horizontal strips.

Continue taping until most of the ankle, lower leg, and posterior two-thirds of the foot are covered. Conclude with a figure-of-eight wrap around the ankle, heel, and arch to stabilize the arch and provide additional heel stabilization. Then replace the patient's boot on the foot. Usually the patient will need one less sock on the injured foot because of the thickness of the tape. It is less painful to remove the tape if it is peeled off *from top to bottom*.

Injuries to the Head, Spine, Chest, Abdomen, and Pelvis; Multiple Injuries

Rockfall accidents, falls while climbing, and high-speed skiing accidents can cause multiple injuries similar to those seen in motor-vehicle accidents. Serious head, neck, back, chest, abdominal, pelvic, and extremity injuries can occur singly or in various combinations, sorely taxing the emergency care skills of rescuers. The immediate care of these injuries is the same as described in Chapters 5, 8, 9, and 22 and in the chapters on specific injuries. Give the patient oxygen, if available. Antibiotics and intravenous fluids also should be given if trained personnel are available.

It is useful to have the ability to insert an endotracheal tube or to insert a tube into the trachea through the cricothyroid membrane (cricothyroidotomy) when the upper airway cannot be opened by the usual measures described in Chapter 5. However, these skills require special training, licensing, and equipment.

Tension pneumothorax (see Chapter 15) is a lethal complication of chest injuries. The definitive treatment is to decompress the involved side of the chest by inserting a needle equipped with a one-way valve (McSwain dart, Heimlich valve). Rescuers must have special training, licensing, and equipment to perform this procedure.

A loop of bowel protruding through an open abdominal wound can be successfully replaced if discovered and treated *immediately*. Replace the loop as aseptically as possible and tape the wound shut. If much time has elapsed, the loop will swell and be impossible to replace. If this happens, cover the bowel with a clean, preferably sterile, cloth moistened with warm physiological saline solution, if available (Fig. 16.2). Otherwise, use the cleanest water possible and add half a teaspoon of salt per liter. All solutions used to keep the dressing moist should first be warmed to body temperature.

Do not move patients with serious injuries, especially head and spine injuries, without proper equipment. If proper equipment is unavailable, make the patient as comfortable as possible while someone goes for help.

Shock

In the wilderness, shock is most often caused by one of the following:
1. Loss of whole blood because of:
   a. Severe or uncontrolled external bleeding.
   b. Bleeding from a fractured femur, fractured pelvis, or multiple injuries.
   c. Internal bleeding, caused by a bleeding ulcer, rupture from an ectopic pregnancy, etc.
2. Loss of the fluid part of the blood because of:
   a. Severe vomiting or diarrhea.
   b. Extensive burns.
3. Heart attack.
4. Spinal cord injury.

These are all serious conditions for which there is no good field emergency care except for controlling external bleeding and replacing fluids lost by vomiting or diarrhea. The care given is designed to buy time until the patient can reach a hospital. When the patient has a condition commonly known to cause shock, anticipate shock and evacuate the patient before it actually develops, if possible.

In the hospital, a patient in shock is treated by replacing whole blood, plasma and fluid, and by correcting the condition that caused the shock. Many rescue groups have members who are trained and licensed to administer intravenous fluids. Although it is rarely possible or practical to transfuse whole blood in the field, rescue groups can carry intravenous fluids. Lactated Ringer's solution is the best standard intravenous preparation to carry for treating shock. In cold weather, intravenous preparations must be protected from freezing. This is frequently done by having rescuers carry the solution inside clothing against the body.

PASGs provide widely distributed direct pressure to control bleeding and redistribute blood volume from the body shell to the core. They are of value in the prehospital treatment of hypovolemic shock. PASGs are most useful in treating shock caused by pelvic fractures, multiple injuries, and intra-abdominal bleeding. Special training and licensing are required to use PASGs.

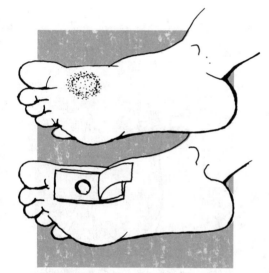

Fig. B.10

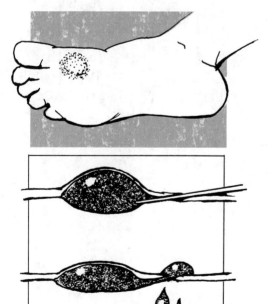

Fig. B.11

Minor Problems

Blisters

Blisters are annoying injuries produced when an ill-fitting boot or a wrinkled sock, for example, rubs repeatedly against the skin. Blisters are most common on the heels, toes, and soles of the feet. The best treatment is prevention. Always wear at least two pairs of socks; preferably a thin pair of polypropylene or silk socks next to the skin with one or two pairs of heavy wool socks over them. Cut the toenails before a trip and wear properly broken-in boots that are correctly fitted for length so that the toes will not jam against the inside of the boot during downhill walking.

Fig. B.12 *Technique of Draining a Subungual Hematoma*

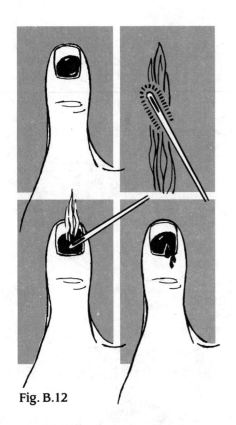

Fig. B.12

If a sore spot develops, immediately remove the boot and sock and look for a reddened area of skin. Overlay this area with four layers of 2-inch-wide tape or a piece of moleskin. Replace the socks, making sure they are not creased or wrinkled, and lace the boot snugly enough to keep the foot and especially the heel from moving around inside.

If a blister has already developed, protect it by overlaying it with several layers of tape. Cut holes slightly larger than the blister in the bottom layers (Fig. B.10). Occasionally, a blister has to be drained. Wash the skin with antiseptic soap, sterilize a needle over a flame, insert the needle under the skin about one-quarter of an inch from the edge of the blister, push it up into the blister, and withdraw it while pressing on the blister (Fig. B.11). After draining the blister, bandage it. Clean and dress a broken blister the same as any other open wound.

Subungual Hematoma

Subungual hematoma, or bleeding under the nail, usually is caused by a hard object such as a hammer striking the fingertip with enough force to break blood vessels underneath the nail. The pressure and consequent severe, throbbing pain of a subungual hematoma can be relieved by draining the hematoma.

Wash the fingertip with soap and water, and heat a piece of thin, rigid metal (e.g., a straightened paper clip or the blunt end of a needle) on a stove or over a candle flame (a match flame is not hot enough) until it is red-hot. Then firmly press the red-hot end into the nail at the center of the hematoma and allow it to burn through the nail (Fig. B.12). Maintain close control so that the hot object does not penetrate too far. A pop and sudden give means that the object is through the nail. When the object is withdrawn, it usually is followed by a drop of blood, and the pain is relieved. Bandage the nail with a Bandaid.

Jewelry Removal

Immediately remove any jewelry from an injured upper extremity. If a ring is not quickly removed and the finger swells, the ring will cause a tourniquet-like effect (Fig. B.13a). Swelling may be so great that the only way to remove the ring will be to cut it off. Fortunately, the following simple technique almost always works.

A small spool of strong thread is needed. Work several inches of the loose end under the ring and pull through. Starting just beyond the ring, wind the thread snugly around the finger, working toward the fingertip (Fig. B.13b). Each turn is made next to the previous one so that the finger is wrapped solidly from the ring over the next joint distally down to the midpoint of the next phalanx (Fig B.13c). Cut the thread at the spool end, leaving three or four inches of loose thread. Next, lubricate the finger with soapy water. Then pull the cut end in the direction of the fingertip (Fig. B.13d), causing the thread to unwind and to pull the ring over the joint and off the finger.

Fishhook Removal

There are two techniques for removing a fishhook embedded in the skin. If a wire cutter or heavy pair of scissors is available, the barbed end of the hook can be pushed up through the skin and cut off, allowing the hook to be backed out of the hole (Fig. B.14).

The second method consists of disengaging the barb of the hook from the tissues so that it can be directly backed out of the hole. This technique, recommended by expert fly fisherman Dr. Ron Loge of Dillon, Montana, has the advantage of not damaging a valuable fly.

First, loop a long piece of fishing line or other thin, strong line around the bend of the hook. Next, determine the exact location of the hook and the direction of penetration by rocking and rotating the hook gently, trying to find the position of least resistance. Then, while holding the hook in this position, apply very firm downward pressure on the shank of the hook directly over the barb and simultaneously push up on the eye of the hook. While maintaining pressure on the shank, release the eye and quickly pull on the looped line horizontally or at a slightly upward angle, to remove the hook. If the eye of the hook has broken off, remove the hook using a pair of pliers instead of a loop of line. Then, clean the wound with germicidal soap. The patient should receive tetanus prophylaxis as soon as possible.

This technique is unsuitable when a hook is imbedded in an area of the body where it is difficult to apply strong downward pressure on the shank, e.g., the sides of the neck, earlobes, and around the eyes. A hook cannot be removed by this method when the barb has already come through the skin. If the hook is in the eyeball itself, cut off the line at the base of the hook and take the patient to an ophthalmologist as soon as possible.

Skin Cracks

Small, painful skin cracks are annoyances that mainly affect the fingertips. Common in the winter and in dry climates, skin cracks can be prevented to some extent by liberal use of hand cream and by avoiding frequent hand washing.

A thick grease such as petrolatum (Vaseline) or Chapstick will speed healing. A more effective treatment is to squeeze the crack shut and apply a small amount of Super Glue or a similar product to seal the crack and protect the area while it heals. This type of glue is waterproof and difficult to remove. The glue will have to be reapplied every day or two because it eventually falls off as the surface area of skin is shed normally.

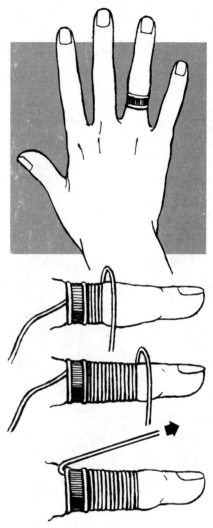

Fig. B.13 *Technique of Removing a Ring from a Swollen Finger*

Fig. B.14 *Fishhook Removal Technique*

Fig. B.13

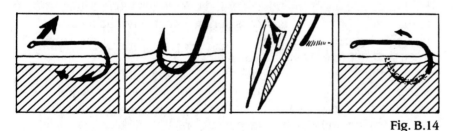

Fig. B.14

USE OF PRESCRIPTION DRUGS

Federal and state laws as well as National Ski Patrol policy prohibit laypeople from dispensing prescription drugs. Prescribing, dispensing, transporting, and/or using the prescription drugs described in this appendix may be illegal under various state and/or federal statutes. Criminal sanctions may apply, unless the drugs in the individual's possession have been prescribed for him or her by a physician and this fact is documented by labels that give the person's name, the physician's name, and directions for use.

Under certain conditions the proper drug may prevent serious illness or even loss of life. For this reason, wilderness travelers may wish to become familiar with the carefully selected drugs described in this appendix and possibly obtain these drugs by prescription from their physicians for inclusion in first aid kits for personal use. Prescription drugs should not be offered to patients. No one should take a drug to which he or she has a known allergy.

Cold Injuries

The prevention and emergency care of cold injuries are discussed in Chapters 1 and 19. The current recommendation for emergency care of a patient with frostbite is to leave blisters unopened and protect them from damage. However, blister fluid contains prostaglandins, thromboxane, and other substances that cause tissue damage. In the future, sterile aspiration of blister fluid with a syringe and needle may be recommended. There is some evidence that prostaglandin inhibitors such as ibuprofen (Advil, Nuprin, Motrin) may be beneficial in preventing some of the tissue damage associated with frostbite. Advil and Nuprin can be purchased in 200-milligram (mg) tablets without prescription. For greatest benefit, immediately begin taking the product in a dosage of two tablets four times daily if hazardous environmental conditions exist.

Diseases of Altitude

The prevention and care of altitude diseases are discussed in Chapter 19. A number of drugs have been advocated as having some use in preventing or treating acute mountain sickness. Medical oxygen is probably the most useful treatment. If available, give oxygen by mask at a rate of 4 to 8 liters per minute. Because oxygen supplies are always finite, simultaneously begin preparations for descent. Acetazolamide (Diamox), a carbonic anhydrase inhibitor, has definite value in preventing acute mountain sickness but is less useful in treating all but mild cases. It is particularly useful for preventing acute mountain sickness in rescuers who do not have time to ascend slowly. The dose is 250 mg by mouth every 12 hours (or one long-acting 500-mg capsule daily) for three to four days during ascent. Start the medication 24 hours before ascent or at the first sign of discomfort, which usually occurs by 10,000 to 12,000 feet (3,048 to 3,658 meters).

For mild acute mountain sickness or severe altitude sickness, take aspirin or acetaminophen with codeine for headache, plus 250 mg of acetazolamide every eight hours for two to three days to speed acclimatization. For nausea and vomiting, take 10 mg orally of prochlorperazine (Compazine) every four hours or take 25 mg by rectal suppository every four hours. Because prochlorperazine also stimulates breathing, it is preferred over triethylperazine (Torecan).

In treating severe acute mountain sickness, acetazolamide is of no value, but the other drugs listed above are useful. In addition, furosemide

(Lasix) can be taken orally or intravenously every 12 hours in 40-mg doses, unless the patient's blood pressure is low. However, although furosemide dehydrates the body overall, it may not relieve lung or brain congestion. Morphine sulfate in intravenous or intramuscular doses of 2 to 5 mg may be useful for high altitude pulmonary edema but should not be taken if there is any sign of cerebral edema. The dose can be repeated every four hours if it seems to be helping. Dexamethasone, taken in oral or intramuscular doses of 4 to 6 mg every six hours, is helpful for patients with cerebral edema.

It cannot be emphasized too strongly that *no* drug should be relied on to correct acute mountain sickness; the definitive treatment is *rapid descent*.

Use of Antibiotics

Because infectious diseases can occur in the wilderness, it is wise for travelers who expect to be very far from the roadhead to carry antibiotics and have some idea of the indications for their use. Under ideal circumstances, the offending bacterium should be identified in each illness, and its sensitivity should be tested so that the correct antibiotic can be chosen. However, the wilderness traveler does not have this luxury and must rely on a small number of carefully selected antibiotics and some general rules of thumb in choosing the best drug based on the signs and symptoms of a given illness, the organism most likely responsible, and the known spectrum of activity of each drug. Fortunately, this process is not difficult.

Many different antibiotics are available and are quite safe when used intelligently by people *who are not allergic to them*. The traveler who will be out a week or more and will be more than two or three days from the roadhead should carry two separate antibiotics: a synthetic penicillin, erythromycin, or a cephalosporin; and tetracycline or a tetracycline derivative.

Together, these two groups of drugs have the greatest likelihood of controlling any infection that may be contracted in the wilderness in temperate latitudes. Large expeditions or rescue groups may wish to include additional antibiotics, including parenteral (injectable) forms for patients who are vomiting or who cannot swallow.

Ampicillin, a semisynthetic penicillin, is taken in 250-mg doses four times daily. If one of the party members is allergic to penicillin, erythromycin can be substituted; the dosage of the ethyl succinate form is 400 mg four times daily. Good but more expensive alternatives are the cephalosporins, cefaclor (Ceclor, dosage 250 mg, three times daily) and cephalexin (Keflex, dosage 250 mg, four times daily).

Tetracycline is taken in a dosage of 250 mg four times daily, at least one hour before or two hours after eating. Avoid milk and milk products while taking tetracycline. Pregnant women or young children should not take this drug.

Because tetracycline deteriorates, supplies should be replaced yearly (fortunately, it is inexpensive). Long-acting tetracyclines such as doxycycline are more convenient and probably more effective, at least for patients with severe diarrhea. The dosage is 100 mg taken twice the first day, then once daily. Patients taking tetracycline, especially doxycycline, occasionally experience severe sun reactions, which can be prevented to some extent by wearing protective clothing and liberally applying a sunscreen with a high SPF value.

To obtain drugs with the longest shelf life, tell the pharmacist that the drugs are to be used in a first aid kit. Ask the druggist to type the expiration date on each label. Try to protect drugs from temperature extremes.

Ampicillin, erythromycin, or a cephalosporin should be taken for severe colds, coughs and sore throats, especially if the patient is producing yellow or green material from the chest or nose or has white spots on the tonsils, earache, a high fever, or sore neck glands beneath the mandible. These antibiotics also should be taken for suspected pneumonia or pleurisy, when wounds are large and/or heavily contaminated, and for skin and wound infections, open wounds of the chest and abdomen (if the patient is able to swallow), and open fractures. A tetracycline (preferably doxycycline) or ampicillin should be taken for suspected urinary or prostate infections and for severe diarrhea (see **Stomach and Bowel Problems**, below). If there is no improvement after 48 hours of treatment with an antibiotic from one group, substitute a member of the other group. Continue taking antibiotics that are producing the desired improvement for a minimum of five days.

The quinolones, a new group of oral antibiotics that includes norfloxacin (Noroxin) and ciprofloxacin (Cipro), recently have become available. They are strongly active against a wide range of bacteria. Unfortunately, they are quite expensive, and it is still undetermined whether they will replace current antibiotics in treating wilderness infections.

Treat abscesses and wound infections with hot packs as well as antibiotics. A wound that becomes swollen, hot, red, tender, and painful is probably infected, especially if there is pus draining out of it. If the wound has been taped closed, remove the tape and allow the wound to drain. Apply hot, wet packs to the wound for half an hour, four times daily to speed healing. A hot pack is made by boiling cloths to make them at least semisterile. Test the temperature of the hot pack against your own skin to make sure that it will not burn the patient.

Suspect an abscess in any patient with fever who has a hot, swollen, red, tender area in the skin or muscles. Apply hot packs as described above to speed the formation of pus, which will collect in a tense, shiny, yellow or reddish spot on the surface of the abscess. To allow pus to drain, clean this spot with antiseptic soap and nick it with a razor blade or sharp knife sterilized over a flame. Continue applying hot packs to promote drainage and speed healing.

Treat small, infected cuts by applying an antibiotic ointment such as Neosporin topical-ophthalmic or Garamycin ophthalmic ointment three times daily. These ointments also can be used in the eye for conjunctivitis, which is characterized by a red, sore eye that may discharge pus. Unless conjunctivitis clears rapidly, evacuate the patient.

Stomach and Bowel Problems

The type of food usually consumed in the wilderness (freeze-dried food, candy, nuts, lunch meat, dried fruit, cheese) frequently produces an unusual amount of intestinal gas and softer-than-normal stools. Individuals may experience cramps, usually in the lower abdomen. Gas may accumulate in the left upper abdomen, causing pressure and/or sharp pains in the chest that can be mistaken for more serious illnesses. These symptoms usually disappear when the offending foods are removed from the diet.

Occasionally, patients with altitude sickness, headache, food poisoning, or gastroenteritis may vomit. Vomiting usually can be controlled with medicated rectal suppositories such as thiethylperazine (Torecan) in 10-mg doses or prochlorperazine (Compazine) in 25-mg doses, inserted every four hours as necessary.

Mild diarrhea, often caused by food or gastroenteritis, can be controlled by taking one 2.5-mg tablet of diphenoxylate/atropine sulfate (Lomotil) every four hours as needed. An alternative is to take one 2-mg capsule of loperamide (Imodium) every four to six hours. Patients with diarrhea accompanied by chills, fever, severe cramps, and blood or pus in the stools should not use these drugs. Patients with these signs and symptoms should start taking a tetracycline or ampicillin and should be evacuated.

Bismuth subsalicylate (Pepto-Bismol) also is quite useful in treating mild to moderately severe diarrhea. The dosage is two tablespoons or two tablets four times a day.

A recent study done in Mexico found that trimethoprim/sulfamethoxazole (Septra, Bactrim) is an effective empiric treatment for travelers' diarrhea in 95 percent of cases. Travelers to developing countries are advised to obtain this medication on prescription from their physicians and use it for moderate to severe diarrhea. The dose is one DS (double strength) tablet (containing 160 mg trimethoprim and 800 mg sulfamethoxazole) twice daily for at least five days. People who are allergic to sulfa should not use this medication.

The new quinolones mentioned above also seem to have value in the empiric treatment of travelers' diarrhea.

Giardiasis is a hazard for wilderness travelers in temperate as well as tropical climates. Infestation with the protozoan *Giardia lamblia* causes gastric distress, mild diarrhea, and foul-smelling flatus. Giardiasis does not respond to any of the antibiotics mentioned above but can be effectively treated with metronidazole (Flagyl), an agent mentioned in **Special Problems of Women**, below. Fortunately, giardiasis usually develops slowly enough to allow the patient to be evacuated for definitive medical care.

When patients with any kind of stomach or bowel disturbance are able to eat, they should be given a light diet consisting of simple carbohydrates such as broth, bland soup, tea, gelatin, pudding, and toast. They should avoid milk, spices, rich foods, and fruit juices at first. Dehydration should be corrected as discussed earlier.

Promptly evacuate any patient with persistent or severe abdominal pain.

Proper sanitation and attention to water and food supplies often will prevent much gastrointestinal misery. Always wash the hands after defecation and before eating. When washing dishes, *thoroughly* rinse off soap to avoid future gastrointestinal irritation. Native food should be avoided in developing countries, unless it has been well cooked and is still hot, or it can be peeled. Do not eat raw vegetables, unpeeled fruit, and cooked food that has cooled. Avoid iced drinks because the ice may be contaminated. Drink only bottled, boiled, or disinfected water.

Respiratory Problems

People with respiratory infections should avoid wilderness trips because the stressful environment may bring on complications such as pneumonia or a sinus infection. Suspect pneumonia or pleurisy in people who have a cough with fever or chest pain, especially pain in the side of the chest underneath the armpit or beneath the scapula that is aggravated by deep breathing and coughing. Patients with suspected pneumonia or other severe respiratory infections should take ampicillin, erythromycin, or a cephalosporin.

Urinary Problems

Symptoms of urinary tract infection include painful urination, frequent voiding of small amounts of urine, a feeling that the bladder has not been emptied, chills, fever, and backache in the costovertebral angle. The patient should drink plenty of fluids and take a tetracycline or ampicillin. The double-strength size of Trimethoprim/sulfamethoxazole also is very effective. It should be taken twice daily for 10 days.

Special Problems of Women

Wilderness travel without the customary amenities of civilization may pose special problems for women. Vaginal infections that may occur can be divided into two general types for purposes of treatment. Yeast infections, characterized by thick, whitish discharge and severe itching, usually respond promptly to miconazole vaginal suppositories (Monistat 7), inserted once daily at bedtime for seven days. Other types of vaginitis commonly involve a thinner, yellowish discharge, sometimes with an objectionable odor. These infections most likely are caused by *Trichomonas vaginalis* or *Gardnerella vaginalis*. They usually respond, at least partly, to one 250-mg tablet of metronidazole (Flagyl) taken three times daily for seven days. If there is no response to Flagyl after two to three days, change the medication to two 250-mg capsules of Ampicillin taken four times daily for 10 days. While taking Flagyl, the patient should *not* drink alcohol: the combination produces symptoms similar to those associated with Antabuse (flushing, copious sweating, severe headache, vomiting, dyspnea, and heart irregularities).

Women who customarily have menstrual cramps usually have a prescription medicine for cramps that they can bring. Otherwise, 200-mg tablets of ibuprofen (nonprescription Advil, Nuprin, etc.) usually are effective. Prescription pain pills such as acetaminophen with codeine (Tylenol with codeine) and propoxyphene with acetaminophen (Darvocet) also can be used.

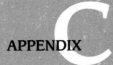

Emergency Care Kits

RECREATIONAL EMERGENCY CARE KIT

The amount of equipment carried in an emergency care kit depends on the length of the planned trip and the difficulty of access to medical help. The requirements of a one-day recreational trip obviously are different from those of a four-week Alaskan expedition. The following lists are suggestions only and can be modified to suit individual needs. Prescription medicines are marked with an asterisk except where listed as part of a physician's kit.

A basic kit is suitable for a day trip or to be carried by each member of a party on a multi-day trip.

Contents of a Basic Kit

Items	Comments
2 cravats	Use for bandage, sling, etc.
1 roll of 3-inch or 4-inch self-adhering roller bandage (e.g., Kling)	Bandaging material.
1 roll of 2-inch adhesive tape	Can be torn in half lengthwise to make 1-inch wide tape. Small strips can be torn off to make butterfly bandages.
4 sterile gauze compresses, 3-inch × 4-inch or 4-inch × 4-inch (nonadhesive Telfa or equivalent)	Can be cut up and used with pieces of tape to make small bandages (regular Bandaids also can be carried).
20 0.3-gm aspirin or Tylenol (acetaminophen) tablets	For headache and other mild pain, 1 to 2 every 3 hours as needed.
Sunscreen or sunblock	See Chapter 19.
Lip salve	Preferably a type that stays relatively soft in cold weather. Use proper SPF number (see Chapter 19).
Swiss army knife with scissors and tweezers	
Safety pins	Various uses, including to improvise upper-extremity splint by pinning sleeve to front of jacket.
Plastic sandwich bags	Fill with snow to improvise cold pack, various other uses.
Personal medications, if any	
Water purification equipment (Potable Aqua tablets, First Need filter, etc.)	
Optional: Bandaids, moleskin	

For Multi-day Trip, Add:

*Sleeping pills of choice, if desired, with directions for use	Try these out at home to be certain they are effective. Use with caution above 12,000 feet (3,658 meters)

A master kit is designed for multi-day recreational tours. A party should carry one master kit.

Contents of a Master Kit

Items	Comments
Extra cravats to provide at least 6 per party	At least 6 are needed to rig an improvised Thomas splint.
3-inch wide rubberized bandage	
6-inch dowel or 30 inches of ⅛- to ¼-inch diameter nylon cord	Use in setting up a Spanish windlass or pulley traction.
Seam ripper	
Sewing needle	Can be part of a sewing kit.
Small bottle of antiseptic cleanser (Betadine, Phisohex)	
Thermometer	Low-reading thermometer may be preferred.
Single-edge razor blade, or packaged sterile #15 scalpel blade	For incising and draining abscesses, etc.
2 pairs of disposable rubber gloves	Use when dressing open wounds or to avoid contact with body fluids.
Pocket mask with one-way valve or mouth shield	To increase effectiveness of rescue breathing and avoid contact with patient's saliva.
Notebook and pencil	To record vital signs and other accident data.

Medications

5-gm tube *Neosporin or *Garamycin ophthalmic ointment	Can be used in eyes or on skin for eye infections, infected cuts, etc. Apply 3 times daily.
24 25-mg or 12 *50-mg Benadryl (diphenhydramine hydrochloride) capsules. Alternatives: *Pyribenzamine (tripelennamine), *Polarimine (dexchlorpheniramine), *Seldane (terfenadine), etc.	For itching, hives, drug reactions, 1 50-mg or 2 25-mg capsules every 4 hours as needed. The 25-mg size is nonprescription.
12 30-mg *Tylenol with codeine (acetaminophen with codeine) tablets. Alternative: *Darvocet N 100 (propoxyphene napsylate and acetaminophen), 1 every 3 hours	For pain, 1 to 2 every 3 hours. Codeine-containing drugs also can be used for diarrhea, 1 every 3 hours.

Optional

12 2.5-mg *Lomotil (diphenoxylate with atropine sulfate) tablets. Alternative: 2-mg capsules of *Imodium (loperamide)	For diarrhea, 1 to 2 every 3 hours

6 10-mg *Torecan (thiethylperazine) rectal suppositories. Alternative: 25-mg *Compazine (prochlorperazine) suppositories — For vomiting, insert 1 every 3 hours as needed. Prochlorperazine is preferred at high altitude.

Additional Considerations

12 100-mg *Demerol (meperidine) tablets. Alternative: *Tylox (oxycodone and acetaminophen) capsules — For severe pain, ½ to 1 every 3 hours as needed. These are prescription narcotics.

For Extended Trips into Remote Country, Add:

20 500-mg capsules *ampicillin capsules. Alternatives: *erythromycin, *Ceclor (cefaclor) — See Appendix B for details.

20 250-mg *tetracycline capsules. Alternative: 8 100-mg *doxycycline tablets — Do not take tetracycline with milk or dairy products or close to meals. See Appendix B for further details.

Optional for High Altitude

12 or more 250-mg *Diamox (acetazolamide) tablets — See Appendix B for details.

30 4-mg *Decadron or *Hexadrol (dexamethasone) tablets — For cerebral edema. Begin with 2 tablets; then, 1 every 6 hours. See Appendix B.

Optional for Underdeveloped Countries

20 *Septra DS or *Bactrim DS (trimethoprim/ sulfamethoxazole) tablets — See Appendix B.

Optional for Women

7 *Monistat 7 (miconazole nitrate) vaginal suppositories — Insert 1 at bedtime for 1 week. See Appendix B.

21 250-mg tablets *Flagyl (metronidazole) tablets — Take 1 tablet 3 times daily for a week. See Appendix B.

Optional for Snake Country

Sawyer extractor — A powerful suction syringe for injected poisons. See Chapters 23 and 24.

WILDERNESS SEARCH AND RESCUE (SAR) EMERGENCY CARE KIT

Dressings, Bandages, and Wound Care

10 3-inch × 4-inch nonadhesive gauze compresses
4 ABD Pads, 2 medium, 2 large
4 self-adhering roller bandages, 2 2-inch, 2 3-inch
2 packs Betadine pledgets
1 500-ml bag (with IV tubing) of sterile saline for wound irrigation
Sterile 20-cc syringe for wound irrigation
2 packets Vaseline gauze
1 roll 2-inch adhesive tape
6 feet of plastic wrap such as Saran, folded or rolled
24 Bandaids
1 3-inch rubberized bandage
1 2-inch rubberized bandage
12 plastic storage bags, 6 small, 6 medium
4 pairs disposable rubber gloves

Splints

Extrication collar (Stifneck or improvised from SAM splint)
Sager splint or Kendrick traction device
Pneumatic splint for lower extremity, long size
Kendrick extrication device or Oregon spine splint
6 cravats
2 ladder or SAM splints

Cardiorespiratory

3 oral airways, 1 each of 3 sizes
Pocket mask with one-way valve and oxygen intake nipple
Suction apparatus (Vitalograph emergency aspirator, AMBU foot-operated suction device, turkey baster, bulb syringe, etc.)
Bag-mask

Drugs

Same as drugs suggested above in the master kit. Add epinephrine autoinjection kit (*Epipen, *Ana-Kit, etc.) for anaphylactic reaction to bee stings, and instant glucose (Glutose, etc.) for insulin shock (hypoglycemia).

Other

Lightweight stethoscope	Hypothermia thermometer
Blood pressure cuff	Safety pins
Tweezers	Notebook and pencil
Bandage scissors	Tags
Urinal or pee bottle	Penlight
Razor blade, single-edge	Seam ripper
Clinical thermometer	Steel sewing needle

Additional Items for Hypothermia

Rewarming equipment such as chemical heating pads, Heat-pac, hydraulic sarong, device for heating inspired air (UVIC Heat Treat, APPLINC Saving Breath, etc.). See Chapter 19.
Extra sleeping bag and tent

PHYSICIAN/PARAMEDIC KIT

Lightweight stethoscope
Blood pressure cuff
Small otoscope/ophthalmoscope with several tongue blades
Cricothyroidotomy set or endotracheal intubation kit
Heimlich valve or McSwain dart (can improvise using 16-gauge needle and a finger cut from sterile surgical glove, with pinhole in tip to form flutter valve)
Intravenous Fluids:
    Liter bags of lactated Ringer's/5-percent glucose solution
    Liter bags of 10-percent glucose/½-percent physiological saline solution
    Liter bags of physiological saline solution
IV administration sets
18-gauge Intracath needles
1-inch adhesive tape
Alcohol swabs
Tourniquets
Drugs:
Tubex hypodermic syringe and empty tubes for injecting:

Meperidine	Thiethylperazine or
Naloxone	prochlorperazine
Diphenhydramine	Atropine
Lidocaine hydrochloride	Digoxin
Adrenalin 1:1000	Aminophylline
Diazepam	(requires a 50-cc syringe)
Dexamethasone	Furosemide

Foley catheter (18 French) with bag and clamp
Sterile gloves
Lubricant
Betadine swabs

SKI PATROL EMERGENCY CARE EQUIPMENT

Recommended Minimum Contents for Alpine Patrol Belt

4 triangular bandages folded as cravats
9 assorted sterile compresses, 3 each of 3 sizes
6 Bandaids
2 rolls self-adhering roller gauze, 1 each of 2 sizes

1 roll 2-inch adhesive tape
Pocket knife
4 large safety pins
Pad and pencil
Bandage scissors
Release of Responsibility form

Highly Recommended

Pocket mask or disposable mouth shield with one-way valve
1 pair disposable rubber gloves

Additional considerations

1 tube instant glucose (Glutose)
Flashlight
Plastic storage bags, several sizes
Screwdriver, pliers, small wrench
Matches in waterproof container
Map of ski area
Wire splint or SAM splint
3 oral airways, 1 each of 3 sizes

Ankle hitch (EZ-TRAC) with 30 inches of ⅛- to ¼-inch cord for traction
6-inch dowel for Spanish windlass
Seam ripper
Avalanche transceiver (or avalanche cord) (Note: avalanche transceiver is preferred, especially at ski areas with high avalanche hazard)

Recommended Minimum Contents for Nordic Patrol Emergency Care Kit

4 or more cravats
2 rolls self-adhering roller bandage, 1 each of 2 sizes
1 roll 2-inch adhesive tape
Sterile nonadhesive gauze compresses, assorted
4 ABD pads, 2 medium, 2 large
Bandaids
Betadine pledgets
Vaseline gauze
6 feet of plastic wrap (folded or rolled), or 4 large plastic storage bags
1 3-inch rubberized bandage
1 pair disposable rubber gloves
SAM splint
3 oral airways, 1 each of 3 sizes
Pocket mask with one-way valve and oxygen intake nipple

Tweezers
Bandage scissors
Single-edge razor blade or #15 scalpel blade in sterile packet
Low-reading clinical thermometer for hypothermic patients
4 large safety pins
Notebook and pencil
Flashlight
Seam ripper
Steel sewing needle
Spreader for ski pole splint
Ankle hitch (EZ-TRAC) with 30 inches of nylon line for traction
6-inch dowel for Spanish windlass
Rewarming device for hypothermic patient (Heatpac, chemical heating pads, hot air inhalation device)

Optional

12 50-mg *Diphenhydramine capsules
20 aspirin or Tylenol (acetaminophen) tablets
12 doses pain medicine such as 30-mg *Tylenol with codeine (acetaminophen with codeine) or *Darvocet N 100 (propoxyphene with acetaminophen, 100 mg)
1 tube instant glucose (Glutose)

Additional Considerations

*Sterile saline for irrigating
Sterile 20-cc syringe for irrigating
Pneumatic splints
*Bee sting kit (Ana-Kit, EpiPen)
12 2.5-mg *Lomotil (diphenoxylate with atropine sulfate) tablets

2 anti-vomiting suppositories such as *Torecan (thiethylperazine) or *Compazine (prochlorperazine)
12 100-mg *Demerol (meperidine) tablets
*Antibiotics
*High-altitude drugs
Urinal or pee bottle

Toboggan Pack

Piece of Ensolite to pad bottom of toboggan
Blankets or sleeping bag
Quick splint or cardboard splint

Cravats and padding material
Waterproof cover for pack
Canvas stretcher

Additional Considerations

(usually kept at top of hill)

Long and short spine boards
Traction splint
Portable oxygen equipment

Vacuum splints
Extra sleeping bags and toboggan packs

Patrol First Aid Room

The following are recommended minimum items. Final selection should be based on local needs and consultation with area management and the patrol medical advisor.

Basic Equipment

Cots or beds
Warming mechanism: infrared lamps, electric blanket, hot water bottles, etc.
Portable screen or curtains for privacy
Sink with running water, soap, towels
Toilet
Waste receptacles
Telephone and radio

Bed pan and urinal
First aid cabinet
Oxygen equipment
Suction equipment
Bag-mask
Pocket mask with one-way valve
Pipe cutter
Large container for rapid rewarming of frostbitten hand or foot in warm water

Contents of First Aid Cabinet

Self-adhering roller bandages
Cravats
Sterile dressings, assorted sizes
Bandaids, butterfly bandages, or Steristrips
Adhesive tape, assorted widths
Antiseptic soap
Compound tincture of benzoin
Bandage scissors
Rubbing alcohol
Washpan, large metal or plastic
Laboratory thermometer, to measure water temperature

Clinical thermometer
Low reading clinical thermometer
Tweezers
Plastic bags (add snow to make cold packs)
Single-edge razor blades
Sewing kit
Safety pins
Disposable paper cups
Accident report forms and pencils
Emesis basin
Disposable rubber gloves
Stethoscope
Blood pressure cuff

Medical Kit for Physician or Paramedic*

The following are suggested items. Final determination should be made through consultation with area management and the patrol medical advisor.

Intravenous fluids, IV sets, IV needles
Cardiac monitor-defibrillator
PASG
Intubation kit with endotracheal tubes
Drugs (see above under physician/paramedic and SAR kits)
Heimlich valve or McSwain dart
Stethoscope
Blood pressure cuff

*Consider Banyan self-contained kits, available from Banyan International Corporation, PO Box 1779, Abilene, TX 79604)

GLOSSARY

abandonment—failure to continue care until the patient is transferred to the care of another qualified person.

abdomen—the part of the body that lies between the chest and the pelvis and contains the abdominal cavity.

abdominal cavity—the cavity in the lower part of the trunk that contains parts of the digestive and urinary tracts and associated organs.

abduct—to draw away from the midline.

abrasion—a superficial injury caused by moving contact between the skin and a parallel rough surface.

absorption—the transfer of digested substances through the intestinal wall into the blood.

acclimatization—the process by which the body adjusts to a new environment.

acetabulum—a cup-shaped depression at the point where the three pelvic bones are joined laterally. The acetabulum forms the socket of the hip joint into which the head of the femur fits.

acetazolamide (Diamox)—a prescription drug that improves acclimatization in people going to high altitude.

Achilles tendon—the tendon that joins the calf muscles to the heel of the foot.

acid—a substance that forms hydrogen ions in solution.

acidosis—abnormal acidity of the blood.

acromioclavicular (AC) joint—the joint between the clavicle and the acromion of the scapula at the point of the shoulder.

acromion—the lateral extension of the spine of the scapula, which forms the highest point of the shoulder.

acute abdomen—a surgical emergency marked by abdominal pain without diarrhea lasting more than eight hours.

acute mountain sickness (AMS)—a condition that can occur at altitudes above 7,500 feet caused by the effects of hypoxia on the brain and lungs.

addiction—a state that includes tolerance, physical dependence, and psychological dependence on a drug.

adduct—to draw toward the midline.

advanced cardiac life support (ACLS)—techniques used by paramedics, nurses, or physicians using equipment such as heart monitors, electrical defibrillation equipment, and intravenous drugs to treat patients who have suffered cardiac arrest.

agitation—restlessness and increased activity accompanied by fear or anxiety.

AIDS (acquired immune deficiency syndrome)—a universally fatal infectious disease caused by a virus that attacks the body's immune system, leading to a chronic wasting disease accompanied by the development of unusual infection and malignant tumors. Most cases have been associated with sexual intercourse and/or sharing intravenous drug apparatus.

AIDS-related complex (ARC)—illness in a patient with antibodies to the human immunodeficiency virus who does not fulfill the criteria for diagnosis of AIDS.

air embolism—an illness caused by blockage of small blood vessels by air bubbles. When a scuba diver is ascending, over-expansion of the lungs causes alveoli to rupture, forcing air bubbles into the circulation via the pulmonary capillaries.

airway obstruction—complete or partial blockage of the airway by a foreign body, vomitus, blood clots, the tongue, or by swollen or relaxed soft tissues of the throat.

alcohol—a liquid obtained by fermentation of carbohydrates with yeast.

alcoholism—addiction to alcohol.

alignment—the process of correcting the deformity of a fractured limb.

alkali—a substance that forms hydroxyl ions in solution; a base.

allergy—a state of hypersensitivity to a specific substance so that reexposure causes reactions in the skin, respiratory tract, and/or gastrointestinal tract.

altitude sickness—distressing symptoms experienced by unacclimatized individuals who ascend rapidly to altitudes over 8,000 feet.

alveoli—the smallest air sacs in the lungs.

amniotic sac—the fluid-filled sac within which the fetus grows and develops.

amphetamines—highly addictive stimulant drugs once used in medicine as mood elevators and appetite suppressants. Side effects of amphetamine use include rapid pulse, elevated blood pressure, excitement, agitation, insomnia, irritability, and inability to concentrate.

amputation—the complete tearing away of a body part from the body.

AMS—see **acute mountain sickness**.

analgesic—an agent that alleviates pain without causing loss of consciousness.

anaphylactic shock—shock caused by an immediate and overwhelming allergic reaction.

anatomic position—the position in which the patient is standing erect, facing the examiner with arms at the side and palms facing forward.

anatomy—the science of the structure of the body and the relation of its parts.

anemia—a condition characterized by too few red blood cells or a decrease in the amount of hemoglobin in the red cells.

aneurysm—a bulging weak spot on a blood vessel that can rupture and cause internal bleeding.

angina pectoris—a pain of characteristic type and location that occurs in patients with coronary artery disease.

Angle of Louis—see **sternal angle**.

ankle joint—a hinge joint formed by the lower ends of the tibia and fibula proximally and the talus bone of the foot distally.

anterior—nearer the front surface of the body.

antibiotics—chemical substances produced by microorganisms that have the capacity to kill other microorganisms. Some antibiotics are used in the control of infectious diseases.

anticholinergic—an agent that blocks the action of acetylcholine, its derivatives, and the parasympathetic nervous system.

antidepressant—a drug that prevents or relieves depression.

antidote—a remedy for counteracting a poison.

antihistamine—a drug that counteracts the action of histamine and relieves allergic symptoms.

anus—the terminal opening of the alimentary canal.

aorta—the major artery of the body into which blood is pumped from the left ventricle of the heart.

apex—the top or highest point.

appendicitis—inflammation or infection of the appendix.

appendicular skeleton—the bones of the upper and lower limbs and the pelvis (see **axial skeleton**).

appendix—a worm-sized organ with no obvious useful purpose that is attached to the beginning of the large bowel.

aqueous humor—the watery fluid contained in the anterior compartment of the eyeball in front of the lens.

arachnoid—the middle of the three layers of meninges that cover the brain and spinal cord.

ARC—see **AIDS-related complex.**

arch—the portion of the foot made up of the calcaneus, talus, and tarsal bones.

arterial blood—oxygenated blood flowing through the arteries to the tissues.

arteriole—the smallest size of artery.

arteriosclerosis—a disease characterized by the stiffening and narrowing of arteries because of fatty deposits and scar tissue within the arterial walls.

artery—a tubular vessel that carries blood from the heart to the body tissues.

artificial kidney—a mechanical device used in patients with kidney failure to remove wastes from the blood that are ordinarily excreted in the urine.

aspiration—the act of sucking in. Aspiration usually refers to sucking foreign matter into the airway.

assessment—examination of the patient.

asthma—a chronic or recurrent condition in which the small bronchi go into spasm.

ataxia—loss of muscle coordination leading to difficulty in maintaining balance.

atrium—either of the two upper chambers of the heart.

aura—a peculiar sensation, which can be a sound, sight or smell, that signals the onset of a generalized (grand mal) epileptic seizure.

auscultation—listening for sounds within the body.

autonomic nervous system—the system that is composed of the sympathetic and parasympathetic nervous systems and controls the activity of the cardiac muscle, smooth muscle and glands, and other automatic functions of the body.

avulsion—a body part torn loose from underlying tissues and left hanging by a flap.

axial skeleton—the skull, spine, ribs, and sternum (see **appendicular skeleton**).

axial traction—a pull parallel to the long axis of a body part.

axilla—the armpit.

axon—the long process of a neuron.

---

back carry—an emergency one-rescuer technique for moving a conscious patient short distances over very rough terrain or for belaying both the patient and rescuer over a short distance vertically. The technique involves fashioning a seat from a climbing rope or sling.

bag-mask—a device consisting of a mask and a squeezable oxygen reservoir bag that is used for delivering oxygen to patients who are not breathing.

"bag of waters"—the sac containing the amniotic fluid that supports and protects the fetus.

bandage—the material used to hold a dressing or compress in place.

bandaging—the process of applying a dressing (or compress) and bandage to a wound.

barbiturates—a class of sedative drugs that depress the nervous system. Barbiturates are used in sleeping pills (e.g., secobarbital, amobarbital, chloral hydrate, methaqualone) and tranquilizers (Valium, Librium, Xanax, Ativan).

basic life support—techniques of rescue breathing, cardiopulmonary resuscitation, and clearing upper airway obstructions that can be used to treat patients who have collapsed because of airway obstruction, cessation of breathing, and/or cardiac arrest.

Battle's sign—ecchymosis at the tip of the mastoid process, a sign of internal bleeding from a skull fracture.

Betadine—the brand name of a povidone-iodine antiseptic solution used for sterilizing instruments and cleaning wounds.

biceps muscle—the major muscle of the anterior upper arm, which flexes the elbow.

bilateral symmetry—the state of each body half being a mirror image of the opposite half.

bile—a substance produced by the liver and stored in the gallbladder that contains an emulsifying agent that prepares fat for digestion.

bilirubin—a byproduct of the normal breakdown of the red blood cells.

bladder—a hollow organ with muscular walls that stores urine before it is passed out of the body through the urethra. The bladder lies in the pelvic cavity.

bleb—a congenital, small, blister-like swelling on the lung surface.

blink reflex—an instantaneous blink that helps keep objects out of the eye.

blood—thick fluid made up of plasma; red cells, which carry oxygen; white cells, which fight infection; and platelets, which aid in blood clotting. The blood carries oxygen and nutrients to the cells of the body and removes carbon dioxide and waste materials.

blood pressure—the pressure transmitted to the walls of the arteries by the blood as it is propelled by the rhythmic contractions of the heart.

blood pressure cuff—the part of a sphygmomanometer that goes around a patient's arm.

blood volume—the quantity of blood in the circulatory system.

body—any mass of matter that is distinct from other masses of matter.

boot-top fracture—a fracture of the tibia and/or fibula at the level of the top of the ski boot.

Bourdon gauge flowmeter—a pressure gauge calibrated to record flow rate when attached to a tank of compressed gas.

brachial artery pulse—a pulse that can be felt beating against the humerus on the inside of the upper arm, midway between the shoulder and elbow.

brachial plexus—the origination of major nerves of the upper extremity, including the radial, ulnar, and median nerves. The brachial plexus lies in the neck behind the clavicles.

brain—the portion of the central nervous system contained within the cranium.

brain contusion—bruising of brain tissue.

brain stem—the most inferior portion of the brain. Centers in the brain stem help regulate breathing, heart function, and blood pressure. Long nerve fibers from upper parts of the brain pass through the brain stem to the spinal cord, to which it connects.

breach—failure to perform a duty.

breathlessness—the absence of spontaneous lung action.

bronchi—the tubular air passages of the lungs.

bronchioles—the smallest bronchi.

burn—a type of wound caused by excessive thermal, electrical, or radiant energy, or a similar injury caused by certain chemicals.

bursa—a fluid-filled sac that is located between moving body parts and acts to decrease friction.

bursitis—inflammation or infection of a bursa.

Calamine—the brand name of a soothing nonprescription lotion used for symptomatic relief of insect bites.

calcaneus—the heel bone.

callus—the calcified tissue formed during the process of bone healing.

cancer—a malignant tumor that tends to become progressively worse and can cause death because of invasion or spreading.

cantharidin—an irritating substance excreted by blister beetles.

capillary—a tiny blood vessel that connects an arteriole to a venule and has thin walls that allow the interchange of substances between the blood and tissue cells.

capillary refill—the ability of the circulatory system to refill small vessels after blood has been squeezed out of them.

carbohydrate—organic compounds composed of carbon, hydrogen, and oxygen present in food mainly as sugars and starches.

carbon monoxide—a colorless, odorless, poisonous gas that causes asphyxiation by combining irreversibly with the blood hemoglobin, thus blocking the transport and use of oxygen.

cardboard splint—an effective, disposable, easy-to-apply, fixation splint often used to replace a quick splint before the patient leaves the first aid room.

cardiac arrest—any condition where blood circulation stops because the heart malfunctions.

cardiac monitor—an electronic device that records and displays on a screen the electrocardiogram pulse rate, blood pressure, and other important data related to the state of the heart.

cardiac output—the quantity of blood pumped by the heart.

cardioaccelerating center—an area in the brain that receives signals from pressure monitors in the circulatory system and responds by increasing heart rate and blood vessel tone to counteract a fall in blood pressure.

cardiogenic shock—shock occurring when the heart is unable to purge a normal amount of blood.

cardioinhibitory center—an area in the brain that tends to slow the heart rate in response to elevated blood pressure.

cardiopulmonary resuscitation (CPR)—a technique of resuscitating victims of cardiac arrest by using rescue breathing to restore ventilation and external chest compressions to maintain blood circulation.

carotid arteries—the two arteries that supply blood to the head and neck. The pulses can be felt between the sternomastoid muscles and the larynx.

carotid veins—the veins that carry blood away from the head and neck.

carpal bone—the wrist bone.

cartilage—a specialized fibrous connective tissue that covers opposing bony surfaces (riding surfaces) of joints and forms the anterior portions of the ribs and parts of the nose and ears.

cecum—the pouch-like first part of the large intestine.

cell—the basic unit of all living matter.

central nervous system—the brain and spinal cord.

cerebellum—the portion of the brain that lies below and to the rear of the cerebrum and regulates posture, balance, muscle tone, and body movement.

cerebral hemispheres—the largest part of the brain, the cerebral hemispheres control conscious functions including voluntary movement and the sensations transmitted by the sensory organs for sight, hearing, touch, taste, and smell.

cerebrospinal fluid—a watery, colorless fluid that bathes the brain and the spinal cord.

cerebrovascular accident—stroke.

cerebrum—the portion of the brain that is composed of the outer right and left cerebral hemispheres and the inner thalamus and hypothalamus, and that controls personality, emotions, visual perceptions, movement, hearing, balance, and speech.

cervical collar—see **extrication collar**.

cervical spine—the uppermost portion of the spine formed by the seven cervical vertebrae in the neck.

cheekbone—the bony ridge of the maxilla below the orbit and above the soft part of the cheek.

chest cavity—see **thoracic cavity**.

Cheyne-Stokes respirations—waxing and waning of the depth of breathing interspersed with regular periods when breathing stops.

choke—to interrupt respiration by obstruction or compression of the airway.

cholecystitis—inflammation or infection of the gallbladder.

cholera—a specific bacterial bowel infection that involves profuse diarrhea, dehydration, and shock, and is caused by the organism Vibrio Cholerae.

cholesterol—a type of fat implicated as a cause of arteriosclerosis.

chondromalacia of the patella—roughening and deterioration of the cartilage of the posterior surface of the patella caused by excessive physical activity with the knee in the partly flexed position.

cirrhosis—chronic inflammation of the liver.

clavicle—the collarbone, which is attached medially to the sternum and laterally to the acromion of the scapula.

cocaine—a widely used illegal drug produced from the coca plant that induces marked euphoria. Overuse can result in convulsions, extreme agitation, and heart irregularities leading to sudden death.

coccyx—the vestigial tail-like structure that is formed by the fusion of the lower four vertebrae and hangs below the sacrum.

"coffee grounds" matter—refers to the appearance of partly digested blood vomited from the stomach.

colic—an intermittent, severe, abdominal pain caused by obstruction of a hollow, muscular organ such as the bowel or ureter.

collateral ligaments—the medial and lateral ligaments that, along with the anterior and posterior cruciate ligaments, are the important ligaments of the knee.

Colles' fracture—a fracture of the distal radius that produces a characteristic "silver fork deformity" resembling an upside-down dinner fork.

colon—the portion of the large intestine extending from the cecum to the rectum.

comminuted—broken or crushed into multiple small fragments.

compress—(see **dressing**).

compression trauma—trauma caused by a wounding object that strikes but does not necessarily penetrate the body.

concussion—a temporary loss of consciousness or other brain dysfunction following a blow to the head.

conductive heat loss—the direct transfer of heat from a warm body to a cooler object it is touching.

condyle—a projection on the end of a bone, usually part of a joint.

conjunctiva—the delicate transparent membrane that lines the eyelids and covers the visible part of the sclera.

conjunctivitis—inflammation or infection of the conjunctiva.

consciousness, level of—the ability of the patient's mind to respond to external stimulation. The range is from normal to complete unconsciousness in which only the activity of the circulatory and respiratory systems can be detected.

consolidation of the lung—stiffening of the lung segments of pneumonia patients, caused by the air spaces filling with fluid.

constipation—the passage of hard, dry stools at less than normal intervals.

constrict—to narrow or decrease in size.

contrecoup injury—an injury to parts on the side opposite the primary injury, such as when the brain is forced against one side of the skull by a blow to the opposite side.

contusion—a bruise.

convective heat loss—the transfer of heat to air moving across the body's surface.

convulsion—an involuntary contraction or series of contractions of the skeletal muscles.

core—the central nervous system, heart, lungs, liver, and other important internal organs of the body (see also **shell**).

core temperature—the temperature of the body core (central nervous system, heart, lungs, liver and other important internal organs), usually measured with a rectal thermometer.

coronary arteries—the arteries that supply blood to the heart.

coronary artery disease—arteriosclerosis of the coronary arteries.

coronary veins—the veins that carry blood away from the heart.

costal arch—the arch formed by the cartilage that connects the sixth through tenth ribs to each other and to the base of the sternum.

costovertebral angle—the triangular space on each side of the back between the lowest rib and the spine.

cough—a sudden, noisy expulsion of air from the lungs.

CRAMS scale—a triage device useful in assigning patients to a high mortality group (score of 6 or less) or a low mortality group (score of 7 or more).

cranial nerves—the nerves that arise directly from the brain, including nerves responsible for sight, hearing, taste, and smell, and nerves that supply sensory and motor fibers to the head.

cranium—the part of the skull that encloses the brain.

cravat—a long bandage, several inches wide, made by folding a triangular bandage lengthwise.

crepitus—a grating sensation caused by broken bone ends grinding together.

cricoid cartilage—a ring-like cartilage that forms the lowest part of the larynx.

cricothyroid membrane—a ligament that connects the thyroid and cricoid cartilages and can be felt as a soft spot between the thyroid and cricoid cartilages at the front of the neck.

crossed-finger technique—a technique for opening the patient's mouth, used when necessary to open the airway for rescue breathing.

crown—the topmost part of the tooth that is covered with enamel.

cruciate ligaments—the anterior and posterior ligaments of the knee that originate in the groove between the femoral condyles, cross each other, and insert in the middle of the tibial plateau. Along with the medial and lateral ligaments (collateral ligaments), the cruciate ligaments make up the four important ligaments of the knee.

crushing injury—an injury caused by compression that involves both direct tissue injury and injury secondary to circulatory disturbance caused by pressure on the blood vessels.

cutaneous system—the system made up of the skin and subcutaneous tissues that protects the internal body parts, controls body temperature, and contains special organs responsible for sensations of pain, touch, and temperature. The cutaneous system protects the body from dehydration and infection, and regulates body temperature by producing sweat and adjusting surface blood flow.

cyanosis—a bluish discoloration of the skin, fingernails, and mucous membranes that occurs because the blood is not adequately oxygenated.

cyst—a congenital swelling of any closed cavity or sac, especially one containing liquid or semisolid material.

deceleration trauma—trauma from dissipation of kinetic energy caused by rapid slowing of the body, such as when a skier collides with a tree.

decompression sickness—an illness that involves the formation of nitrogen bubbles in various body tissues and is caused by dissolved nitrogen coming out of solution faster than it can be excreted by the lungs. Decompression sickness results from too-rapid ascent from a deep dive.

decongestant—a substance that reduces enlargement or swelling.

defibrillator—an electronic device used to treat abnormal heart rhythms by applying a brief electroshock to the heart.

definitive medical care—care given in a hospital or physician's office (see also **first aid** and **emergency medical care**).

deformity—malformation, distortion, or disfigurement of the body or its parts.

dehydration—the condition that results from excessive loss of body water.

deltoid muscle—a muscle in the upper extremity that forms the rounded part of the shoulder and is the main muscle that lifts the upper extremity up and outward.

dendrites—the short processes of a neuron.

dermis—the inner layer of the skin that contains hair follicles, oil glands, sweat glands, blood vessels, nerves, and the sensory organs that perceive pain, touch, and temperature.

deviation—a turning away from the regular standard or course.

diabetes mellitus—a metabolic disorder in which the ability to use carbohydrates as fuel is lost because of an absolute or relative insufficiency of insulin.

diabetic coma—unconsciousness caused by loss of fluid and increased acidity that occurs in people with previously undiagnosed diabetes mellitus and in known diabetics who have taken insufficient insulin. Signs and symptoms include confusion, stupor, or coma; rapid, deep respirations; flushed, dry, warm skin; weakness; and fatigue. The patient's breath has a fruity odor and there may be signs of shock.

diabetic ketoacidosis—a serious condition occurring in patients with severe, uncontrolled diabetes. The condition is caused by a lack of insulin, which results in the inability to metabolize glucose and the accumulation of acidic breakdown products of fat in the blood and other body tissues.

diagnosis—identification of a disease or injury based on the results of examination.

diaphragm—the muscular partition separating the abdominal and thoracic cavities.

diarrhea—the passage of soft or liquid stools with abnormally high frequency.

diastolic blood pressure—the lowest point of the blood pressure curve.

digestion—the breakdown of food into simpler substances that can be more easily absorbed into the bloodstream.

digestive system—the system that consists of the digestive tract—a tube that conducts food through the body from mouth to anus—and associated organs that produce substances to aid digestion. This system ingests, digests and absorbs food and fluid, and eliminates wastes.

dilate—to enlarge.

direct ground lift—a technique in which three or four rescuers lift and move an injured patient.

direct pressure—a technique to reduce external bleeding by applying manual pressure over a compress placed directly on a wound.

disc—the doughnut-shaped ring of fibrous cartilage that separates the vertebrae.

discharge—an excretion of material from a body orifice.

disease—any deviation from or interruption of the normal structure or function of the body as manifested by a characteristic set of symptoms and signs.

disinfection—the removal of disease-causing organisms by means of chemical treatment.

dislocation—a disruption of a joint that occurs when the joint is forced to move beyond its normal range.

disorientation—a state of mental confusion regarding time, location, or identity.

dissipation—the dispersal of the energy from a moving object through deformation of body tissues. The amount of injury is roughly proportional to the amount of energy that has to be dissipated.

distal—closer to the tips of the extremities.

distention—the state of being swollen or enlarged.

diuretic—an agent that promotes the excretion of urine.

Diving Accident Network (DAN)—an organization that provides assistance in locating hyperbaric chambers and advice on emergency care of scuba-related medical problems. (Telephone: (919) 684-8111.)

dorsalis pedis pulse—the pulse felt on the top of the foot between the first and second metatarsals.

dorsiflex—to flex the foot upward, or dorsally.

dressing—a sterile cloth material placed directly on a wound.

drowning—death by suffocation after being submerged in water or another liquid.

drug—any substance that alters mental or physical function when introduced into the body.

duodenum—the first portion of the small intestine, which connects the stomach to the jejunum.

dura mater—the outermost of the three layers of meninges that cover the brain and spinal cord.

dysentery—a severe bowel infection causing profuse diarrhea, chills, fever, and prostration. Blood and pus typically are present in the stools.

dysphagia—difficulty in swallowing.

dyspnea—difficult or labored breathing.

dysuria—painful urination.

ear—the organ of hearing and equilibrium.

ear canal—the portion of the ear that is surrounded by the pinna (external ear) and leads to the middle and inner ear.

ecchymosis—a blue or purplish spot in the skin or mucous membranes caused by bleeding; a bruise.

ectopic pregnancy—a pregnancy in which the fetus develops outside of the uterus, usually in the fallopian tube.

edema—the escape of fluid from vascular or lymphatic spaces into tissues, causing local or generalized swelling.

egg—the female germ cell.

ejaculation—sudden, forceful expulsion.

elbow joint—the joint that connects the humerus proximally with the radius and ulna distally.

electrocution—death caused by high-voltage electrical current passing through the body.

electrolytes—ionic components of inorganic salts found in cells and body fluids.

elimination—the expulsion of indigestible residues through the feces.

embryo—the developing unborn offspring between the second and eighth weeks of pregnancy (the period of most rapid growth).

emergency medical care—more sophisticated than first aid, emergency care techniques are used when interaction with the Emergency Medical Services (EMS) system may be delayed (see also **definitive medical care** and **first aid**).

Emergency Medical Services (EMS) system—an interconnected network of hospitals, emergency departments, and emergency vehicles manned by physicians, nurses, and trained emergency medical technicians.

emergency medical technician (EMT)—an individual who has passed a basic or advanced EMT course sanctioned by a state and the United States Department of Transportation. EMTs work in the Emergency Medical Services (EMS) system and are trained to reach patients rapidly, provide emergency care, and transport them to a hospital.

emphysema—a chronic, progressive, obstructive pulmonary disease, often caused by cigarette smoking, that involves the loss of some alveoli in the lungs, enlargement of other alveoli, and narrowing of the bronchi. Patients have a barrel-chested appearance, their breath sounds are quieter than normal, and exhalations are prolonged.

emphysema, subcutaneous—an injury to the air-containing parts of the respiratory tract in the chest or neck that allows air to escape into the subcutaneous tissues, producing a unique crackling sensation similar to Rice Krispies under the skin.

endogenous—developing or originating within the body.

endotracheal intubation—opening and maintaining an airway by inserting an endotracheal tube through the nose or mouth or directly through the larynx between the vocal cords into the trachea.

endotracheal tube—a breathing tube inserted through the mouth or nose into the trachea.

energy—the capacity for doing work. Energy can be either potential, which is derived from the position of a body in a gravity field, or kinetic, which is created by motion.

engorgement—excessive fullness of an organ, vessel, or tissue because of the accumulation of blood or other fluids.

enzyme—a substance that is produced by the body and controls cellular chemical reactions.

epicondyle—a bony projection located above a condyle or a bone.

epidermis—the outer layer of skin composed of many layers of flat, closely adhering cells, the innermost layer of which is the germinal layer that constantly multiplies to renew the outer layers.

epiglottis—a thin, lid-like cartilage flap overhanging the entrance to the larynx that allows air to pass into the trachea but prevents food or liquid from entering the respiratory tract.

epiglottitis—inflammation or infection of the epiglottis, which occasionally causes swelling sufficient to obstruct the upper respiratory tract.

epilepsy—recurrent episodes of seizures caused by an abnormal focus of activity within the brain that may be manifested as impaired consciousness, abnormal movement, or psychic or sensory disturbances.

epinephrine (adrenalin)—a hormone normally produced by the adrenal gland that stimulates the sympathetic nervous system and the heart muscle, raises blood pressure, and relaxes bronchial smooth muscle.

erection—enlargement and hardening of erectile tissue filled with blood.

esophageal varices—large, dilated veins in the upper stomach and lower esophagus in patients with chronic liver disease. Rupture of these vessels can cause severe hemorrhage.

esophagus—the tubular organ that connects the oropharynx with the stomach.

eustachian tube—the channel that connects the tympanic cavity of the ear with the nasopharynx and serves to adjust the pressure of the air in the cavity to the external pressure.

evaporative heat loss—loss of heat when water or another volatile liquid on the body's surface is converted into vapor.

exhalation—breathing air out of the lungs.

expressive aphasia—a characteristic speech impairment marked by ability to understand but inability to choose the right words to reply.

extend—to straighten a joint.

extremities—the arms and legs.

extremity, lower—each lower extremity consists of the femur (thigh), the tibia and fibula (lower leg bones), and the foot.

extremity, upper—the shoulder, arm (upper arm), forearm, wrist, and hand.

extremity lift—a method of moving a patient with a splinted lower extremity from the first aid room to a nearby vehicle.

extrication—the process of moving a patient from an awkward, unusual, or poorly accessible situation or position.

extrication collar—a device that limits head and neck motion when applied to the neck of a patient with an actual or suspected neck injury (formerly called a cervical collar).

eye—the organ of vision.

eyeball—a hollow globe about 1 inch in diameter that lies in the eye socket of the skull and is connected with the brain by the optic nerve that passes through the back of the socket.

eyes-front position—when the head is in a natural position relative to the rest of the body.

---

fallopian tubes—the tubular structures through which the ovum passes from the ovary to the uterus.

false motion—limb motion where there is no joint, a sign of bone fracture.

fast-twitch fibers (type I fibers)—muscle fibers that are capable of rapid contraction, tend to rely on anaerobic metabolism, and readily form lactic acid (see also **slow-twitch fibers**).

fat—organic compounds that are composed of carbon, oxygen, and hydrogen and are stored in fatty tissue.

fat, polyunsaturated—fat that contains fewer hydrogen atoms than normal and is found in fish oil and vegetable products.

fat, saturated—fat that contains normal numbers of hydrogen atoms and usually is of animal origin.

fatigue—a state of discomfort and decreased efficiency resulting from prolonged or excessive exertion.

fatigue fracture (stress fracture)—a bone fracture caused by the strain of repeated stresses such as prolonged walking or exercise.

febrile illness—an illness with fever.

feces—the residue remaining in the bowel after digestible material has been removed.

femoral artery pulse—the pulse that can be felt just below the midpoint of the inguinal ligament, which lies between the anterior superior iliac spine and the pubis.

femoral condyles—the two rounded projections of the distal end of the femur.

femoral nerve—a major nerve of the lower extremity that enters the front of the thigh lateral to the femoral artery and provides sensation to part of the front of the thigh and the inner leg, as well as supplying the muscles that flex the hip and extend the knee.

femur—the thigh bone.

fetus—the developing unborn offspring between the eighth week of pregnancy and birth.

fever—an increase in body temperature of more than 1°F (0.5°C) above normal.

fibrillation—rapid, uncoordinated heart beat.

fibrin—an insoluble protein that forms the essential part of a blood clot.

fibula—the lateral of the two bones of the lower leg.

filtration—a method of purifying water using substances that contain microscopic pores through which most microorganisms can not pass.

finger sweep—the technique of using a hooked finger to clear a foreign body lodged in the mouth of an unconscious adult or older child.

fireman's carry—an emergency, one-rescuer technique for moving a patient unlikely to have a spine injury.

fireman's drag—an emergency, one-rescuer technique for moving a patient unlikely to have a spine injury.

first aid—simple emergency care techniques that require little equipment and rely on speedy coordination with the Emergency Medical Services (EMS) system (see also **definitive medical care** and **emergency care**).

fissure—a crack or small ulcer.

fixation splint—a splint that prevents motion at the site of a fracture or other injury when it is applied tightly to an extremity above, below, and across the injury site.

flail ankle—an injured ankle that is abnormally mobile.

flail chest—a loose section of the chest caused by multiple adjacent rib fractures.

flank—the part of the side of the body below the ribs and above the ilium of the pelvis.

flat bones—bones found in the skull and pelvis, as opposed to long bones, found in the limbs, and irregular bones, such as the vertebrae.

flatus—gas expelled through the anus.

flex—to bend a joint.

floating ribs—the eleventh and twelfth pairs of ribs, which lack a connection at the front of the chest.

"floor burn"—a type of abrasion commonly seen in gymnasts.

food poisoning—abdominal pain, vomiting, and/or diarrhea caused by irritating or contaminated food.

foot drop—inability to dorsiflex the foot because of paralysis of the anterior leg muscles.

foramen magnum—a hole at the base of the skull through which the spinal cord passes from the base of the brain to the spinal canal.

force—any action that changes the state of rest or motion of a body to which force is applied; a manifestation of kinetic energy.

fore-and-aft carry—an emergency two-rescuer technique for moving an unconscious patient with no serious injuries.

forearm bones—the radius and the ulna.

forehead—the area of the face above the eyes.

foreskin—a covering of folded skin over the glans of the penis.

fracture—any break in the continuity of a bone.

fracture-dislocation—an injury that includes both dislocation and fracture.

frequency—abnormally frequent urination.

front cradle—an emergency one-rescuer technique for carrying a small patient.

frostbite—damage to tissue caused by low environmental temperature. Before thawing, frostbite is categorized as superficial or deep; following thawing, it is categorized as first-degree, second-degree, third-degree, or fourth-degree based on the extent of blistering, swelling, skin color, and temperature.

---

gallbladder—a reservoir for bile storage located on the undersurface of the liver.

"gamekeeper's thumb"—see **"skier's thumb."**

ganglia—small clusters of autonomic nervous system neurons that lie outside the spinal cord.

gangrene—tissue death usually associated with loss of blood supply followed by bacterial invasion and putrification.

gastric distention—enlargement of the stomach by overfilling with air or another substance.

gastric juice—the liquid secretion of the stomach glands, containing hydrochloric acid and an enzyme that digests protein.

gastroenteritis—inflammation of the stomach and intestines caused by infection, overuse of alcohol, food poisoning, irritating drugs, or emotion.

Gatorade—the brand name of an electrolyte preparation.

genitalia--the male and female reproductive organs, usually referring to the external ones.

genitourinary system—the organs of reproduction together with the organs for the production and excretion of urine.

Giardia lamblia—an organism that is present in the feces of infected animals, often contaminates outdoor water sources, and causes a diarrheal illness.

glottis—the part of the larynx that produces speech, i.e., the vocal cords and the opening between them.

glucose—a simple sugar containing six carbon atoms that is the chief source of energy for living organisms; also known as dextrose.

gluteus muscle—one of the large muscles that form the buttocks and allow extension and abduction of the hips.

glycogen—a complex carbohydrate that is the chief storage form of carbohydrate in animals. It is found in the muscles and liver and is readily broken down into glucose.

goiter—an enlarged thyroid gland.

"golden hour"—the average time before a patient with multiple injuries starts to deteriorate rapidly; for every half hour following the first hour, the patient's chances of survival are cut in half.

gray matter—groups of nerve cells in the brain and spinal cord that derive their name from their color.

greater trochanter of the femur—the prominent knob on the outside of the upper end of the femur.

greenstick fracture—an angulated fracture that passes partway through the shaft of a bone.

groin—the region where the abdomen joins the thigh.

gross negligence—injury to another person caused by failure to provide even the degree of care that an unreasonable or imprudent person would exercise in similar circumstances. (see also **negligence** and **willful negligence**).

guarding—tightening of abdominal muscles overlying a tender area.

gurney—an adjustable, wheeled stretcher developed for ambulance use.

hallucination—a perception by the brain of a sight, sound, smell, touch, or taste that has no origin in an external stimulus.

hallucinogen—a drug such as LSD, psilocybin, mescaline, and peyote that alters perceptions of the environment, sometimes producing hallucinations or delusions.

hamstring muscles—the major muscles of the posterior thigh, which flex the knee.

hamstring tendons—the tendons of the muscles that flex the knee joint and can be felt on either side of the popliteal fossa behind the knee.

Hare splint—a commercially available modification of the Thomas traction splint that replaces cradle hitches with Velcro straps and uses a mechanical ratchet device to provide traction.

hay fever—an allergic condition of the upper respiratory tract that causes symptoms similar to those of a head cold.

head-tilt/chin-lift—a method of opening the airway by tilting the head back and lifting the chin with the fingers.

heart—the hollow, muscular organ that maintains the circulation of the blood by functioning as a pump.

heart attack—a term commonly used for any sudden episode caused by malfunction of the heart (see also **acute myocardial infarction**).

heart disease—any organic, mechanical, or functional abnormality of the heart.

heart failure, chronic—a clinical syndrome that is caused by the inability of the heart to pump an adequate amount of blood, and characterized by shortness of breath, weakness, and swelling of the abdomen and legs.

heartburn—a burning sensation in the epigastric area or beneath the sternum, often accompanied by increased saliva production.

heat cramps—cramping in active muscles that results from excessive loss of fluid and electrolytes because of perspiring in the heat.

heat exhaustion—a form of hypovolemic shock caused by either excessive sweating or the inadequate replacement of water and electrolytes lost by sweating.

heat syncope—a mild form of hypovolemic shock that resembles simple fainting. Heat syncope can result from sitting or standing for long periods in the direct sun or in hot weather.

Heatpac—the brand name of a lightweight stove fueled by a charcoal cartridge.

heatstroke—an illness characterized by prolonged elevation of the body core temperature above 104 to 105°F (40 to 40.6°C).

Heimlich maneuver—a technique of relieving upper-airway obstruction in adults and children (but not infants) that uses a sudden push on the abdomen or chest to expel residual air in the lungs and remove a foreign object blocking the upper airway.

hematoma—a localized tumor-like collection of blood within an organ or tissue.

hematuria—blood in the urine.

hemopneumothorax—air and blood in the pleural space.

hemoptysis—blood coughed up from the lungs.

hemorrhage—profuse bleeding.

hemorrhagic shock—the sudden collapse of heart function caused by blood loss.

hemorrhoid—an enlarged vein in the anal area.

hemothorax—blood in the pleural space.

hepatitis—an inflammatory or infectious disease of the liver, usually caused by a virus.

hernia—the abnormal protrusion of an organ or tissue through an opening.

high altitude cerebral edema (HACE)—a type of acute mountain sickness characterized by swelling of the brain.

high altitude pulmonary edema (HAPE)—a type of acute mountain sickness characterized by filling of the lungs with edema fluid.

hip fracture—a fracture of the upper end of the femur.

hip joint—a ball-and-socket joint formed by the acetabulum proximally and the head of the femur distally.

histology—the branch of anatomy that deals with the minute structure, composition, and function of the tissues.

hoarseness—a rough, low-pitched quality of the voice.

homeotherm—a human or other warm-blooded animal that maintains a relatively constant body temperature despite changes in environmental temperature.

hooked-finger technique—a method of clearing solid debris from the oral cavity.

hormones—organic compounds that are produced by glands and regulate the activity of other organs.

humerus—the upper arm bone.

hydraulic sarong—an apparatus for rewarming a hypothermic patient that uses a backpacking stove to heat a pot of water and a bilge pump to circulate the water through plastic tubes sewn into a blanket that can be wrapped around the patient's trunk.

hyperbaric chamber—a pressure chamber used for recompression of patients suffering from air embolism and decompression sickness.

hyperflexion trauma—a type of bending trauma.

hyperpigmentation—abnormally increased pigmentation.

hyperpnea—an increase in breathing depth.

hyperthermia—see **heatstroke**.

hyperventilation—deep, rapid breathing; a common, benign form of respiratory distress that starts with an increase in the rate and depth of breathing, which produces an excessive loss of carbon dioxide, making the blood more alkaline.

hypervitaminosis—a toxic condition caused by excess intake of vitamins.

hypoglycemia—low blood sugar.

hypothalamus—the portion of the cerebrum of the brain that controls automatic functions such as the regulation of the heart, circulation, digestion, and blood pressure, as well as water balance, sexual function, sleep, appetite, and body temperature.

hypothermia—a fall in the body core temperature to below 95°F (35°C).

hypovolemic shock—shock caused by a decrease in circulating blood volume that results from the loss of whole blood or a decrease in the fluid portion of the blood secondary to dehydration from vomiting, diarrhea, or severe burns.

hypoxia—insufficient oxygen for normal tissue function.

ileum—the distal portion of the small intestine, extending from the jejunum and connecting to the large intestine at the cecum.

iliac arteries—the arteries that supply blood to the lower extremities.

iliac crest—the long curving portion of the ilium.

iliac veins—the veins that carry blood away from the lower extremities.

iliopsoas muscle—one of the two muscles that lie at the back of the abdominal and pelvic cavities on either side of the spine and flex the hip joints.

ilium—the most lateral of the three fused bones making up the pelvis.

illness—a condition marked by deviation from the normal healthy state; sickness.

implied consent—the legal presumption that a patient (or the parent or guardian if present) would consent to accepting care if able to do so in situations where care is urgently needed for life-threatening or serious illness or injury and the patient is unconscious, irrational, or a minor.

incision—a type of laceration caused by a knife or other sharp object.

incontinence—the uncontrolled passage of urine or feces.

indigestion—disturbance of the normal function of the stomach, producing symptoms such as heartburn, pain, nausea, and vomiting.

infection—the invasion and multiplication of microorganisms (e.g., viruses, bacteria, or parasites) in body tissues.

infectious disease (communicable disease)—a disease that is caused by bacteria, viruses, and other microorganisms and can be transmitted from person to person by transfer of the causative microorganism.

inferior—nearer the soles of the feet.

inflammation—a condition caused by injury or infection and marked by swelling, pain, heat, redness, and loss of function.

ingestion—to take into the body.

inguinal hernia—a hernia in the groin.

inhalant—a substance such as the fumes of gasoline, organic solvents, and glue inhaled for its central nervous system depressant effects.

inhalation—breathing air into the lungs.

injury—damage to the body, usually inflicted by an external source.

insidious—of gradual and subtle development.

insomnia—the inability to sleep.

insulin—a hormone that is produced by the pancreas and is essential for use of glucose as fuel by the cells. Insulin quantities are deficient in patients with diabetes.

insulin shock—an abnormally low blood glucose level in a patient with diabetes mellitus, usually caused by too much insulin or insufficient food. Insulin shock is manifested by an alteration of the mental state, progressing from personality changes and confusion to stupor or coma.

intensive care unit—a hospital unit using special equipment and skilled personnel to care for seriously ill patients who require immediate and continuous attention.

intercostal muscles—the muscles between the ribs.

intercostal spaces—the spaces between the ribs.

interspaces—see intercostal spaces.

intestine (bowel)—the part of the digestive tract that extends from the distal opening of the stomach to the anus. The small intestine is the proximal portion of the bowel, while the large intestine is the distal portion.

iris—the muscle behind the cornea that dilates and constricts the pupil, regulating the amount of light that enters the eye. The iris forms the colored portion of the eye surrounding the pupil.

irregular bones—bones of irregular shape, such as the vertebrae.

irreversible shock—prolonged shock marked by the production of toxic substances from injured organs, which prevent reestablishment of the circulation despite treatment.

ischial tuberosity—the lowermost knob-like part of the ischium.

ischium—the most posterior of the three fused bones making up the pelvis.

-itis—suffix denoting infection or inflammation, e.g., appendicitis or bronchitis.

IV—intravenous, within a vein.

jaundice—yellowing of the skin and whites of the eyes caused by the accumulation of bilirubin in patients with liver disease and certain types of anemia.

jaw ramus—a process projecting superiorly from the posterior part of either side of the mandible.

jaw-thrust—a method of opening the airway by thrusting the lower jaw forward with the fingers.

jejunum—the portion of the small intestine, extending from the duodenum to the ileum.

joint—the junction between two or more bones.

joint capsule—a sac of fibrous tissue enclosing movable joints.

Kendrick extrication device (KED)—a lightweight, collapsible, short backboard made of nylon strengthened with vertical slats.

Kendrick traction device—a traction splint similar to the Sager splint.

kidney—one of a pair of organs that lie on either side of the spine against the upper part of the posterior abdominal wall. The kidneys filter the waste products of cellular metabolism from the blood and regulate the body's content of water and essential minerals by adjusting salt retention and urine excretion.

kidney stones—stones that pass from the kidney into the ureter where they cause excruciating pain until they enter the bladder.

knee joint—a complex joint that joins the two lower leg bones (the tibia and fibula) distally to the femur proximally.

liver—a large gland essential to life that is located in the upper right quadrant of the abdomen. The liver has many functions, including storage and filtration of blood, secretion of bile, excretion of bilirubin and other substances formed elsewhere in the body, and numerous metabolic functions including assistance in fat metabolism, detoxification of drugs and other substances, conversion of sugars to glycogen, and storage of glycogen.

"lockjaw"—see tetanus.

logroll—a technique used to move a patient without causing bending or twisting of the spine.

long bones—one of the three major types of bones (the others are flat bones and irregular bones), long bones are found in the limbs.

LSD—lysergic acid diethylamide, a commonly used hallucinogenic drug.

lumbar spine—the five lumbar vertebrae.

Lyme disease—a tick-born infectious arthritis caused by a spirochete.

labor—the process by which a baby is forced from the uterus through the vagina to the outside world.

laceration—a tear in the skin.

lactic acid—an intermediate product of carbohydrate metabolism that accumulates in the blood during exercise and normally is metabolized to carbon dioxide and water if sufficient oxygen is available.

ladder splint—a fixation splint made of heavy, rigid wire.

large intestine—see **colon**.

larynx—the organ that connects the pharynx with the trachea and contains the vocal cords responsible for production of the voice.

lateral—farther from the midline of the body.

lateral malleolus—the outer portion of the ankle joint formed by the distal end of the fibula.

latissimus dorsi muscle—the muscle that extends like a wing from each shoulder girdle to the spine and adducts the upper arm. The muscle can be felt as it extends downward from the armpit to the side of the chest; it is attached to the humerus laterally and the spinous processes of the thoracic vertebrae medially.

Law of Conservation of Energy—energy can neither be created nor destroyed but may be changed from any form to any other form.

lens—the transparent biconvex body that forms part of the optics of the eye. The lens is located behind the cornea and separates the anterior compartment of the eye from the posterior compartment.

leprosy—a chronic infectious disease that is caused by Mycobacterium leprae and affects the skin and peripheral nerves.

ligament—a band of thick, strong, fibrous tissue that connects bones or cartilages. A ligament may be a localized thickening of the joint capsule.

"magic" mushroom (Psilocybe mexicana)—the source of psilocybin, a commonly used hallucinogenic drug.

malaria—a mosquito-borne tropical disease caused by protozoa of the genus Plasmodium. The organism is a parasite of red blood cells. Symptoms include cyclic fever, chills, and fatigue.

malleable metal splint—a fixation splint made of soft sheet metal padded with thin sheets of foam.

mammalian diving reflex—slowing of the heart rate, cessation of breathing, and diversion of blood flow from the shell to the body core in response to immersion of the face in cold water. The reflex acts to conserve vital oxygen for the most important tissues.

mandible—the lower jaw, containing the lower teeth.

manual stabilization—using the rescuer's hands to stabilize the head and neck of a patient with a possible neck or back injury.

manual traction—traction using the hands alone.

marijuana—a product of the Indian hemp plant Cannabis sativa, marijuana causes mild euphoria, relaxation, and drowsiness when ingested or smoked.

mass-casualty incident (MCI)—a disaster that initially overwhelms the resources of the community and requires triage to ensure that the greatest good is done for the greatest number.

masseter muscle—one of the two large, powerful muscles that close the jaws (see **temporalis muscle**).

mastoid process—the sharp tip of the mastoid part of the temporal bone that can be felt just behind the ear.

maxilla—the upper jaw, containing the upper teeth.

medial—nearer to the midline of the body.

medial malleolus—the distal end of the tibia that forms the inside part of the ankle joint.

median nerve—a major nerve of the upper extremity that supplies sensation to the lateral side of the ring finger, most of the thumb, and the first two fingers.

median plane—an imaginary plane separating the body into right and left sides.

mediastinum—the space in the chest that separates the two thoracic cavities and contains the heart and other important structures.

meninges—the three layers of protective membranes that cover the brain and spinal cord.

meningitis—inflammation of the meninges.

meniscus—a cushion of cartilage that fills up a space between bones and aids in the gliding motion of a joint; e.g., the medial and lateral menisci atop the tibial plateau that cushion the knee joint.

menstrual period—the normal, cyclic discharge consisting of blood and mucosal tissue from the lining of the uterus, which normally occurs every 28 days in a nonpregnant woman of reproductive age.

mescal cactus (Lophophora williamsii)—the source of mescaline and peyote, two commonly used hallucinogenic drugs.

mesenteric arteries—the arteries that supply blood to the digestive tract.

mesenteric veins—the veins that carry blood away from the digestive tract.

mesentery—a thin sheet of connective tissue that attaches the organs of the abdominal cavity to the body wall.

metabolism—the oxygen-requiring chemical reactions by which the body produces or uses energy.

metacarpal bones—the five bones found in the palm of the hand that form a base for the fingers and thumb and connect with the eight carpal bones that form the wrist.

metatarsal bones—five long, slender bones that form the arch of the foot and are located between the tarsals proximally and the digits distally.

micron—a unit of measurement equalling 0.000039 inches or 0.001 millimeter.

midclavicular line—an imaginary line running perpendicular to the midpoint of the clavicle.

midline—the intersection of the median plane with the body surface in front and in back.

migraine—a recurrent, throbbing, one-sided headache accompanied by nausea and preceded by abnormal visual phenomena such as blurred vision or bright, moving lights.

minerals—inorganic elements and compounds that are found in the earth's crust. Many minerals are necessary for normal metabolic body functioning.

miscarriage—the spontaneous expelling of the fetus from the pregnant uterus before the fetus is capable of life outside the uterus.

monitor—to check constantly or repeatedly on a condition or phenomenon, i.e., the vital signs of a patient.

motor area—the part of the cerebral cortex of the brain that controls the movement of the voluntary muscles.

motor fibers—fibers composed of nerve cell axons that regulate muscle motion.

motor nerves—nerves that transmit impulses to the skeletal muscles.

mouth-to-mouth breathing—see **rescue breathing**.

mouth-to-nose breathing—a rescue breathing technique used in infants, small children, patients with facial injuries or mouths that cannot be opened, or when it is difficult to achieve a tight seal around the patient's mouth.

mucoid—mucus-like.

mucous membrane—a thin, moist mucous-producing tissue that lines the mouth, nasal cavity, and other body cavities.

mucus—the slimy material that is found on the mucous membranes and lubricates body openings; the secretions of the mucous glands.

muscle—a special tissue composed of cells that can shorten, or contract, and lengthen, or relax.

muscle tension headache—a headache caused by chronic contraction of the muscles of the head and/or neck.

myelin—a fatty substance that encloses the axons of the neurons and acts like the insulation that prevents short circuits in electric wires.

myocardial contusion—a bruise of the heart.

myocardial infarction—death of the heart muscle caused by lack of oxygen, usually because of a blood clot or sudden narrowing of an artery in a patient with coronary artery disease.

narcotic—a pain-relieving drug that suppresses the central nervous system, producing stupor, insensibility, or sound sleep. Narcotics are derived from the opium poppy or a similar chemical manufactured synthetically, e.g., heroin, codeine, Methadone, Demerol, and Dilaudid.

nasal cavity—the interior cavity of the nose, separated into two halves by the nasal septum.

nasal septum—the thin partition that divides the nasal cavity into two nostrils and is composed of membrane, cartilage, and bone.

NATO position—the semiprone or stable side position recommended for all unconscious or semiconscious patients without neck or back injuries.

nausea—an unpleasant sensation in the upper abdomen that often leads to vomiting.

navel—the umbilicus; a depression in the abdominal wall marking the site of attachment of the umbilical cord in the fetus.

near-drowning—survival, at least temporarily, after submersion in water.

negligence—injury to another person caused by failure to provide the degree of care that any reasonable and prudent person would provide in similar circumstances (see also **willful negligence** and **gross negligence**).

neoplasm—new growth; a benign or malignant tumor.

nervous system—the system of nerve cells and their supporting structures that collects and processes stimuli from the environment and coordinates the activities of the other major organ systems.

neurogenic shock—shock that is secondary to dilation of the blood vessels and is caused by the nervous system.

neurons—the primary cells of the nervous system.

Newton's First Law of Motion—a body at rest will tend to remain at rest, and a body in motion will tend to remain in motion unless acted upon by an outside force.

nicotine—a poisonous alkaloid in tobacco that accounts for the addictive nature of cigarette smoking.

nipple—the pigmented projection on the anterior surface of the breast.

nitrogen narcosis ("rapture of the deep")—an effect similar to alcohol intoxication that is caused by breathing nitrogen at depths below about 90 feet (27 meters).

nitroglycerin—a medication dispensed as a small white tablet that is placed under the tongue to treat patients with angina pectoris. Nitroglycerin relaxes vascular smooth muscle and increases blood flow and oxygen supply to the heart muscle.

non-rebreather mask—a transparent mask fitted with a plastic reservoir bag and one-way valve that allows the patient to inhale oxygen from the bag but prevents exhalation into the bag.

nostrils—the external openings of the nasal cavity; the nares.

numbness—a lack of or decrease in sensation in a part.

occiput—the back of the head.

olecranon of the ulna—the bony projection of the ulna at the elbow, to which the triceps muscle tendon is attached.

olfactory organ—the part of the nose that contains the end organs for smell.

ophthalmologist—a physician specializing in the treatment of eye disease and injury.

optic nerve—one of the paired cranial nerves that transmits visual sensations generated by light-sensitive retina cells to the brain.

oral airway—a curved device designed to keep the tongue of an unconscious patient from falling back and occluding the upper airway.

orbit—the bony socket that contains and protects the eye.

Oregon spine splint—the brand name of a portable short backboard similar to the Kendrick extrication device.

oropharynx—the portion of the pharynx between the soft palate and the upper edge of the epiglottis.

orthopedics—the branch of surgery concerned with the preservation and restoration of the function of the skeletal system, its articulations, and associated structures.

osmotic pressure—pressure exerted by a solution in direct proportion to the number of particles dissolved in it.

ovary—one of the two female gonads, which produce sex hormones and eggs.

ovum—an egg.

oxygen (O^2)—a gas that makes up 21 percent of air and is necessary for normal metabolism.

oxygen debt—a buildup of lactic acid in the blood and muscle tissues during exercise because of a relative lack of oxygen.

oxygen poisoning--convulsions caused by breathing pure oxygen below 33 feet (10 meters) or breathing compressed air below 297 feet (90 meters).

---

packaging—the process of securing a patient to a device such as a spine board, litter, or toboggan, and otherwise preparing the patient for transport after initial emergency care has been given.

palpation—feeling; examining by touch.

pancreas—the organ that aids in digestion and makes the fuel-regulating hormone insulin, which is necessary for the metabolism of glucose, the body's chief source of energy.

pancreatic juice—a fluid produced by the pancreas that contains enzymes that aid in the digestion of fat, starch, and protein.

pancreatitis—inflammation or infection of the pancreas.

pant leg pinch lift—a technique used to lift a patient's lower extremity onto a quick splint by grasping the clothing rather than the extremity itself.

paradoxical motion of the chest wall—a condition in which a flail section of the chest wall moves in instead of out with inhalation and out instead of in with exhalation.

paralysis—inability to move.

paranoia—a psychiatric disorder marked by delusions of grandeur or persecution.

parasympathetic nervous system—one of the two parts of the autonomic nervous system, the parasympathetic nervous system has many functions, including constriction of the pupils, slowing of the heart rate, and relaxation of body sphincters.

paravertebral muscles—the generic name given to a number of different muscles lying on either side of the spine.

partial pressure of oxygen—the percentage of total atmospheric pressure accounted for by oxygen. At sea level, oxygen partial pressure is 160 mm Hg (21 percent of 760 mm Hg).

PASG (pneumatic antishock garment)—a form of pneumatic counterpressure device.

patella—the kneecap.

patellar ligament—the continuation of the quadriceps muscle tendon that extends from the patella to the tibial tuberosity.

patient—an ill or injured person who requires emergency care.

pectoralis muscle—one of the two muscles beneath the breasts that help adduct the upper extremities.

pelvic cavity—the cavity located in the lowest part of the trunk that is continuous with the abdominal cavity. It contains the bladder, rectum, and female reproductive organs.

pelvis—a cone-shaped, bony ring made up of the right and left pelvic bones joined in front at the pubis and in back to the sacrum at the sacroiliac joints. Each pelvic bone is made up of three fused bones—the ilium, ischium, and pubis. The pelvis contains the bladder, rectum, and female reproductive organs.

penetration trauma—trauma caused by a sharp object moving at a moderate to high speed, or by a moving body striking a narrow, pointed object.

penis—the male organ of sexual intercourse.

Pepto-Bismol—the brand name of a nonprescription bismuth preparation useful in controlling diarrhea.

pericardial tamponade—the failure of heart action because of fluid accumulation in the pericardium that leads to increased pressure, which interferes with the heart's ability to relax between contractions and refill with blood.

pericardium—the fibrous sac that surrounds the heart and the roots of the great vessels.

perineum—the area between the pubis anteriorly and the coccyx posteriorly.

periodic breathing—Cheyne-Stokes respirations.

peripheral nervous system—the portion of the nervous system consisting of the nerves and their branches and the special sensory organs lying outside the brain and spinal cord.

peristalsis—the worm-like movement by which the alimentary canal propels and mixes its contents.

peristaltic activity—the contraction of the muscles in the walls of the small and large intestines that mixes and propels their contents forward.

peritoneal cavity—the abdominal cavity.

peritoneal dialysis—dialysis using the peritoneum as a dialyzing membrane, with the dialyzing solution being introduced and removed from the peritoneal cavity.

peritoneum—a thin membrane that lines the abdominal cavity and is continuous with the outer coverings of the organs within the cavity, forming a closed sac similar to the pleural cavity. A continuation of the peritoneum lines the pelvic cavity.

peritonitis—inflammation caused by irritation or infection of the peritoneum.

peroneal nerve—one of the branches of the sciatic nerve, the peroneal nerve winds around the head of the fibula before entering the lower leg where it divides into superficial and deep branches. It supplies sensation to the top of the foot and helps move the ankle.

perspiration—the liquid excreted by the sweat glands.

phalanges—the small bones that make up each finger and toe.

pharynx—the cavity that is continuous with the nasal cavities and mouth in front and the larynx and the esophagus below.

phenothiazines—a group of tranquilizing drugs.

phrenic nerves—nerves that originate in the cervical part of the spinal cord and pass down through the chest to supply the diaphragm.

physical dependence—physiological changes in response to a drug, so that suddenly stopping its use causes well-defined symptoms of withdrawal.

physiological saline solution—also called normal saline, a 0.9-percent solution of table salt in water with the same osmotic pressure as normal human tissue, used to irrigate an open wound or keep tissue moist.

physiology—the branch of biology dealing with the function of the living organism and its parts.

pia mater—the innermost of the three layers of meninges that cover the brain and spinal cord.

pinna—the external ear, which is made of cartilage covered by skin and surrounds the ear canal.

"pitting edema"—a type of swelling characterized by a depression or pit that remains after a finger is pressed into a swollen area.

pituitary gland—a gland at the base of the brain that controls the male and female reproductive systems, thyroid, adrenal cortex, body growth, and other body functions.

placenta (afterbirth)—an organ that attaches to the lining of the uterus and contains special tissues through which the blood of the mother and fetus are brought in close proximity so that oxygen, nutrients, waste products, and other substances can be exchanged.

plantarflex—to bend the foot downward, in the direction of the sole of the foot.

plasma—the fluid component of blood. Plasma transports the blood cells and contains a large variety of dissolved minerals and inorganic and organic compounds. The compounds include nutrients, waste products, and components involved in immunity and blood clotting.

pleura—a thin membrane that lines the inner wall of each thoracic cavity and covers the outer surface of each lung.

pleural space—a potential rather than actual space between the pleura lining the rib cage and the pleura covering the outside of the lung; the pleural space is normally filled with a thin film of fluid.

pleurisy—inflammation of the pleura.

pneumatic counterpressure device—an inflatable splint used to stabilize fractures and provide direct pressure to extensive or internal areas of bleeding.

pneumonia—an infection or inflammation of the lung alveoli that causes consolidation and results in shortness of breath and lowered arterial blood oxygen.

pneumothorax—air in the pleural space caused by an abnormal passage that connects the pleural space with the outside air, either through the chest wall or within the lung.

poison—any substance that impairs the functioning of the body through chemical action that interferes with normal metabolic processes.

polycythemia—an increase in the numbers of red blood cells that can occur in association with certain diseases and as an adaptive response to living at high altitude.

popliteal fossa—the area behind the knee bordered by the hamstring tendons.

position of function—the position in which an immobilized body part functions best.

posterior—nearer to the back surface of the body.

posterior tibial artery pulse—a pulse that can be felt just below and behind the medial malleolus.

potentiator—an agent that enhances another agent so that the combined effect is greater than the sum of each agent alone.

predisposition—a latent susceptibility.

pregnancy—the condition of carrying a developing offspring inside the body.

pressure point—a point where a major artery lies close to the skin and over a bone. Pressure at this point is sometimes used as an aid to control severe bleeding.

priapism—a long-lasting, painful erection of the penis.

progressive—advancing, increasing in strength or severity.

process—a projection of bone or tissue.

prone—lying face down.

prostate gland—a small gland that lies at the base of the bladder and surrounds the male urethra. It produces part of the seminal fluid.

protein—compounds composed of chains of amino acids made up of nitrogen, sulfur, and phosphorus in addition to carbon, hydrogen, and oxygen.

proximal—closer to the trunk of the body.

psychological dependence—a state in which a drug user becomes obsessed with taking a drug and continues to take it despite obvious physical, mental, or social harm.

psychosomatic illness—an illness with bodily symptoms but an emotional or mental cause.

pubic bone—see **pubis**.

pubis—the most anterior of the three bones that make up the pelvic bone.

pulmonary artery—the major artery leading from the right ventricle of the heart to the lungs.

pulmonary contusion—a bruise of the lung.

pulmonary edema—the abnormal accumulation of fluid in the tissues and air spaces of the lung.

pulmonary embolus—a blood clot that has broken loose and traveled to the lung.

pulmonary emphysema—a chronic obstructive lung disease involving dilation and/or destruction of the alveoli.

pulmonary fibrosis—a condition that leads to thickening of the walls of the alveoli in the lungs because of increased fibrous tissue in their walls.

pulse—the rhythmic, expanding tap felt when the fingers are placed over an artery lying close to the body surface. The pulse represents the pressure wave produced each time the heart beats.

pulselessness—absence of a heart beat.

puncture—a deep wound with a small entrance caused by a sharp, narrow object or by a high-velocity blunt object.

pupil of the eye—the opening in the center of the iris of the eye through which light enters.

pupils, reaction of—ability of the pupils of the eyes to respond to light and other stimulants by enlarging or decreasing in size.

pus—a thick, yellowish or greenish liquid made up of white cells and fluid, produced in response to inflammation.

quadriceps—the major muscle of the anterior thigh, which allows extension of the knee.

quick splint—a splint made of plywood padded with foam, designed for rapid application so that a chilled patient can be quickly evacuated.

rabies—a universally fatal disease of the central nervous system that is caused by a virus present in the saliva of infected animals and is transmitted through biting or licking.

"raccoon eyes"—ecchymosis in the skin around the eyes, a sign of internal bleeding from a skull fracture.

radial artery pulse—a pulse felt anterior to the radial styloid process proximal to the base of the thumb.

radial nerve—a nerve that winds around the humerus at its midpoint, carrying sensations to the back of the hand and controlling extension of the hand at the wrist.

radiating—characterized by divergence from a common center.

radiation heat loss—heat transferred by infrared waves emanating from the body.

radius—the lateral of the two forearm bones when the palms are held facing forward.

reclining—lying down.

rectum—the distal portion of the large intestine ending at the anal canal.

rectus muscle—one of the two strap-like muscles covering the front of the abdomen that provide support for the abdomen and allow flexion of the lumbar spine.

red cell sludging—clumping together of red cells within blood vessels.

reduce—to restore the normal relationship of parts, e.g., to reduce a fractured bone.

reflex arcs—short connections between motor and sensory nerve fibers within the spinal cord that bypass the brain and provide an immediate reaction to noxious stimuli, i.e., pulling a hand away from a hot stove.

regulator—the name given to the device that contains a pressure-reducing valve, pressure gauge and flowmeter, and is attached to the outlet of a gas cylinder.

regurgitation—backward flowing, e.g., the casting up of undigested food.

renal arteries—the arteries that supply blood to the kidneys.

renal pelvis—the funnel-shaped upper portion of each ureter.

renal veins—the veins that carry blood away from the kidneys.

reproductive system—the system of organs that provides the means of producing successive generations of offspring.

reproductive system, female—the ovaries, fallopian tubes, uterus, vagina, and associated glands.

reproductive system, male—the testicles, vasa deferentia, seminal vesicles, prostate gland, and penis.

rescue breathing—mouth-to-mouth breathing performed after opening the airway of a breathless patient.

rescuer—a ski patroller, backcountry search and rescue group member, leader of a backcountry recreational party, or any other person who provides care in an emergency.

respiration—breathing.

respiration heat loss—heat lost as inhaled air is warmed to body temperature before being exhaled.

respiratory center—the brain center that controls the depth, rate, and rhythm of breathing.

respiratory distress—an abnormal rate of breathing that includes dyspnea (difficulty in breathing), tachypnea (increase in the breathing rate), and hyperpnea (increase in the breathing depth).

retina—the lining of the inner surface of the sclera of the eye, which contains light-sensitive cells.

rewarm—to raise the body temperature of a patient with hypothermia, or to raise the temperature of a part affected with frostbite.

rhonchi—coarse sounds produced by air moving through larger air passages partly blocked by sputum or other secretions (see also **wheezes** and **stridor**).

rib—one of 24 paired, curved bones that form and support the chest wall.

rigor mortis—the stiffening of a dead body.

"road burn"—a type of abrasion commonly seen in cyclists.

Rocky Mountain spotted fever—a severe febrile illness accompanied by a rash that is caused by the parasite Rickettsia rickettsii and is carried by certain wood ticks.

---

sacroiliac joint—the joint between the sacrum medially and the ilium laterally.

sacrum—a flat, triangular bone formed from the five sacral vertebrae fused together to form a single bone that can be felt below the lumbar vertebrae and above the sharp coccyx.

Sager splint—the brand name of a small, lightweight, device used for applying traction to the lower extremity.

salicylate—a compound such as aspirin that is a salt of salicylic acid.

saliva—the liquid secretion of the glands of the mouth that serves to moisten and soften food and initiate the digestion of starch.

SAM splint—the brand name of a malleable metal splint padded with thin sheets of foam.

Sawyer extractor—the brand name a small, powerful suction pump for removing injected poisons.

scalp—the part of the skin of the head that is normally covered by hair.

scapula—the shoulder blade; a large, flat, triangular bone lying against the posterior chest wall.

sciatic nerve—the largest nerve in the body; the sciatic nerve provides sensation to the lateral leg and foot, and supplies the muscles that extend the hip, flex the knee, and move the ankle and foot. In the back of the thigh, the sciatic nerve branches into the tibial and peroneal nerves.

sclera—the dense tissue that forms the posterior five-sixths of the globe of the eye. The visible part of the sclera is called the white of the eye.

scoop stretcher—a lightweight aluminum frame that breaks apart lengthwise. Each side is inserted beneath a patient until the two sides meet in the middle.

scrotum—the sac that contains the testicles and their accessory organs.

seated carries—emergency two-rescuer techniques for moving conscious patients without spinal injuries by carrying them in the seated position.

seizure—a sudden, transient alteration of normal brain function.

semen—the fluid that contains sperm and the secretions of the prostate and seminal vesicles and is discharged at ejaculation.

seminal fluid—see **semen**.

seminal vesicles—outpouchings of the vasa deferentia that store the sperm.

sensory fibers—fibers that are composed of nerve cell axons and carry sensation to the brain from the organs of touch, pain, and temperature in the skin and muscles.

sexually-transmitted infection—an infectious disease transmitted by sexual contact.

shell—the skin, muscles, and extremities of the body (see also **core**).

shivering—an involuntary method of heat production that involves involuntary trembling or quivering of the body caused by contraction or twitching of the muscles.

shock—a form of acute failure of the blood circulation.

short spine board—a device developed to evacuate patients with spine injuries from wrecked automobiles and other confined spaces.

shoulder girdle—the clavicle, scapula, humerus, sternoclavicular joint, acromioclavicular (AC) joint, and shoulder joint.

shoulder joint—a ball-and-socket joint in the shoulder girdle where the humerus connects distally with the scapula proximally.

side crutch support—an emergency technique for assisting a conscious patient to walk to safety with the support of one or two rescuers.

sign—an important characteristic of an illness or injury that the observer notes by looking, feeling, listening, or smelling (see also **symptom** and **vital signs**).

silent—producing no detectable signs or symptoms.

simple fainting—a common, benign form of collapse caused by temporary slowing of the circulation because of loss of blood vessel tone and slowing of the heart rate.

skeletal system—made up of 206 bones and their associated ligaments, the skeletal system provides a rigid framework to protect and support the soft tissues, gives form to the body, and, together with the muscular system, allows body movement.

"skier's thumb" ("gamekeeper's thumb")—a ligament at the base of the thumb caused when the skier tries to break a fall with an outstretched hand while holding a ski pole, which bends the thumb backward on impact.

skin—the largest organ in the body, made up of the epidermis and the dermis.

skull—the bones of the head, including the eight bones of the cranium, the mandible, and the facial bones.

sling—a triangular bandage tied around the neck to support the weight of the upper extremity (see **swathe**).

slow-twitch (Type I) fibers—muscle fibers designed for sustained, slow contractions that rely mainly on aerobic metabolic processes (see also **fast-twitch fibers**).

small intestine—the segment of bowel from which most digested food is absorbed before the undigested residue is passed to the large intestine.

smallpox—an acute infectious disease caused by a virus and characterized by a severe pustular rash.

snowblindness—sunburn of the conjunctiva of the eye.

socket—a hollow or depression into which a corresponding part fits, e.g., the socket of a tooth or joint.

soft fixation splint—a splint made of soft material, i.e., an air splint, splints improvised from folded parkas, blankets or pillows, and the sling and swathe.

somatic nervous system—the system that controls voluntary activities such as eating, walking, and talking.

Spanish windlass—a device that provides traction through tightening a twisted cravat.

sperm—the male germ cell.

sphygmomanometer—an instrument used to measure blood pressure.

spinal canal—the tunnel that is formed by the vertebral arches and contains the spinal cord.

spinal cord—the part of the central nervous system that lies in the spinal canal. The spinal cord is connected to the brain above at the foramen magnum of the skull.

spinal nerves—the 31 pairs of nerves that branch off from the spinal nerve and exit through notches between the vertebrae.

spine—the vertebral column that is composed of 33 vertebrae, forms the main support for the body, and protects the spinal cord.

spine board—a long, rigid board designed to immobilize the body of a patient with a neck or back injury.

spinous processes—the posterior processes of the vertebrae that form the attachment points for ligaments and tendons.

spiral fracture—a fracture in which the fracture line spirals around the shaft of the bone. A spiral fracture usually is caused by a twisting force.

spleen—the organ that filters the blood and lies in the upper-left part of the abdominal cavity.

splint—a device designed to prevent or reduce motion at the site of a fracture or other injury.

splinting—the application of a splint.

spontaneous pneumothorax—air in the pleural space caused by spontaneous rupture of a bleb or cyst of the lung.

sprain—the stretching or tearing of a ligament or tendon.

sputum—mucoid material from the lower respiratory tract (trachea, bronchi, and lungs), usually produced by coughing.

"squeeze" injuries—injuries to certain body areas caused by failure to equalize pressure between the area and the outside water. The middle and inner ears, sinuses, and lungs are most often affected.

standard of care—the common law requirement that care providers perform as any other reasonable, prudent person with similar training and experience would perform under similar circumstances, with due regard for the safety and welfare of both the patient and fellow care providers.

START—Simple Triage and Rapid Treatment, a four-step technique for managing mass-casualty incidents developed by Hoag Memorial Hospital Presbyterian, Newport Beach, California.

sterile—free from living microorganisms.

sterilize—to make sterile or free from bacterial contamination.

sternal angle (Angle of Louis)—a prominent bony ridge at the junction of the upper and lower parts of the sternum.

sternal notch—the notch at the top of the sternum.

sternoclavicular joint—the joint that joins the sternum to the clavicle.

sternomastoid muscle—one of the two strap-like muscles on either side of the front of the neck that are attached above to the mastoid processes and below to the sternoclavicular joints. The sternomastoid muscles help turn the head and flex the neck.

sternum—breastbone.

stethoscope—an instrument used to transmit sounds from the body to the examiner's ears.

stimulant—a drug that excites the mind, increases the heart rate, raises the blood pressure and breathing rate, and provides a sense of euphoria or well-being. Stimulants include caffeine, nicotine, decongestants, and asthma drugs as well as cocaine and amphetamines.

stomach—the sac-like organ between the esophagus and the duodenum where food is mixed with gastric juice to form a semifluid substance that is passed on to the intestine for further digestion.

stomach ulcer—a defect in the inner lining of the stomach caused by destruction from infection, inflammation, or self-digestion.

straddle injury—an injury to the groin or perineum caused by a fall when the patient lands with the legs straddling an object such as a fence.

straddle slide—a technique for placing a patient on a spine board.

strain—the stretching or tearing of a muscle because of over-stretching or overexertion.

stridor—harsh, high-pitched sounds on inhalation produced by air moving through a narrowed larynx (see also **wheezes** and **rhonchi**).

styloid process—a long, pointed process of a bone.

subclavian arteries—the arteries that supply blood to the upper extremities.

subclavian veins—the veins that carry blood away from the upper extremities.

subcutaneous emphysema—an injury to the air-containing parts of the respiratory tract in the chest or neck that allows air to escape into the subcutaneous tissues, producing a unique crackling sensation similar to Rice Krispies under the skin.

subnormal temperature—an orally measured body temperature below 98°F (36.5°C).

substance abuse—use of mind-altering chemicals without a legal medical purpose.

subtrochanteric fracture—a fracture of the upper part of the femur below the trochanters.

sucking chest wound—an open hole in the chest wall that establishes a connection between the pleural space and the outside air. The lung is collapsed, and when the patient breathes, air moves in and out of the hole in the chest rather than in and out of the lung through the normal airway.

suction apparatus—a mechanical device for sucking liquid and solid foreign matter from the mouth, nose, and throat.

suffocation—stoppage of respiration and the resulting lack of oxygen to the tissues.

sun protection factor (SPF)—a number that refers to how many times longer skin protected by a sunscreen can be exposed to the sun before becoming red compared to unprotected skin.

sunburn—a first- or second-degree skin burn caused by ultraviolet light in the medium-wave range (UVB) with a wavelength of 290 to 320 nanometers.

sunscreen—a preparation that protects the skin from the harmful effects of sunlight. Physical sunscreens block sunlight; chemical sunscreens selectively filter out harmful rays.

superior—nearer to the top of the head.

supine—lying face up.

supracondylar fracture—a fracture of the femur above the knee.

swathe—a cravat that is tied around the trunk and used with a sling to immobilize the upper extremity.

sweat—see **perspiration**.

swelling—a transient enlargement of a body part or area.

swimmer's ear—an infection of the ear canal that occurs in swimmers and divers whose ears are continually wet.

sympathetic nervous system—one of the two parts of the autonomic nervous system, the sympathetic nervous system prepares the body for action in response to stress by causing the pupils of the eyes to dilate, hairs to stand on end, the heart rate to increase, sphincters to tighten, and other reactions.

symptom—an important characteristic of an illness or injury that the patient notes and describes to the observer.

synapse—the site at which neurons connect, allowing nerve impulses to be transmitted from one to another.

syncope—a faint; a temporary loss of consciousness because of insufficient blood flow to the brain.

synovial membrane—the inner lining of the joint capsule which produces the fluid that lubricates and nourishes joint tissue.

syphilis—a contagious venereal disease caused by the spirochete Treponema pallidum. It can involve the central nervous system, skin, heart, and many other organs.

systolic blood pressure—the highest point of the blood pressure curve.

tachycardia—rapid heart beat.

tachypnea—an abnormal increase in the breathing rate.

talus—a bone of the foot that forms the distal portion of the ankle joint.

tarsals—the five small bones of the midfoot located between the calcaneus proximally and the metatarsals distally.

taste buds—the tiny sensory end organs for taste.

tear ducts—the passages on the inner side of the eye along the lower and upper eyelids through which tears drain into the nasal cavity.

tear glands—the glands above the outer part of each eye that produce tears.

tears—fluid that is produced by tear glands and keeps the conjunctiva and cornea moist.

temporal pulse—the pulse of the temporal artery that can be felt just in front of and above the opening of the ear canal.

temporalis muscle—one of the two large, powerful muscles that close the jaws (see **masseter muscle**).

temporomandibular (TM) joint—the joint that connects the mandible, or jawbone, to the base of the skull just in front of the ear on either side.

tenderness—abnormal sensitivity to touch or pressure.

tendon—a tough fibrous cord that attaches a muscle to a bone.

tension pneumothorax—a serious complication of pneumothorax that occurs when a defect simulating a one-way valve develops at an injury site and allows air to enter but not escape the pleural space. The pressure in the pleural space increases with each breath until it compresses the lung and interferes with the function of the heart and the opposite, normal lung.

testicle (testis)—the male gonad, one of a pair of egg-shaped glands normally located in the scrotum that contain specialized cells that produce hormones and sperm.

testis—see **testicle.**

tetanus—a disease caused by a soil bacterium that grows in open soft tissue wounds and produces a toxin that provokes serious muscle spasms and interferes with breathing.

tetanus prophylaxis—immunization to prevent tetanus. A full protective course is given in infancy followed with boosters every 10 years or following an open wound if a booster has not been given within five years.

thalamus—a portion of the cerebrum of the brain that contains centers for temperature, touch, and emotion.

thermometer—an instrument for recording body temperature.

Thomas splint—a traction splint for immobilizing a fractured femur that was developed during World War I by Sir Hugh Owen Thomas.

thoracic cage—the hollow cage-like structure formed by the ribs, sternum, and vertebral column that encloses the pleural cavities and mediastinum.

thoracic cavities—the two cavities in the chest that contain the right and left lungs and are separated by the mediastinum.

thoracic spine—the 12 thoracic vertebrae.

thorax—the chest.

thyroid cartilage ("Adam's apple")—the shield-shaped cartilage of the larynx at the front of the neck.

thyroid gland—an endocrine gland consisting of two lobes joined by a narrow passage, with one lobe on each side of the lower larynx and upper trachea. The thyroid gland produces iodine-containing hormones that regulate metabolic rate and calcium metabolism.

tibia—the weight-bearing bone that is the medial of the two bones of the lower leg.

tibial plateau—the concave riding surface of the knee on which the femoral condyles sit.

tolerance—a state in which the body adjusts to the presence of a drug so that increasing amounts are required to produce the desired effect.

"tonsil" tip—see **Yankauer tip.**

tourniquet—a device used to control hemorrhage by exerting circumferential pressure around a limb proximal to the bleeding site.

toxic—poisonous; manifesting the symptoms of severe infection.

toxin—a poison, frequently referring to the highly poisonous proteins produced by some plants, animals, or bacteria.

trachea—the tube that is attached to the larynx above and that branches below to form the two main bronchi.

tracheostomy—an incision made through the neck into the trachea to allow insertion of a tube to relieve upper airway obstruction and aid ventilation.

traction—the action of drawing or pulling on an object.

traction splint—a splint that stabilizes a fracture by means of a steady pull on the limb.

tranquilizer—a drug used for treating patients with anxiety states, neuroses, and other mental disorders.

transient ischemic attacks (TIAs)—minor transient strokes (cerebrovascular accidents) that occur when blood flow through a narrowed brain artery is temporarily inadequate to support the function of the brain area supplied.

trapezius muscle—one of the two muscles that form the web of the neck and are attached to the scapula laterally and to the spinous processes of the cervical and upper thoracic vertebrae and the base of the skull medially. These muscles strengthen the shoulder girdles and lift the shoulders.

trauma—the end effect of a force applied to the body, often used interchangeably with injury; a physical or psychological wound or injury.

tremor—the involuntary shaking of a body part.

triage—the technique of handling a disaster when limited resources do not allow everything possible to be done for every patient; also, the technique of determining the proper order in which to treat each injury in a patient with multiple injuries.

triceps muscle—the major muscle of the posterior upper arm, which extends the elbow.

tuberculosis (TB)—a chronic infectious disease caused by Mycobacteria and characterized by the formation of granular tumors in many organs, particularly the lungs.

turgor—the normal consistency of living tissue.

---

ulna—the medial of the two forearm bones when the palm is held facing forward.

ulnar nerve ("crazy bone")—a nerve lying in the groove behind the medial epicondyle at the lower end of the humerus that controls most of the muscular function of the hand and the sensation over the ring and little fingers. Bumping this nerve causes a tingling sensation in the medial forearm and hand.

umbilical cord—the cord-like structure that connects the fetus with the placenta.

umbilicus—see **navel.**

unconscious—incapable of responding to sensory stimuli.

ureter—a muscular tube that drains urine from the kidneys into the bladder. The ureters lie behind the abdominal and pelvic cavities against the back muscle.

urethra—the tube that passes urine from the bladder out of the body. In males, the urethra passes through the penis; in females the urethra opens above the entrance to the vagina.

urinary system—the system that consists of the two kidneys; the two ureters, which drain the urine from the kidneys; the bladder, which stores urine; and the urethra, which drains urine from the body. The urinary system removes waste products of cellular metabolism from the bloodstream and excretes them in the urine.

urine—a fluid excreted by the kidneys that contains water and the waste products of cellular metabolism.

uterus—the muscular organ within which the unborn offspring is nourished.

vacuum splint—an airtight plastic or rubber splint filled with small plastic pellets. After being fitted to the body part, it becomes rigid after air is evacuated with a pump.

vacuum spine board—a spine board based on the same principles as the vacuum splint.

vagina—the canal in the female that connects the uterus with the external female genitalia; it receives the penis during sexual intercourse.

vagus nerves—nerves that originate in the brain and pass through the neck into the chest and abdomen. They help regulate the heart rate and digestive tract function.

vaporization—conversion of water or another volatile liquid into vapor.

vas deferens—one of the two ducts that conduct sperm from the testicles to the urethra.

vascular shock—enlargement and relaxation of the blood vessels caused by failure of the mechanisms that normally control vessel tone.

Vaseline—a brand name for petrolatum or petroleum jelly.

Vaseline gauze—gauze saturated with petrolatum (petroleum jelly).

veins—tubular vessels that carry blood from the tissues back to the heart, venules, and the smallest veins.

vena cava, inferior—the large vein that drains blood from the abdomen, pelvis, and lower extremities.

vena cava, superior—the large vein that drains blood from the head, neck, and upper extremities.

venae cavae—the two large veins that carry blood to the right atrium of the heart.

venous blood—deoxygenated blood that flows from the tissues through the veins.

ventilation—the exchange of air between the lungs and outside air.

ventricle—either of the two lower chambers of the heart.

ventricular fibrillation—a sudden, rapid, irregular, worm-like twitching of the ventricular muscle.

vertebra—one of the 33 bones making up the spine.

vertebral arches—the portion of the vertebrae forming the tunnel that contains the spinal canal.

vertebral column—the spine.

vertigo—dizziness; a sensation of whirling.

vital signs—important characteristics of illness or injury: pulse, respiration, temperature, blood pressure, and level of consciousness (see also **sign** and **symptom**).

vitamins—organic substances necessary in trace amounts for the metabolic functioning of the body.

vitreous humor—a jellylike fluid that fills the posterior compartment of the eyeball behind the lens.

void—to cast out as waste matter.

vomitus—vomited matter.

vulva—the external female genital organs.

"walking wounded"—individuals involved in a mass-casualty incident whose injuries do not present a risk to life and who are ambulatory and can wait several hours before being transported to a hospital.

wheezes—high-pitched whistling sounds produced by exhaled air traveling through small air passages narrowed by swelling or spasm (see also **rhonchi** and **stridor**).

white matter—groups of myelin-covered axons that derive their name from their yellowish-white color.

white of the eye—the visible part of the sclera covered by the transparent conjunctiva.

willful negligence—negligence involving malicious intentions (see also **negligence** and **gross negligence**).

windburn—irritation of the skin that is caused by exposure to wind and resembles first-degree sunburn.

wire splint—a fixation splint made of wire mesh.

wrist joint—the joint between the radius and ulna proximally and the carpal bones distally.

X-rays—electromagnetic vibrations of short wavelength that can penetrate most substances and can affect a photographic plate.

xiphoid process—a cartilaginous process attached to the lower end of the sternum.

Yankauer tip ("tonsil" tip)—a rigid, plastic pharyngeal suction tip attached to the rubber tubing of a mechanical suction device.

Zepharin—the brand name of an antiseptic solution containing benzalkonium chloride.

INDEX

comminuted, 160
displaced, 160
force necessary to cause, 332
greenstick, 160
in spinal cord injured patients, 235
in wilderness, 397
indications of, 161
lower extremity, 203
mechanism of injury, 161
non-displaced, 160
of clavicle, 197
of face, 224
of pelvis, 208
of pelvis/femur, 403
of scapula, 197
open, 159-160
    emergency care of, 166
    medication for, 408
signs and symptoms of, 161
simple, 160
spiral, 160
stress, 160
transverse, 160
upper extremity, 195, 197-200
Frequency, 264
sign of diabetes, 265
Front cradle, 313
Frost tunnel, 15
Frostbite, 289-291
body areas susceptible to, 289
factors contributing to, 289
in wilderness, 390
prostaglandin inhibitors and, 406
Fruit, unpeeled, avoid in developing countries, 409
Full exposure suits, 370
Furosemide (Lasix), 415
for diseases of altitude, 406-407

Gastrointestinal complaints, 261
emergency care of, 264
Gastrointestinal hemorrhage in alcoholics, 281
Gatorade, 394
for heat exhaustion, 299
Gauze, 415
compresses, 415
Gait disturbance, acute effect of hallucinogen use, 283
Gaiters, felt-lined for mountaineering, 21
Gallbladder colic, 263
Gallstone
cause of colic, 263
cause of jaundice, 263
contraindication to wilderness travel, 391
Gamekeeper's thumb, 197
Gangrene
complication of frostbite, 290
of the intestine, complication of cocaine use, 282
Garamycin ophthalmic ointment, 408, 413
Gardnerella vaginalis, 410
Garrick, James, Dr., 330

Gas
intestinal in wilderness, 408
mistaken for severe illness, 408
Gasoline, 16, 283
Gastric distention
complication of CPR, 118
relief of, 118
Gastroenteritis
cause of nausea, 262
vomiting with, 409
Genitalia, female
injuries, 250
Genitalia, male
injuries, 250
Genitourinary complaints, 264-266
Giardia lamblia, 262
hazard for wilderness travelers, 409
symptoms of infestation, 409
Glacier glasses, 304
Glasgow Coma Scale, 85-86, 92, 215, 349
Glove liners, 18
Gloves, 18
Glucose, 274, 394
Glucose
glucose/saline solution, 415
solution, for hypoglycemia, 275
Glue inhalation, 283
Glutethimide (Doriden), 281
Glutose (instant glucose), 414, 415, 416
Goggles, 304, 335
"Golden hour," 348
Good Samaritan laws, 385
"Gooseflesh," sign of narcotic withdrawal, 281
Gore-Tex, 15, 16, 18
Grand mal seizures, 277
Great vessels, injury to, 242
Green triage category, 342, 344
Ground currents, 305
"Guarding," 98
Gurneys, 322, 325
Gymnastics, 30

HACE, see High altitude cerebral edema
Halcion (triazolam), 281
Hallucinations
side effect of inhalant abuse, 283
side effect of marijuana, 282
symptom of alcohol withdrawal, 281
symptom of cocaine use, 282
withdrawal from depressant drugs, 281
Hallucinogens, 283
Halogenated hydrocarbons, 283
Hamstring muscles, 206
Hand
fracture, 200
in alpine skiers, 331
sprain, 197
in alpine skiers, 329, 331
Handball, 30

OTHER PUBLICATIONS AVAILABLE FROM THE NATIONAL SKI PATROL

WEC Instructor's Manual–First Edition (1988)
The principle resource for instructors in the Winter Emergency Care program. This manual is in notebook format to accommodate supplemental materials and includes program administration for courses and refreshers, lesson plans, skill performance guidelines, evaluation principles, and necessary administrative forms.
Cat. No. 551 $19.50

Winter Emergency Care Workbook– Second Edition (1989)
This workbook closely follows the WEC lesson plans using *Outdoor Emergency Care* as the reference textbook. It is included in the WEC trainee packet for new candidates.
Cat. No. 552 $9.00

Winter Emergency Care Annotated Workbook– Second Edition (1989)
Cat. No. 552A $9.00

The Ski Patroller's Manual — Thirteenth Edition (1990)
The definitive source and education tool for ski patrolling. This manual outlines the National Ski Patrol's historical development, organizational and administrative structure, and educational programs. Included is an overview of ski patrol management and area operations. Also contains a study guide for new candidates.
Cat. No. 501 $15.00

The Lift Evacuation Technical Manual — Third Edition (1990)
This manual presents the most recent standards, decisions, and technical efforts of experienced ski industry personnel and corporations throughout the country. Provides detailed, easy-to-understand illustrations, a lift evacuation questionnaire, and guidelines for developing a ski area lift evacuation plan.
Cat. No. 505 $14.50

National Ski Patrol Nordic Manual–First Edition (1985)
Patrol directors and trainers will find this manual a useful guide to training candidate nordic patrollers. It covers the techniques, skills, and knowledge required of all nordic patrollers by the NSP.
Cat. No. 516 $7.00

The National Ski Patrol Ski Mountaineering Manual–
Second Edition (1982)
This manual covers the full spectrum of ski mountaineering from personal survival to the NSP's basic and advanced ski mountaineering courses.
Cat. No. 509 $5.00

Avalanche Instructor's Handbook–First Edition (1987)
A guide to help instructors present better avalanche courses.
Cat. No. 519 $9.50

Classroom Guide for Skier Education–First Edition (1986)
This kit is designed for teachers and NSP members planning to make classroom presentations on skier safety to students in grades 1-4 and 5-8. Group activities and reproducible masters reinforce valuable safety education lessons.
Cat. No. 520M $4.00

The National Ski Patrol: Samaritans of the Snow
Written by Dr. Gretchen R. Besser, NSP historian, this book tells the story of the people who were and are the National Ski Patrol.
Cat. No. 515 $8.50

Please send your order plus a check or money order to: National Ski Patrol, Ski Patrol Building, 133 South Van Gordon Street, Suite 100, Lakewood, CO 80228. Fax your Visa/MasterCard orders to (303) 988-3005.